Introduction to Nuclear Medicine for Trainees in Imaging and Imaging Sciences

Adrien Michael Peters
Manuela Vadrucci

Introduction to Nuclear Medicine for Trainees in Imaging and Imaging Sciences

Springer

Adrien Michael Peters
Department of Nuclear Medicine
King's College Hospital
London, UK

Manuela Vadrucci
Department of Nuclear Medicine
Barts Health NHS Trust
London, UK

ISBN 978-3-032-18363-7 ISBN 978-3-032-18364-4 (eBook)
https://doi.org/10.1007/978-3-032-18364-4

This Springer imprint is published by the registered company Springer Nature Switzerland AG
The registered company address is: Gewerbestrasse 11, 6330 Cham, Switzerland

Foreword

I was delighted to receive a request from Prof Adrien "Mike" Peters to write a foreword to this book. I first met Mike early on in my nuclear medicine career during a training opportunity at the Hammersmith Hospital, London, prior to taking up my consultant appointment in Cardiff in 1991. This was at a time when there were no established nuclear medicine training programmes for radiologists, and I was pleased that my request for training was accepted without hesitation. There followed a very enjoyable and intensive month-long attachment with Mike and Prof Peter Lavender. It became clear to me from the outset that Mike placed great emphasis on a full understanding of the basic physiological principles that underlie common nuclear medicine tests such as MAG 3 renograms, HIDA scans and FDG PET scans, principles that are often overlooked when these scans are performed on a daily basis in imaging departments throughout the world. His teachings have continued over the years, and along with countless publications, he has contributed greatly to the understanding of nuclear medicine techniques and their clinical applications. It is fitting therefore that with help from a consultant colleague Dr Manuela Vadrucci, these principles have been recorded in this book for the benefit of those with an interest in the specialty for years to come. The first two sections cover tracer kinetics and statistics, although following some of the equations will require a good grounding in advanced mathematics! There follows a section on the basic principles of nuclear medicine imaging including gamma camera and PET scanner technology. The latter half of the book is dedicated to a comprehensive review of the various radiopharmaceuticals used in conventional nuclear medicine and PET, their mechanism of action and clinical applications, along with useful pointers on how to interpret the studies. The book will provide an invaluable resource to trainees in radiology, nuclear medicine and basic sciences, as well as practising nuclear medicine specialists who wish to gain a better understanding of the physiological principles underlying commonly performed nuclear medicine tests.

Consultant Radiologist, Department of Radiology
University Hospital of Wales,
Heath Park, Cardiff, Wales

John Rees

Competing Interests

The authors have no competing interests to declare that are relevant to the content of this manuscript.

Contents

About the Authors

Adrien Michael Peters has been a consultant nuclear medicine physician since 1984. He previously held chairs in Diagnostic Radiology at Royal Postgraduate Medical School (and then Imperial College), in Nuclear Medicine at University of Cambridge (Foundation Chair) and in Applied Physiology at Brighton Sussex Medical School. He is currently a nuclear medicine consultant at King's College Hospital, London. He holds an honorary chair in Nuclear Medicine at King's College, London, and is Emeritus Professor of Applied Physiology at Brighton Sussex Medical School. He was awarded the higher doctorate of DSc by the University of Liverpool in 2009, was Nimmo Visiting Professor at the Royal Adelaide Hospital in 2001 and is a Fellow of the Academy of Medical Sciences.

Manuela Vadrucci graduated and completed her specialist training in Nuclear Medicine in Milan, Italy, in 2016. Then, she worked as a research fellow at the European Institute of Oncology IEO in Milan, focusing on molecular imaging in breast and neuroendocrine tumours, before relocating to the UK in 2017. After a few years working as a Locum and then substantive consultant in King's College Hospital, London, in 2020, she joined St Bartholomew's Hospital in the same city.

Her current position as a Nuclear Medicine Consultant in one of the largest teaching hospitals in England enables her to broaden her knowledge on molecular imaging techniques in common and less common oncological and inflammatory diseases, as well as to contribute regularly to the teaching of pre- and post-graduate medical trainees and radiology resident doctors.

She has also shared her experience through several publications, often in collaboration with the co-author of this book.

Part I

Tracer Kinetics

Nuclear medicine is a discipline with a platform of applied physiology and tracer kinetics. Such kinetics determine how tracers accumulate in, and are cleared from, tissues.

1 Mathematical Equations

The following mathematical equations are frequently encountered in clinical and academic nuclear medicine. In general, x is the independent variable in equations, and y is the dependent variable. Therefore, y is described as a function of x. This may be a linear function, exponential function, power function or more. The type of equation to which acquired data most closely conform depends on the physiological context and the closeness with which the data fit the function, determined by the correlation coefficient.

1.1 Linear

$$y = A + Bx \tag{1.1}$$

This is the simplest equation and gives a straight-line graph with gradient of B and y-axis intercept (when x = 0) of A.

When y = 0, x = − A/B.

which is the x-axis intercept (Fig. 1.1).

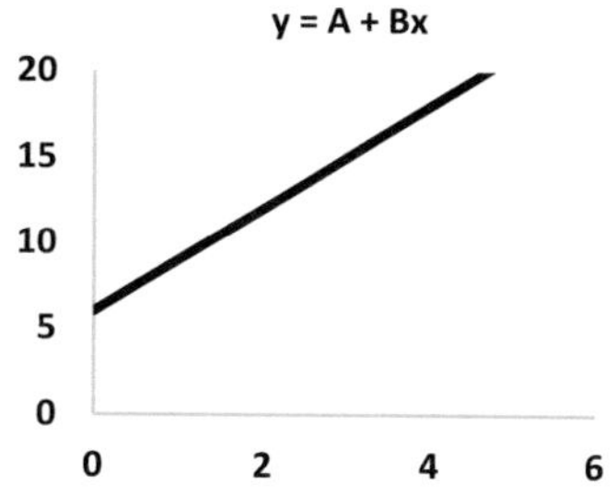

Fig. 1.1 Linear equation

1.2 Polynomial

$$y = A + Bx + Cx^2 + Dx \tag{1.2}$$

Polynomial equations are designated according to the number of terms after A (Fig. 1.2). Thus, a first-order polynomial is identical to a linear equation. A second order polynomial extends to Cx^2 and is the most frequently used in nuclear medicine. Second-order polynomials are

A. M. Peters, M. Vadrucci, *Introduction to Nuclear Medicine for Trainees in Imaging and Imaging Sciences*, https://doi.org/10.1007/978-3-032-18364-4_1

useful for quantifying non-linear relationships between variables that, for example, change from a positive to negative gradient as the x value increases, such as the accumulation of phosphorylated FDG in the liver as a function of blood glucose (see Chap. 28). Measurement of GFR from blood samples taken 2 h post-injection of tracer uses a second-order polynomial to correct for the exclusion of earlier blood samples, as described in Chap. 11. Higher-order polynomials will fit a graph of almost any form and are therefore of little use.

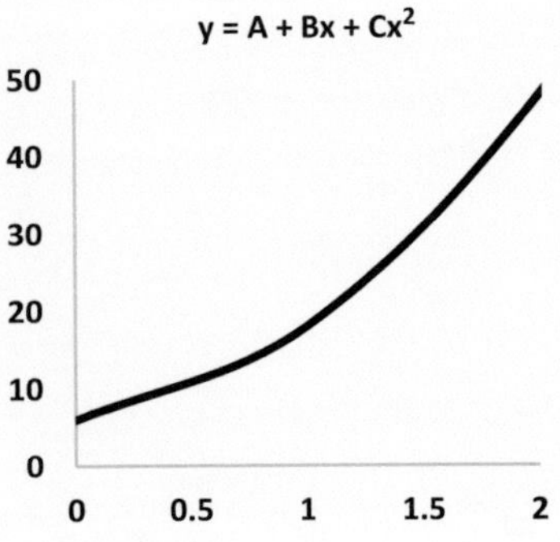

Fig. 1.2 Second-order polynomial equation

1.3 Power

A power equation has y as a function of x raised to a power (Fig. 1.3).

$$y = A.x^{b} \text{ and } y = A.x^{-b} \tag{1.3}$$

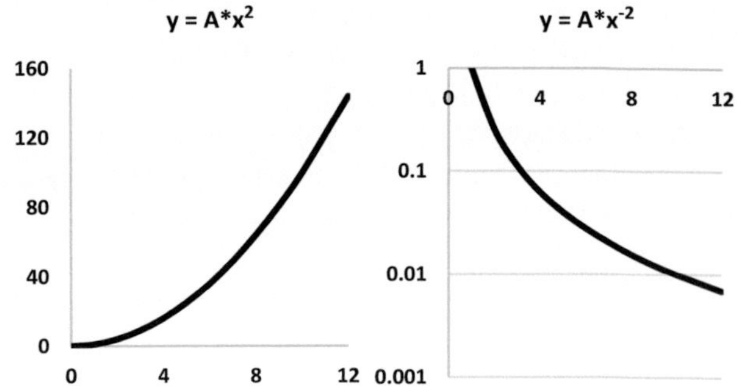

Fig. 1.3 Power functions, positive (left panel) and inverse (right panel)

1.4 Exponential

$$y = A.e^{-kx} \text{ and } y = A.e^{kx} \quad (1.4)$$

Euler's number, e, like pi, is an irrational number equal approximately to 2.72 with an infinite number of decimal places:

$$e = 1 + 1/1! + 1/2! + 1/3! + 1/4! \ldots\ldots 1/n!$$

The *derivative* of a function of x is the rate at which the function is changing at a given value of x; i.e. dy/dx. The function $y = e^x$ is unique in that it has an identical derivative. The introduction of the terms A and k (as in Fig. 1.4) does not change this. Thus, the derivative of $y = 3e^{2x}$, for example, is $6e^{2x}$ or 2y. In contrast, the derivative of the power function $y = 4x^2$ is 8x; i.e. it is a function of x. So, when the rate of change (either increasing or decreasing) of y at a specified value of x is proportional to the amount y at x, then the quantity is changing exponentially. The amount of heat, for example, being lost from a hot drink at temperature H in a carton depends on H; i.e. how hot it is. Theoretically, the temperature never reaches surrounding temperature; in other words, the graph of temperature versus time is asymptotic to the time axis.

So

$$dH/dt = -k.H(t) \quad (1.5)$$

where the constant, k, could, for example, be related to the thickness of the carton. Note that k is negative in this example because the temperature is decreasing.

Integrating Eq. 1.5

$$H(t) = H(0).e^{-kt} \quad (1.6)$$

where H(0) is the starting temperature and t is the elapsed time.

When the y-axis is displayed in orders of magnitude, an exponential function is a straight line (Fig. 1.5).

Plotting ln y against x also gives a straight line with an intercept of ln A and gradient equal to -k (Fig. 1.6).

When x is time, k is called a rate constant. Radionuclides decay exponentially, with k being equal to ln 2 (=0.693) divided by half-life and known as the decay constant.

Declining exponentials are encountered in nuclear medicine more commonly than those that increase. It is worth noting that the total area (i.e. to infinite x) under a declining exponential graph is the y value when x = 0 (i.e., the y-axis intercept of the graph) divided by k. The area up to a specific value of x (AUC_x), rather than to infinity, is the total area to infinite x minus the area to infinite x from the specific value of x. In other words:

$$AUC_x = \frac{y(x=0) - y(x)}{k} \quad (1.7)$$

Frequently, declining double exponentials are encountered, more often the sum than the difference of two exponentials. Thus, for the sum

$$y = A.e^{-k_1 x} + B.e^{-k_2 x} \quad (1.8)$$

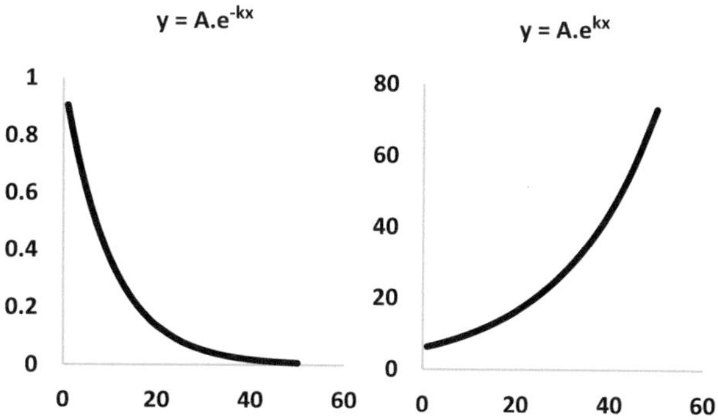

Fig. 1.4 Exponential equations; negative in left panel, positive in right panel

Fig. 1.5 Exponential functions plotted on logarithmic axes

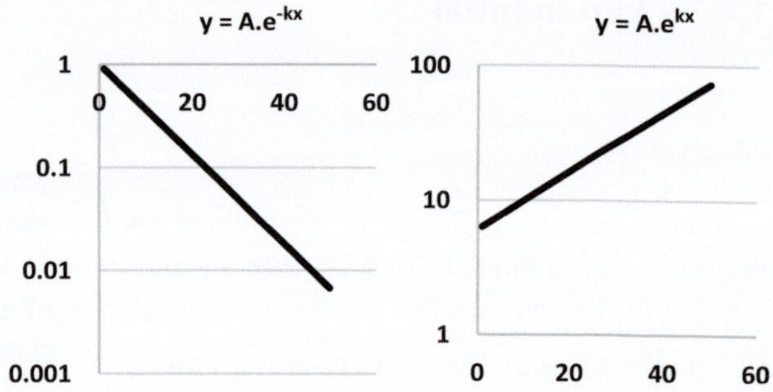

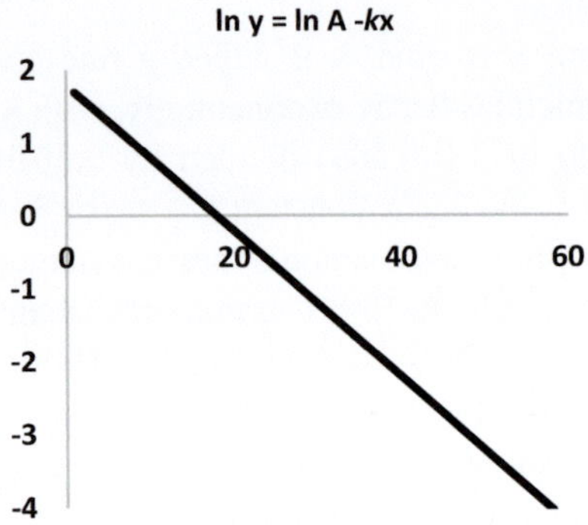

Fig. 1.6 Log transformation of y which has an inverse relationship with x. The gradient is -k

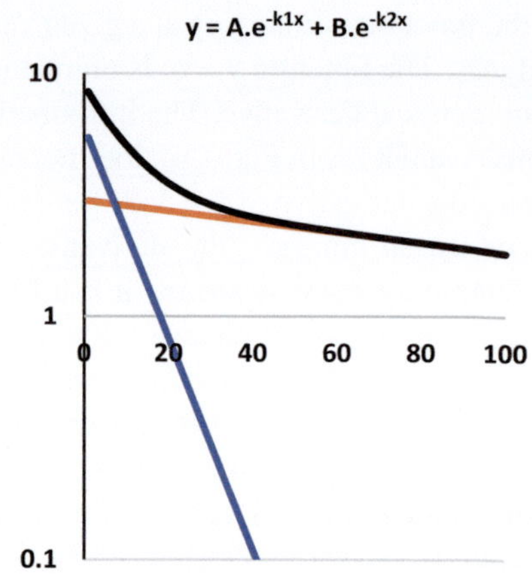

Fig. 1.7 Sum (black line) of two exponentials, one red and one blue

For the difference of two exponentials

$$y = A\left(e^{-k_2x} - e^{-k_1x}\right) \tag{1.9}$$

where, ignoring the minus sign, k_2 is less than k_1. Because y in the recorded curve starts from zero, both exponentials have the same y-axis intercept, A (Fig. 1.8).

The time-concentration curve recorded from the time of injection of Tc-99 m-DTPA, such as for measurement of GFR, conforms to the sum of two exponentials, as do declining blood drug concentration curves when the two exponentials are called alpha and beta phases of drug disappearance. The faster of the two exponentials reflects movement of the drug from blood to the

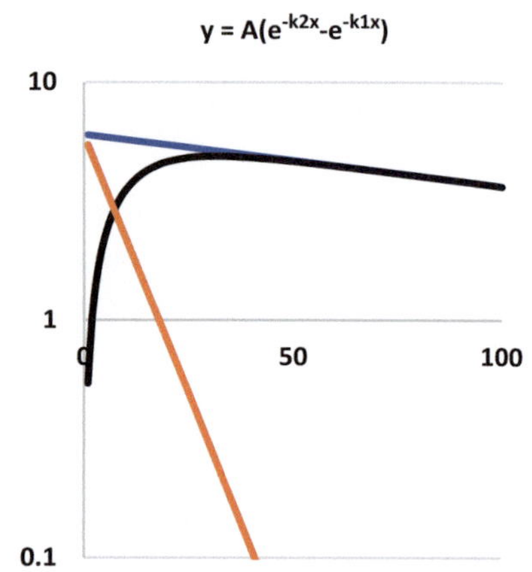

Fig. 1.8 Difference (black line) of two exponentials, one red and one blue

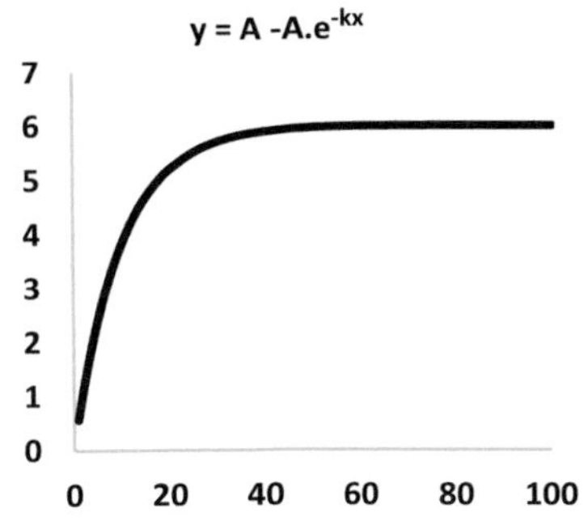

Fig. 1.9 A rising inverse exponential that reflects tracer entering tissue, such as labelled platelets entering the spleen, from another compartment, such as blood, and, through bidirectional transport, reaching equilibration between the two compartments

interstitial space of the whole body, and the slower reflects its disposal by metabolism or excretion. Functions with more than two exponentials are described as multiexponential.

The difference of two exponentials (Eq. 1.9) is typically recorded from a tissue into which tracer is entering from another compartment after injection into that compartment, such as in Tc-99 m-HIDA scintigraphy in which tracer enters the liver (exclusively) from blood exponentially and then leaves the liver rapidly through secretion into the biliary canaliculi. In this situation, the decline in blood concentration is the *sum* of two exponentials with respective rate constants equal to the two rate constants of the hepatic exponential *difference* curve.

A curve that rises exponentially to a plateau (A) can be viewed as an 'upside-down' declining exponential curve, such as when labelled platelets or leucocytes equilibrate between blood and spleen (Chap. 26) or when HIDA equilibrates between blood and liver in situations where no biliary excretion is possible, such as biliary atresia (Chap. 14).

$$y = A - Ae^{-kx}$$

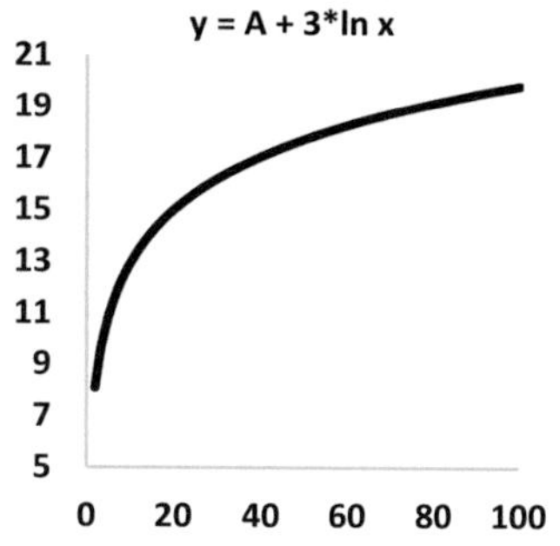

Fig. 1.10 Logarithmic function

$$= A\left(1 - e^{-kx}\right) \tag{1.10}$$

It is a special case of Eq. 1.9 when k_2 is zero and e^{-k2x} is 1 (Fig. 1.9).

1.5 Logarithmic

A logarithmic equation has y as a function of the logarithm of x.

$$y = A + B.\ln x \tag{1.11}$$

Logarithmic equations are seldom used in nuclear medicine but sometimes fit data as well as the rising inverted exponential (Eq. 1.10 and Fig. 1.10).

1.6 Hyperbolic

When a graph is asymptotic to both axes, it is described as hyperbolic.

Thus y = A/x

$$\text{or } 1/y = x/A \tag{1.12}$$

in which case 1/y has a linear relationship with x (Fig. 1.11).

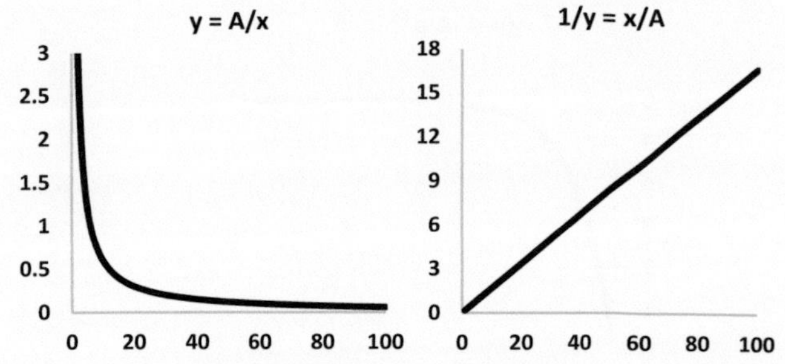

Fig. 1.11 Hyperbolic relationship between y and x. The simplest way to obtain A is to plot 1/y against x, which gives a linear graph with gradient 1/A

An example is the relationship between blood glucose level (x) and fluorodeoxyglucose (FDG) clearance (y) into brain where A is the rate of glucose consumption, which is constant in brain. A hyperbolic function also describes the relationship between GFR (x) and serum creatinine concentration (y).

Further Readings

1. Bröchner-Mortensen J. A simple method for the determination of glomerular filtration rate. Scand J Clin Lab Invest. 1972;30:271–4.
2. Gambhir SS, Hawkins RA, Huang S-C, Hall TR, Busuttil RW, Phelps ME. Tracer kinetic modeling approaches for the quantification of hepatic function with technetium-99 m DISIDA and scintigraphy. J Nucl Med. 1989;30:1507–18.
3. Peters AM, Klonizakis I, Lavender JP, Lewis SM. Use of 111Indium-labeled platelets to measure spleen function. Br J Haematol. 1980;46:587–93.

2 Physiological Equations

There are three physiological equations upon which almost all tracer kinetics relevant to nuclear medicine are based – the Fick, transit time and dilution equations.

2.1 The Fick Equation

The Fick principle states that the rate of accumulation of tracer in a tissue (dM/dt) is equal to the difference between input and output rates. In Fick's day (he published his principle in 1870), the 'tracer' was oxygen, and the tissue was the entire body, but nowadays input and output rates are most often based on blood concentrations of a tracer, such as for the measurement of blood flow to an organ (Q), i.e.

$$\mathrm{dM/dt} = \mathrm{Q.Ca} - \mathrm{Q.Cv}$$
$$= \mathrm{Q.}(\mathrm{Ca} - \mathrm{Cv})$$

and

$$\mathrm{Q} = \frac{(\mathrm{dM/dt})}{(\mathrm{Ca} - \mathrm{Cv})} \quad (2.1)$$

where Ca and Cv are arterial and venous tracer concentrations. It also applies to other situations not involving blood flow, for example imaging regional lung ventilation with Kr-81 m (Chap. 23). Fick's principle is the basis of measurement of tissue clearance from Patlak-Rutland graphical analysis (described below under clearance).

2.2 The Transit Time Equation

$$\mathrm{T} = \mathrm{V/Q} \quad (2.2)$$

where T is the mean transit time of tracer through, or mean waiting time in, a tissue compartment and V is the volume of the compartment within which the tracer is distributed. The equation assumes a well-mixed compartment. Examples include measurement of tissue perfusion, Q, with Xe-133 when T is tracer residence time in the tissue; measurements of GFR with Tc-99 m-DTPA where T is residence time in the extracellular fluid volume and Q is GFR; and renography, where T is residence time in the renal pelvis, V is pelvis volume and Q is urinary flow rate.

2.3 The Dilution Equation

$$\mathrm{C} = \mathrm{M/V} \quad (2.3)$$

where C is tissue or compartment tracer concentration and M is the amount of tracer in the compartment of volume V. This equation is used to measure volumes such as blood volume with

A. M. Peters, M. Vadrucci, *Introduction to Nuclear Medicine for Trainees in Imaging and Imaging Sciences*, https://doi.org/10.1007/978-3-032-18364-4_2

radiolabelled red cells or plasma volume with labelled human serum albumin.

In relation to these equations and more complex equations derived from them, a useful tip to help understand them is to inspect the units on either side of the equation and confirm that they cancel out. For example, take Eq. 2.1. The left side has units of ml/min. The right side has units of MBq/min divided by MBq/ml, giving ml/min.

Further Readings

1. Mullani NA, Gould KL. First-pass measurements of regional blood flow with external detectors. J Nucl Med. 1983;24:577–81.
2. Peters AM. Expressing glomerular filtration rate in terms of extracellular fluid volume. Nephrol Dial Transplant. 1992;7:205–10.

3 Clearance, Blood Flow and Extraction Fraction [or Efficiency (%)]

Tissue blood flow (Q), tissue tracer clearance (Cl) and tracer extraction fraction (E) are related in the following equation

$$\mathrm{Cl} = \mathrm{E} * \mathrm{Q} \tag{3.1}$$

3.1 Extraction Fraction

This is the proportion of a tracer or marker arriving in tissue via its blood flow that is extracted by the tissue and is equal to the arteriovenous concentration difference across the tissue divided by the arterial concentration.

$$\mathrm{E} = \frac{(\mathrm{Ca} - \mathrm{Cv})}{\mathrm{Ca}} \tag{3.2}$$

3.2 Blood Flow

Blood flow to an organ can be expressed in absolute terms (whole organ blood flow; ml/min) or as tissue perfusion (blood flow per unit of tissue; ml/min/ml or ml/min/g), depending on how it is measured. The term blood flow is used in a general sense to include both. Organ blood flow can also be measured as fraction of cardiac output received.

3.3 Clearance

The concept of clearance is of fundamental importance in nuclear medicine. It is defined as the virtual volume from which a marker or tracer is cleared in unit time, which can be appreciated from its units of ml/min. There are several variants of clearance.

3.3.1 Tissue Clearance

Clearance of tracer from plasma into a tissue (tissue clearance) is the equivalent plasma flow from which the tracer is extracted in a single pass through the tissue. For example, if tissue plasma flow is 100 ml/min and 50% of the tracer is extracted, then tissue plasma clearance is 50 ml/min (Fig. 3.1). Tissue clearance from plasma of tracers that do not enter red cells can be converted to clearance from whole blood by dividing by (1- haematocrit).

3.3.2 Urinary and Biliary Clearance

With respect to the kidney, some or all of the cleared marker or tracer may enter the urine. Say, in the above example, 50% of the tracer cleared

A. M. Peters, M. Vadrucci, *Introduction to Nuclear Medicine for Trainees in Imaging and Imaging Sciences*, https://doi.org/10.1007/978-3-032-18364-4_3

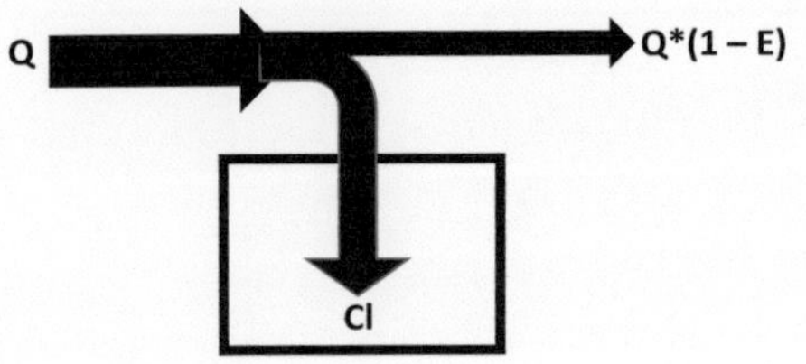

Fig. 3.1 Blood flow (Q), clearance (Cl) and extraction fraction (E = Cl/Q). Width of arrows represents tracer movement

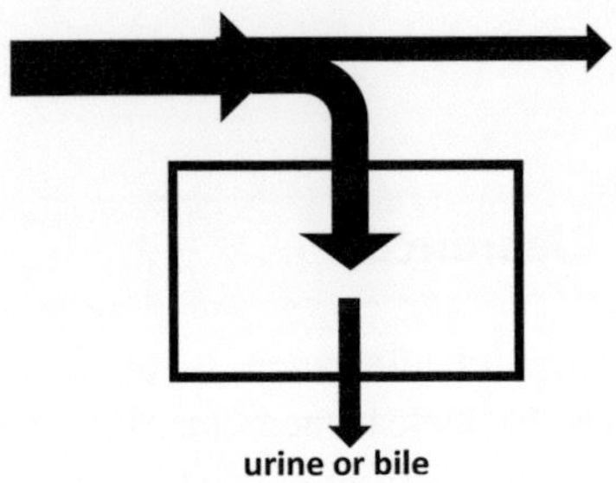

Fig. 3.2 Urinary and biliary clearance

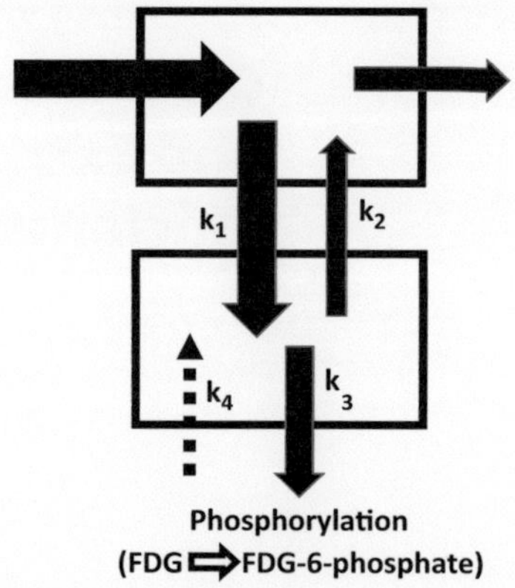

Fig. 3.3 A more complex model of clearance for tracers that display bidirectional movement between blood and tissue (e.g., Tc-99 m-HIDA and F-18FDG in the liver) and at the same time some is fixed within (e.g., FDG) or excreted from (e.g., HIDA) the tissue. There are, therefore, two clearances to consider, firstly into the tissue (K_1) and secondly into the non-reversible state (K_i), which is equal to $K_1.k_3/(k_2 + k_3)$. Liver and kidney both possess glucose-6-phosphatase, so k_4 is active and the model even more complex. k_4 does not exist for Tc-99 m-HIDA

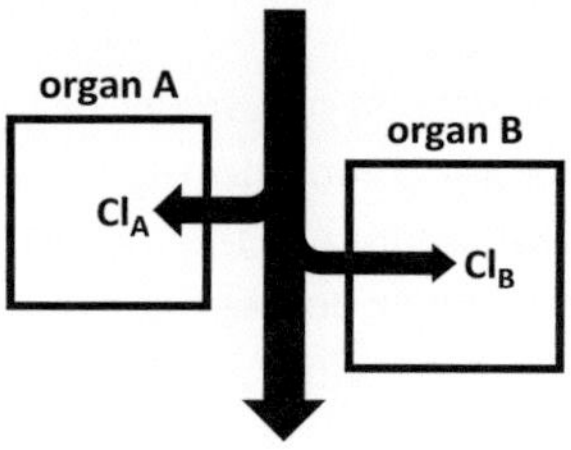

Fig. 3.4 Plasma (whole body) clearance is equal to the sum of individual organ clearances (Cl_A plus Cl_B)

into the kidney from plasma entered urine, then urinary clearance would be 25 ml/min. The same principle applies to biliary clearance of tracers excreted in bile (Fig. 3.2).

A more complex situation exists when a tracer is cleared into a tissue from which it can readily move back into blood because of bidirectional transport between tissue and blood. Examples are FDG and HIDA in the liver. Thus, some FDG is phosphorylated and retained in the cell (Fig. 3.3), while some HIDA is irreversibly excreted into bile. So, both tracers have extraction efficiencies and clearances describing their *irreversible* movement from blood to phosphorylation and excretion, respectively, as well as their *unidirectional* extraction efficiencies from blood to cell, which approach 100% for both tracers.

3.3.3 Plasma Clearance

The rate at which a tracer leaves plasma is plasma clearance. Again, it is the virtual volume from which the tracer is cleared in unit time. Tracers such as Tc-99 m-DMSA or F-18-FDG that enter multiple tissues have a plasma clearance equal to the sum of the individual organ clearances (Fig. 3.4).

Dividing plasma clearance by (1—haematocrit) gives blood clearance of tracers that do not enter circulating erythrocytes. Approximate clearance values are shown for some radiopharmaceuticals in Table 3.1.

3.3.4 Clearance from Tissue and Between Compartments in a Tissue

The clearance of a tracer *from* a tissue, into plasma for example, is usually expressed as the proportion of tracer leaving the tissue in unit

Table 3.1 Approximate clearance values (Cl; ml/min) for some radiopharmaceuticals

	Plasma Cl	Target organ/Cl	Renal Cl	Urinary Cl	Biliary Cl
Tc-99mO_4	20	Salivary glands, thyroid, stomach	10	10	<5
DTPA	100	Kidney/100	100	100	0
MAG3	275	Kidney/250	250	250	25
DMSA	50	Kidney/30	30	10	0
HIDA	*1225	Liver/1200	25	25	**350
Colloid	1500	Liver/1200	0	0	0
MIBI	>1500	Multiple	100	50	200
MDP	250	Bone/100	100	50	0
FDG	*>1000	Multiple	100	80	0

*K_1; **Ki (see Fig. 3.3)

time. If this is exponential, it is given as the rate constant of disappearance from the tissue. When the tracer is cleared from one compartment to another within a tissue, its rate constant of clearance (min^{-1}) from the compartment is equal to the clearance (ml/min) divided by the volume (ml) of the compartment. In this situation the reciprocal of mean residence time, which is what is measured, is often misquoted as clearance.

3.4 Measurement of Clearance

3.4.1 Tissue Clearance

Tissue clearance is equal to plasma clearance if the tracer is taken up in a single tissue. GFR, for example, is measured as the plasma clearances of inulin or Tc-99 m-DTPA, both of which are cleared from plasma exclusively by glomerular filtration.

For tracers entering multiple organs, clearance measurement into a specific tissue requires imaging. This is best achieved using a technique called graphical analysis, originally described by Michael Rutland for I-131 renography and later elaborated for PET by Clifford Patlak, and therefore generally known as Patlak-Rutland graphical analysis.

In single-photon nuclear medicine, Patlak-Rutland analysis cannot measure tissue clearance in absolute units but is useful for measuring relative clearances, such as in Tc-99 m-MAG3 renography, for which the technique is the optimal method for measuring split renal function. Tissue clearance of PET tracers, however, can be measured because absolute tissue and blood concentrations of tracers can be measured with PET/CT.

Firstly, from the Fick principle (Eq. 2.1), we can show that the rate of uptake of tracer in the tissue, dM/dt, is the product of clearance (Cl) and the arteriovenous tracer concentration difference (Ca – Cv). Thus

$$\mathrm{dM/dt = Q.(Ca - Cv)}$$

where Q is blood flow.

Now Cl = Q. E.

$$\text{and } \mathrm{E = \frac{(Ca - Cv)}{Ca}}$$

So

$$\mathrm{dM/dt = \frac{Q[(Ca - Cv)/Ca] \times (Ca - Cv)}{(Ca - Cv)/Ca}}$$

$$\mathrm{= \frac{Cl \times (Ca - Cv)}{(Ca - Cv)/Ca}}$$

$$\mathrm{= Cl \times Ca} \tag{3.3}$$

Integrating Eq. 3.3:

$$\mathrm{M(t) = Cl.\int Ca(t).dt} \tag{3.4}$$

In other words, the amount of tracer accumulated in the tissue at time t after injection is equal to the area under the arterial time-concentration curve up to t multiplied by tissue clearance.

As well as M(t), the activity recorded in the ROI (or VOI for multiple slices) includes a signal, B(t), that comprises tracer in tissue cells that has not been irreversibly bound and tracer in blood in the VOI. So, B(t) is added to both sides of Eq. 3.4.

$$M(t)+B(t)=Cl.\int Ca(t).dt+B(t)$$

Dividing both sides by Ca(t)

$$\frac{M(t)+B(t)}{Ca(t)}=\frac{Cl.\int Ca(t).dt}{Ca(t)}+\frac{B(t)}{Ca(t)} \quad (3.5)$$

So, the Patlak-Rutland technique involves two crucial steps: firstly, the addition of the unbound tracer to both sides of Eq. 3.4, and secondly, division throughout by Ca(t).

The term (∫Ca(t).dt)/Ca has units of time. It is not, however, 'clock' time but instead greater or less, depending on whether Ca(t) is decreasing or increasing over time, and is called normalised time (Table 3.2 and Fig. 3.5).

Equation 3.5 is the Patlak-Rutland equation, which can be seen to be linear. Plotting the left side of the equation against normalised time gives Cl as the gradient and B(t)/Ca(t) as the intercept. It is important to appreciate that the clearance measured is that of tracer that is irreversibly bound. For example, in Fig. 3.3, Patlak-Rutland analysis would give the clearance of FDG to phosphorylation. The plot in this example would only become linear once the tracer had completely mixed between blood and the cells of the tissue, which for FDG is generally rapid. A critical assumption required by the technique is that once cleared into the tissue, the tracer remains within it. So, for example, in Tc-99 m-MAG3 renography, the plot is only linear until the tracer leaves the ROI and enters the proximal ureter, which takes about 2 min from tracer injection, after which the analysis breaks down.

How the equation is used differs between single-photon nuclear medicine and PET/CT. In the former, the variables cannot be measured in absolute units and can only give relative clearance values. The intercept in Tc-99 m-MAG3 renography portrays the blood pool activity in the ROI—predominantly the blood in the kidney but also the blood in the non-renal background tissue included in the ROI. In PET/CT, on the other hand, M(t) is given as the tissue tracer concentration, and the plot gradient gives clearance with units of ml/min/ml (like perfusion). Is the measured clearance tissue plasma clearance or blood clearance? If blood concentration (Ca) is mea-

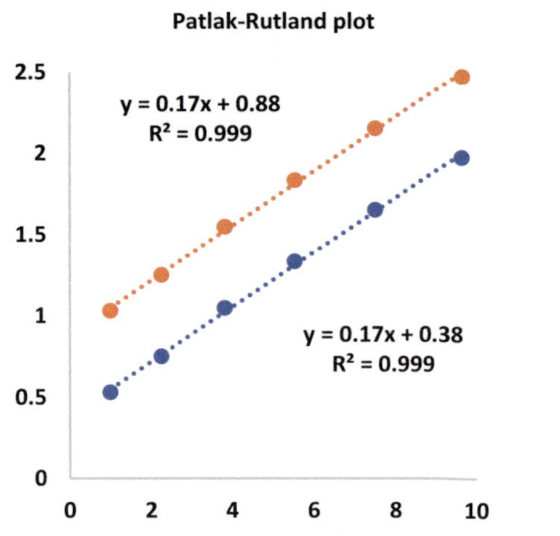

Fig. 3.5 Blue dots: Patlak-Rutland plot from data in Table 3.2. x is normalised time (min) and tissue clearance is 0.17 ml/min/ml. Red dots: B(t) has been doubled—intercept increases but no change in plot gradient

Table 3.2 Worked example of Patlak-Rutland plot

	x-axis					y-axis
Ca(t)	∫Ca(t).dt	∫Ca(t).dt/Ca(t)	M(t)	B(t)	M(t) + B(t)	[(M(t) + B(t)]/ Ca(t)
100	100	1	3	50	53	0.53
80	180	2.25	20	40	60	0.75
64	244	3.81	35	32	67	1.05
54	298	5.52	45	27	72	1.33
46	344	7.48	53	23	76	1.65
40	384	9.6	59	20	79	1.98

sured from an ROI over the left ventricular cavity or aorta, then tissue *blood* clearance is obtained. If, in contrast, Ca is measured in sampled plasma, then it is tissue *plasma* clearance. For tracers that freely enter erythrocytes, which is almost the case for FDG, plasma and blood clearances are the same.

The intercept in PET/CT is the concentration ratio of tracer in the tissue and tracer in arterial blood and is called the distribution volume. Like the term on the left of Eq. 3.5, distribution volume is unitless and expressed as ml per ml of tissue. 'True' distribution volume would be unbound intracellular tracer concentration divided by plasma concentration. In the liver, for example, FDG that has not been phosphorylated freely exchanges between hepatocytes and sinusoidal plasma, and the distribution volume approaches 1 ml/ml. Distribution volume in practice, however, is more complex and effectively a virtual volume that depends on fraction of tissue volume occupied by blood (e.g., 25% in the liver), haematocrit and whether the denominator is plasma or blood concentration.

3.4.2 Plasma Clearance

Plasma clearance of a tracer or marker can be measured at *non-steady state* from plasma sampling after intravenous bolus injection and is equal to the ratio of amount of injected tracer or marker to the total area (i.e. to infinity) under the plasma time-concentration profile. It has already been shown above in Eq. 3.3 that uptake rate of a tracer into a tissue is the product of arterial concentration and clearance. This equation can also be applied to tracer leaving a compartment, in this case plasma. Thus

$$dM(t)/dt = Cl * Ca(t)$$

where M(t) is tracer *remaining* in plasma at time t after injection and Cl is plasma clearance. Integrating and rearranging

$$Cl = M(t)/\int Ca(t).dt$$

Taking Ca(t) to infinite time gives the total area (AUC) of the plasma concentration-time curve. Therefore

$$Cl = M(0)/AUC \tag{3.6}$$

Where $M(0)$ is amount of administered tracer

The terminal part of the concentration-time curve needs to be mathematically definable—for example, as a rate constant—to enable estimation of the area to infinite time. This is the gold standard approach to measuring GFR with a suitable filtration marker like inulin and is a widely used equation because it is relevant to the plasma clearance of any substance, including drugs.

Plasma clearance can be measured at *steady state* as the ratio of infusion rate of tracer (MBq/min) to the steady-state plasma or blood concentration (MBq/ml), but this is seldom performed in nuclear medicine because it is cumbersome.

3.4.3 Urinary Clearance

Urinary clearance, Cl_U, is measured at *steady state* using the classical equation in renal physiology,

$$Cl_U = UV/P \tag{3.7}$$

where U and P are urinary and plasma tracer concentrations, respectively, and V is urine flow rate recorded at steady state during continuous infusion of the tracer. This has mostly been applied to the measurement of GFR with inulin and has historical importance in renal physiology. Because only the kidney clears inulin and there is no tubular reabsorption, inulin has plasma, renal and urinary clearances that are identical.

3.5 Measurement of Blood Flow

There are many different methods for measuring blood flow. Although some are more relevant to nuclear medicine than others, a 'global' understanding of the kinetic principles of blood flow measurement is desirable. Units of whole organ blood flow are ml/min and those of perfusion are ml/min/ml, or, if tissue density is known, ml/min/g. Blood flow can also be expressed as fraction of cardiac output.

3.5.1 Indicator Dilution

The indicator dilution technique for the measurement of blood flow (ml/min) is based on both the transit time and dilution equations. The principle of the technique is to measure the dilution of tracer or marker (which can include cold saline) as it passes through the organ of interest from the site of injection to the sampling point. This is the classical technique for measuring cardiac output where the injection site is a peripheral vein, and the sampling site is any artery. For organ blood flow measurement, the injection site is any artery supplying the organ, and the sampling site is any draining vein. Because it is invasive, the technique is rarely used, but you may come across it in research papers.

So, substituting for V in the transit time (2.2) and dilution (2.3) equations

$$T * Q = M / C$$

So

$$Q = M / (T * C) \tag{3.8}$$

T*C is the time concentration curve in blood from which the tracer is sampled.

Indicator dilution is the classical method with which to measure cardiac output (CO) from the following equation

$$CO = M(0) / AUC_1 \tag{3.9}$$

Where M(0) is the amount of tracer administered by bolus IV injection and AUC_1 is the total area under the first-pass blood time-concentration curve (measured from any artery) corrected for tracer recirculation. The validity of Eq. 3.9 can be checked from the units. Thus, T*C and AUC_1 both have units of min*MBq/ml, so dividing into MBq (administered activity) gives ml/min.

3.5.2 Inert Gas Clearance

The classical tracer used for measuring tissue perfusion from inert (noble) gas clearance is Xe-133. Following bolus injection of Xe-133 in solution into an artery supplying an organ, the tracer rapidly diffuses throughout the tissue of the organ because of its high lipid solubility and reaches equilibrium between tissue and blood almost instantaneously. It is then washed out of the organ by incoming blood at a rate depending on tissue perfusion (ml/min/ml). Thus, from Fick, tissue clearance rate is

$$dM / dt = -Q \,.\, Cv$$

where Cv is outflowing venous concentration.

However, because of rapid equilibration,

$$Cv = Ct$$

$$= M(t) / V$$

so

$$dM / dt = \frac{-Q \,.\, M(t)}{V} \tag{3.10}$$

As dM/dt is proportional to M(t), the count rate from the organ declines exponentially (hence the negative sign). The time-activity curve recorded by an external detector, known as the impulse response function (IRF), displays a brief plateau that reflects the minimum intravascular transit time. If there are two tissue compartments within the detector's field of view, such as white and grey matter in the brain, a double exponential is recorded, each giving white and grey matter perfusion, respectively.

An attraction of Xe-133 is that it does not recirculate because 95% enters pulmonary alveoli on reaching the lungs and is expired. Its disadvantage is that it requires arterial injection, although it has been given IV with the aim of exploiting the 5% that recirculates. Perfusion of just about every tissue in the body has at some time been measured with Xe-133. Kr-81 m, another inert gas, has also been used to measure perfusion, but because of its ultra-short half-life of 13 s, the kinetics, although still based on Fick, are different, as described in Chap. 23.

3.5.3 Plethysmography

Plethysmography measures the rate of change in volume, usually of a limb, over a few seconds, following abrupt occlusion of the venous outflow with a cuff raised to a pressure between venous and arterial. This gives ml/min but can be converted to perfusion by dividing by the volume of the limb.

3.5.4 As Plasma Clearance

When a tracer or marker is cleared from blood by a single organ, the rate of clearance gives blood flow to the organ (ml/min) *if the extraction efficiency is 100%*. The value of 100% is seldom achieved by any organ/tracer combination but may closely approach it. An example that has been very widely used, mainly in research, is renal clearance of para-amino-hippurate (PAH) by the kidney, which gives 'effective' renal plasma flow (ERPF) – 'effective' being introduced in recognition of the assumption of 100% extraction efficiency. Liver blood flow can also be measured using the organic anions, a group of substances that includes Tc-99 m-HIDA that are cleared from blood exclusively into the liver.

3.5.5 From First-Pass

Measurement of blood flow from the first pass of tracer in a tissue makes use of the Fick principle where Cv = 0. Thus, dM/dt in Eq. 2.1 is captured in the brief period following intravenous injection during which tracer has entered the tissue but not yet entered the venous outflow, giving

$$Q = \frac{dM/dt}{Ca(t)} \tag{3.11}$$

Integration gives

$$Q = M(t) / \int Ca(t).dt \tag{3.12}$$

where t is less than the minimum intravascular transit time.

This technique (Fig. 3.6) cannot give blood flow in absolute units (ml/min/100 ml) from single photon emitters, but it can from dynamic PET/CT (with any PET tracer) because tissue tracer concentration can be measured.

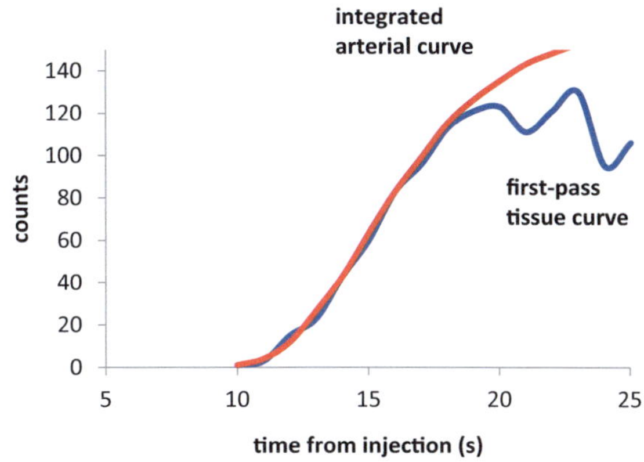

Fig. 3.6 First-pass data following intravenous injection of any radiopharmaceutical. For a PET tracer, tissue and blood concentrations can be measured and applied to Eq. 3.11, which shows that Q is equal to the ratio of first-pass tissue curve (blue line) and the integrated arterial curve (red line). Q is therefore equal to the scaling factor applied to the integrated arterial curve to make it parallel to the tissue curve. The tissue curve has been shifted to the left to allow the two curves to be superimposed, facilitating the derivation of the scaling factor. For a single photon emitting tracer, the plateau of the integrated recirculation-corrected arterial curve indicates the level of activity that an organ would have reached if all the activity arriving in it on first pass was retained. Combining this, with quantification of the activity in the organ, determined from quantitative imaging, and the administered activity gives the fraction of cardiac output serving the organ

Dynamic contrast-enhanced perfusion CT (DCT) uses the same theory, taking Ca(t) as the peak height of the arterial curve and dM/dt as the maximum gradient of the tissue curve. The tissue concentration of contrast is given as Hounsfield units, so dynamic CT, like PET/CT, gives perfusion in absolute units. However, because it needs a higher bolus volume and uses fewer data points (limited by radiation exposure), DCT is inferior to dynamic PET/CT as a measure of tissue perfusion.

The transit time equation can be used to estimate roughly the minimum intravascular transit time for a particular tissue. For example, renal Q is about 300 ml/min/100 ml and renal blood volume about 25 ml/100 ml, so mean intravascular transit time is about 5 s. Hepatic blood volume is also 25 ml/100 ml. Tracer arriving in the liver on the first pass is in the hepatic artery, not portal vein which delivers tracer later, but is washed out by total hepatic blood flow (100 ml/min/100 ml), so intravascular transit time is 25/100 min, or 15 s, which makes hepatic arterial perfusion easier to measure on the first pass.

3.5.6 As a Fraction of Cardiac Output

When a particulate tracer such as Tc-99 m-macroaggregated albumin (MAA; Chap. 21) that is too large to traverse a blood capillary is injected into the left ventricle, it is distributed to organs in proportion to the organ's share of cardiac output. Measurement of activity in the organ as a proportion of administered activity gives the organ's fraction of cardiac output. Typical approximate values are 10% for each kidney, 4% for spleen, 15% for brain and 5% for myocardium (at rest). For the liver, only hepatic arterial fraction is given (7%) because portal venous blood has been freed of particles. Using any single photon emitting tracer, organ blood flow can be measured non-invasively from quantitative imaging as a fraction of cardiac output by estimating the activity delivered to the organ on first pass as a fraction of administered activity (Fig. 3.6). Fractionation is less relevant to PET because absolute concentrations can be measured.

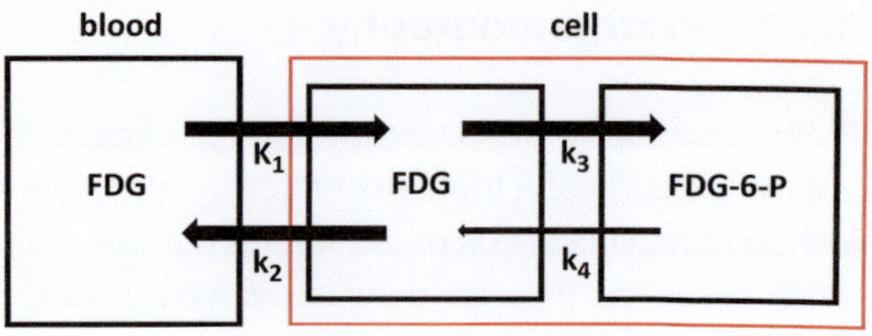

Fig. 3.7 Model depicting FDG transport in tissue. For most tissues, FDG extraction efficiency into the cell is almost 100%, so K_1 is close to blood flow and given upper case K; lower case k are rate constants (clearance from compartment divided by compartment volume). FDG-6-P undergoes dephosphorylation but only in liver and kidney because these are the only two tissues containing glucose-6-phosphatase—liver to maintain fasting blood glucose and kidney to reabsorb filtered glucose

3.5.7 Computerised Modelling

In PET/CT, unlike single photon imaging, tissue and blood tracer concentrations can be measured in absolute units. Models depicting pathways of movement of tracer between compartments can be constructed, and, using complex computerised techniques (the description of which is beyond the scope of this text), these pathways can be quantified. The most widely used model is shown in Fig. 3.7. K_1 is blood flow. The other pathways depict rate constants with values given with k in lower case.

3.6 Measurement of Extraction Fraction

Simultaneous measurement of clearance and blood flow yields extraction fraction. A convenient technique not requiring blood flow or clearance in absolute units and therefore applicable to single photon tracers is to combine first-pass data (Eq. 3.8) with clearance from Patlak-Rutland analysis (Eq. 3.5) in the same ROI. Photon attenuation is the same in both phases, so it cancels out.

Extraction fraction can also be measured using a technique called deconvolution analysis. Understanding the reverse of deconvolution, namely convolution, helps understand the technique. Imagine following IV injection that a tracer arrived in a tissue as an infinite series of sequential tiny parcels via an artery supplying the

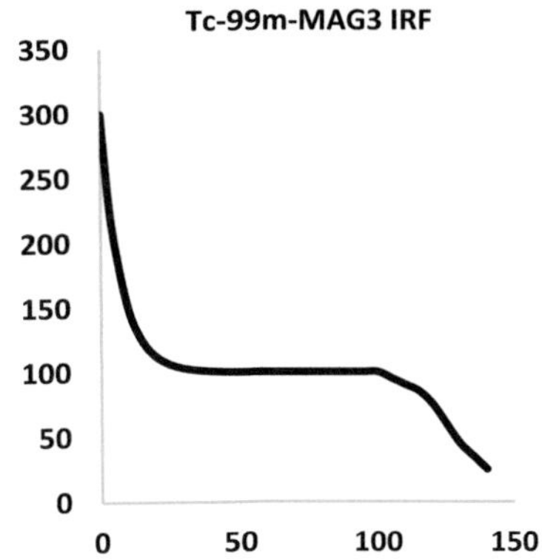

Fig. 3.8 Deconvolution analysis applied to Tc-99 m-MAG3 (y-axis: arbitrary units of activity; x-axis: time (s)). 300 units of tracer arrive in the kidney via the renal artery. 100 units are extracted in the proximal tubular epithelium and make their way through the renal tubules to the collecting system over a period of ~2 min and depart the kidney. 200 units are not extracted, remain within the renal circulation, and depart the kidney via renal vein over ~20 s. The extraction fraction is 0.33

organ. If you were able to image the tissue time-activity curve resulting from an individual parcel, you would record the impulse response function (IRF). Applied to renography, for example, Tc-99 m-MAG3 would give an infinite number of miniature IRFs, which when all added up, would be the same as the recorded renogram. Using the recorded renogram and blood time-concentration curve, deconvolution analysis performs this process in reverse to generate the Tc-99 m-MAG3 IRF (Fig. 3.8). The sharp downslope reflects unextracted tracer leaving via the renal vein. The duration of the plateau reflects the time it takes for extracted tracer in proximal tubular lumen to reach the collecting system. The extraction fraction is given as the ratio of the initial height of the IRF and the plateau.

Deconvolution analysis is also performed to measure unidirectional hepatic extraction fraction of Tc-99 m-HIDA. The time-activity curve generated in a tissue following arterial injection of Xe-133 is an IRF because the tracer does not recirculate. Convolution and deconvolution analyses are used in a less transparent fashion in computerised PET modelling for the measurement of clearance and blood flow.

Further Readings

1. Peters AM. Graphical analysis of dynamic data: the Patlak-Rutland plot. Nucl Med Commun. 1994;15:669–72.
2. Wicks S, Levart D, Conway L, Heraghty H, Peters AM. Noninvasive measurement of tracer extraction efficiency in tissue, illustrated with Tc-99m-MAG3. Nucl Med Commun. 2024;45:519–25.
3. Hollenberg NK, Meggs LG, Williams GH, Katz J, Garnic JD, Harrington DP. Sodium intake and renal responses to captopril in normal man and in essential hypertension. Kidney Int. 1981;20:240–5.
4. Brown PH, Juni JE, Lieberman DA, Krishnamurthy GT. Hepatocyte versus biliary disease: a distinction by deconvolutional analysis of technetium-99m IDA time-activity curves. J Nucl Med. 1988;29:623–30.

4 Distribution Volume and Mean Transit Time

4.1 Distribution Volume (Vd)

Vd is the volume of any compartment that a tracer enters. It determines the concentration of tracer in the compartment. A simple example is blood volume, which can be measured from dilution in blood of a known amount of radiolabelled red cells administered i.v., or plasma volume from Tc-99 m-labelled human serum albumin.

Vd may be virtual as in the measurement of GFR from a single blood sample (the current method recommended by the British Nuclear Medicine Society) when it is expressed as the ratio of the amount of injected Tc-99 m-DTPA to plasma concentration at any time following injection. As the concentration falls over time, the virtual Vd increases at a rate reflecting GFR and approaches infinity.

4.2 Mean Transit Time

Mean transit or residence time (T) is the ratio of the volume of a compartment (V) to the rate of tracer flow through the compartment:

$$T = V / \text{flow} \tag{4.1}$$

The inverse of T gives a rate constant, k (min^{-1}).

Flow could be blood flow, as in the measurement of perfusion with Xe-133, or the flow of a tracer through a compartment, such as Tc-99 m-MAG3 through the renal pelvis in renography.

Further Readings

1. Koff SA, Binkovitz L, Coley B, Jayanthi VR. Renal pelvis volume during diuresis in children with hydronephrosis: implications for diagnosing obstruction with diuretic renography. J Urol. 2005;174:303–7.
2. Boer P. Estimated lean body mass as an index for normalization of body fluid volumes in humans. Am J Phys. 1984;247:F632–6.
3. Durand E, Blaufox MD, Britton KE, et al. International Scientific Committee of Radionuclides in Nephrourology (ISCORN): consensus on renal transit time measurements. Semin Nucl Med. 2008;38:82–102.

A. M. Peters, M. Vadrucci, *Introduction to Nuclear Medicine for Trainees in Imaging and Imaging Sciences*, https://doi.org/10.1007/978-3-032-18364-4_4

5 Blood Capillary Function

5.1 Permeability-Surface Area (PS) Product

As tracer passes along a tissue capillary, undergoing extraction into the tissue as it progresses, its concentration in the capillary falls exponentially (with distance constant, k cm^{-1}) and its clearance is a function of perfusion and extraction efficiency, as described above. The PS product for the tracer is the clearance that would be achieved were the tracer concentration not to decline along the capillary. PS product is therefore always greater than clearance by an amount that depends on extraction efficiency. When extraction efficiency is high, tracer transport across the capillary is described as perfusion-dependent and when low, as diffusion-dependent.

Thus

$$PS * Cm = Q * (Ca - Cv)$$

where Ca and Cv are the concentrations at the arterial and venous ends of the capillary, and C_m is the average concentration along the capillary.

Rearranging

$$PS / Q = \frac{(Ca - Cv)}{Cm} \tag{5.1}$$

As explained in derivation of Eq. 1.6, the area under the concentration-capillary distance curve up to Cv is (Ca-Cv)/k.

The area of equal magnitude under the imaginary graph of C_m versus distance, d, is C_m*d, so

$$(Ca - Cv) / k = Cm * d$$

and (Ca − Cv)/kd = Cm.

Therefore, substituting for C_m in Eq. 5.1

$$PS / Q = \frac{(Ca - Cv).kd}{(Ca - Cv)}$$

$$= k * d$$

Now (Cv/Ca) = e^{-kd} and ln(Cv/Ca) = − kd

But

$$E = 1 - (Cv / Ca)$$

so

$$Cv / Ca = 1 - E$$

Therefore

$$PS / Q = -\ln(1 - E)$$

and

$$PS = -Q.\ln(1 - E) \tag{5.2}$$

A. M. Peters, M. Vadrucci, *Introduction to Nuclear Medicine for Trainees in Imaging and Imaging Sciences*, https://doi.org/10.1007/978-3-032-18364-4_5

Equation 5.2, separately developed by the microvascular physiologists Eugene Renkin and Christian Crone, describes capillary permeability of specific solutes in tissues.

Re-arrangement of Eq. 5.2,

$$E = 1 - e^{-PS/Q}$$

and

$$Ki = \left(1 - e^{-PS/Q}\right).Q \tag{5.3}$$

shows the relationship between tracer clearance into tissue, Ki, and blood flow for a given PS product. In the measurement of blood flow—for example myocardial blood flow (MBF) with Rb-82 using a modelling approach rather than first-pass—Eq. 5.3 is used to convert Ki to blood flow. In the context of MBF, the response to stress (Chap. 16) needs to consider capillary recruitment so an additional variable, A, is inserted to give

$$Ki = \left(1 - A.e^{-PS/Q}\right).Q$$

MBF is then calculated from Ki and values of PS and A pre-determined in control subjects using a 'gold standard' method of blood flow measurement. There are several publications in the literature giving values for A and PS, and they largely agree.

5.2 Reflection Coefficient

Reflection coefficient is a concept relating to the movement of macromolecules, such as albumin, across capillary endothelial membranes. Because of their molecular size, this is by convection rather than diffusion; in other words, macromolecules are 'dragged' through the tiny pores of the capillary endothelium by the movement of water. The flow of water, summarised in the Starling Eq. (5.3), is determined by the filtration coefficient, K_f, capillary surface area (A) and two pressure gradients between the capillary (i) and interstitial space (e)—firstly, the hydrostatic pressure, P, which is higher in the capillary and pushes water out of the capillary, and secondly, colloid oncotic pressure, Π, which is also higher in the capillary and draws water back in.

$$J = K_f.A.\left[\left(P_i - P_e\right) - \sigma.\left(\pi_i - \pi_e\right)\right] \tag{5.3}$$

The reflection coefficient, σ, the value of which varies between 0 and 1, determines the effectiveness of the oncotic pressure difference. For example, hepatic sinusoids have wide pores to allow protein movement into and out of hepatocytes, and the reflection coefficient is therefore almost zero, effectively disabling oncotic pressure. In contrast, in muscle and skin capillaries, it approaches unity, and the oncotic pressure gradient is fully active.

5.3 Quantification in Nuclear Medicine (Table 5.1)

An important rule when reporting nuclear medicine studies is to form your first impression from the images and to then confirm it from quantification. Allow the quantification to override the impression from imaging only with caution.

Table 5.1 Normal ranges or limits of organ-specific clinical measurements. p.i. post-injection

Organ	Tracer	Variable	Normal range/limits
Brain	I-123-ioflupane	Target/background	z score: −2 to +2
Thyroid	Tc-99mO_4	Uptake at 20 min p.i.	1-3%
Lungs	Tc-99 m-DTPA (inhaled)	Clearance half-time	Ill-defined, >60 min
Heart	Tc-99 m-MIBI	LV ejection fraction (EF)	Ill-defined, ~50–75%
	Tc-99 m-erythrocytes	LV EF	Ditto
	I-123-MIBG	Target/background	>1.5
Liver	Tc-99 m-HIDA	Excretion halftime	<30 min
	Tc-99 m-HIDA	Gallbladder EF	Ill-defined, 35–85%
Stomach	Tc-99 m-semisolid meal	Half-emptying time	Ill-defined, 60 min
Intestine	Se-75-HCAT	7-day whole body retention	>15%
Spleen	In-111-platelets	Blood recovery at 30 min	>60%
	Labelled leucocytes.	Blood recovery at 30 min	>40%
Kidney	Tc-99 m-MAG3 or DTPA	Split function	43–57%
	Tc-99 m-DMSA	Split function	44–56%
Lymph	Tc-99 m-nanocolloid	Ilioinguinal uptake	8–30%

See subsequent chapters for explanation of abbreviations

Further Readings

1. Crone C. The permeability of capillaries in various organs as determined by use of the 'indicator diffusion' method. Acta Physiol Scand. 1963;58:292–305. https://doi.org/10.1111/j.1748-1716.1963.tb02652.x.
2. Orntoft NW, Gormsen LC, Keiding S, Munk OL, Ott P, Sorensen M. Hepatic bile acid transport increases in the postprandial state: a functional ^{11}C-CSar PET/CT study in healthy humans. JHEP Rep. 2021;3(3):100288. https://doi.org/10.1016/j.jhepr.2021.100288. eCollection 2021 Jun
3. Kongstad L, Moller AD, Grande PO. Reflection coefficient for albumin and capillary fluid permeability in cat calf muscle after traumatic injury. Acta Physiol Scand. 1999;165:369–77.

Part II

Basic Medical Statistics

In general, nuclear medicine generates continuous data rather than categorical data. This part will describe in brief the statistical tests of continuous data that are mostly encountered in nuclear medicine. The section is obviously not comprehensive but aims to improve the reader's confidence when approaching statistics.

Statistical tests are described as parametric when the data are normally distributed or otherwise as non-parametric, which does not require any specific conformation of data.

Parametric Statistics

6

Terms in parametric medical statistics that you will find helpful to understand are:

- Normal distribution,
- Variance,
- Standard deviation,
- Z score,
- Standard error,
- Degrees of freedom,
- Correlation and regression,
- Null hypothesis,
- Probability (p).

6.1 Normal Distribution

Any quantitative attribute in normal individuals, such as blood pressure (BP), displays biological variation that can be captured in a frequency distribution curve. Such a curve is described as a normal distribution curve (or Gaussian curve) when it is 'bell-shaped' or in other words when it is symmetrical about the mean value, giving median and mean values of the attribute that are the same. When the mean is zero, or the curve scaled to have a mean of zero, the curve is described as a standard normal distribution curve. The numbers of individuals with values lower than the mean and the number higher than the mean are equal, and the area under the curve to the left of mean is equal to the area to the right of mean. BP measured in a cohort of individuals gives the distribution curve for BP to a level of confidence that depends on the number of individuals 'sampled'. The range of values in the sampled cohort is described as the variance.

6.2 Variance

The spread of values of a normally distributed attribute in a sampled cohort is expressed as the variance, V, which is the sum of the squared differences of individual values, y, from the cohort mean divided by the number of individuals, n, in the cohort.

$$\frac{\sum \left(y - y_{mean}\right)^2}{n} \quad (6.1)$$

The individual differences from the mean, known as the residuals, are squared otherwise V would always be zero.

6.3 Standard Deviation

By taking the squares of the residuals, variance gives the units of the variable squared (e.g., for BP, mm Hg^2). To reverse this, the square root of variance is taken, giving the standard deviation (SD). When comparing two cohorts of patients (for example, the same attribute compared between women and men), a pooled SD (based on both cohorts) is calculated (see below).

A. M. Peters, M. Vadrucci, *Introduction to Nuclear Medicine for Trainees in Imaging and Imaging Sciences*, https://doi.org/10.1007/978-3-032-18364-4_6

6.4 Z Score

The x-axis in a normal distribution curve is the attribute of interest, such as BP, and the y-axis is the number of individuals with a specified value of BP. Instead of mm Hg, the x-axis can be expressed in units of SD. The area under the curve, as a proportion of the total area, between say SDs of −1 and +1, gives the proportion of the population that possess BP between these SD limits. The proportion corresponding to these limits is 67%; i.e., 33.5% of individuals have a BP between −1 and 0 SDs and 33.5% have a BP between 0 and +1 SDs. Conversely, 33% would have BP outside these limits. BP that is considered abnormal is assigned to individuals with SD values outside the limits of −1.96 and +1.96 because the area enclosed outside these limits (within the two extreme tails) represents 5% of the population, which is conventionally taken as the cut-off for normality. There are therefore 2.5% defined as having an abnormally low BP (the lower tail of the frequency distribution curve) and 2.5% having an abnormally high BP (the upper tail). When the distribution curve is scaled to make the mean zero (i.e., converted into a standard normal distribution curve), the SD units of the x-axis are given the symbol z. The proportions of the area in a standard normal distribution curve below or above a specific z value can be obtained from the z-distribution table.

In nuclear medicine, the z score is routinely used to identify abnormal I-123-ioflupane (DaT) scans (Fig. 6.1; Chap. 24). The variable (x-axis) in the distribution curve is the count rate recorded in an element of the basal ganglia (e.g., a caudate nucleus) expressed as a ratio with brain background (usually cerebellum). If you have a z score of −1.96, it means you are one of 2.5% of individuals with the lowest ratio and therefore considered abnormal. A z score of −1.64 would still put you in the bottom 5%, but that is not low enough to deem you abnormal in a one-tail test (i.e., considering only the lower end of the curve).

6.5 Standard Error

SD is not dependent on the number of patients in a cohort. Nevertheless, it carries greater confidence in identifying the true spread of values if it is based on, say, 100 individuals (samples) compared with, say, 10. This is addressed by dividing SD by the square root of the number in the cohort to give the standard error (SE).

$$SE = SD / \left(n^{0.5}\right) \tag{6.3}$$

(index 0.5 means square root)

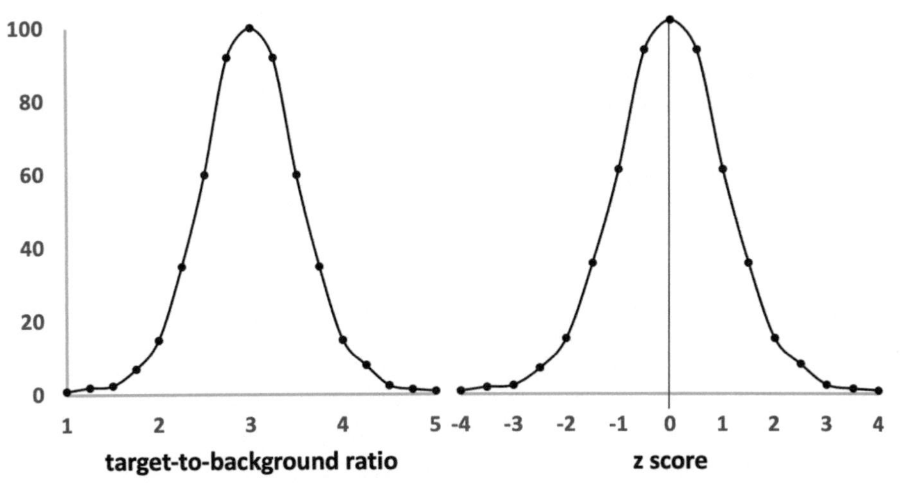

Fig. 6.1 Left panel: normal distribution curve of target (corpus)-to-background (cerebellum) ratio in I-123-ioflupane scintigraphy. Right panel: standard normal distribution curve in which the mean ratio of 3 has been given a z score of 0. A z score of less than −1.96 (essentially 2) is regarded as abnormal

Pooled SE for comparison of two groups is calculated from pooled SD (see below).

6.6 Correlation and Regression

The extent to which two quantitative attributes are associated or correlate with each other is quantified using a value between −1 and +1 called the correlation coefficient. In correlation, one variable is dependent on the other. When expressed graphically, the dependent variable occupies the y-axis, and the independent variable occupies the x-axis, and their relationship is defined by the regression line, which may be linear or non-linear.

Analogous to variance, the difference between a y value and the regression line at the corresponding x value is called a residual. The regression line is defined as that which gives the lowest sum of all the squared residuals, explaining the term 'least squares' fitting. The correlation coefficient is calculated from the variance of the residuals, perfect correlation being −1 for a declining regression slope and +1 for a perfect rising slope. 0 indicates no correlation.

The regression line may take any of several forms according to the nature of the equation relating y to x, as in the mathematical equations described in Chap. 1. It may pass through the origin of the graph or give positive or negative y-axis intercepts.

An infinite number of individuals sampled would give the 'true' relationship between the two attributes. In practice, a limited number of individuals are sampled to predict the true relationship. The more patients in cohort that are sampled, the closer the true relationship will be predicted. Sample number is therefore critical.

6.7 Significance Testing

Using a concept known as the null hypothesis, statistical tests in nuclear medicine in general aim to quantify the significance of

- Differences between groups of patients,
- Differences in individual patients before and after an intervention,
- Correlation between quantitative attributes.

Sample means, differences, regression line gradients and intercepts all have their own SEs, which, along with the sample number in the cohort indicate their statistical significance. An intercept, for example, may have biological relevance, and whether it is significantly different from 0 may be of importance.

6.8 Null Hypothesis

The null hypothesis is that there is no difference between two or more sets of data, or that there is no correlation between two variables. Tests of statistical significance are designed to test the null hypothesis. They determine the probability (p) that the sampled data are consistent with the null hypothesis. A p value of 0.05 stipulates a 1-in-20 chance that there is no difference between the sets of values or no correlation. For p values less than 0.05, the null hypothesis is conventionally rejected.

6.9 Student's T Distribution

Student was the pen name adopted by the statistician who described the t distribution. The standard normal distribution defines, using z, the spread of values of an attribute that exists in a population of infinite size. The accuracy in attempting to reproduce the normal distribution of an attribute, in other words to determine the z distribution, depends on the number of individuals, n, in the sample in whom the attribute is measured. The smaller the number, the lower the confidence you will have in reproducing z. If the sample is very large (≥ 100), t and z will be identical, but as the sample size shrinks, t becomes progressively larger than z (Fig. 6.2). So, to test the null hypothesis when comparing the differ-

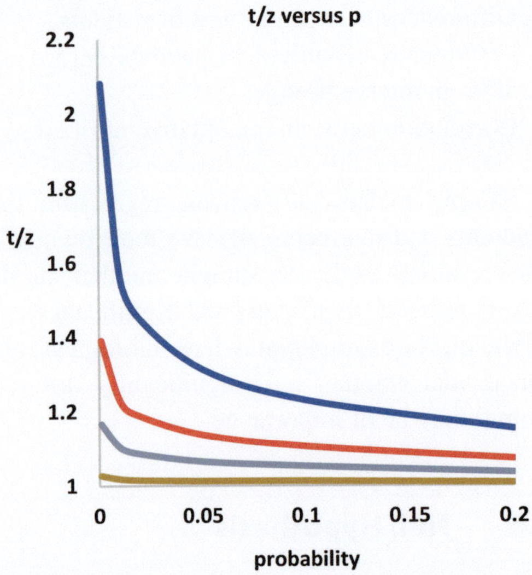

Fig. 6.2 Narrowing of t and z (as t/z in y-axis) as degrees of freedom increase from 5 (blue) through 10 (red) and 20 (grey) to 100 (brown) and as probability (x-axis) increases. Thus, t needs to be about twice z to give the same p value of 0.001 when there are 5 degrees of freedom. In contrast, t and z are almost equal for any p value when there are 100 degrees of freedom

ence between a cohort mean with a fixed value or the difference between the means of two cohorts, t (rather than z) and n are both required. In general, the crucial variable when testing such differences is the SE, which when divided into the mean or mean difference gives the value of t. Using the t-distribution rather than z-distribution, p is then calculated from t and n.

6.10 Degrees of Freedom

As hinted above, the number of degrees of freedom in a test is generally the number of observations, n, that have been made. However, it is n-1, rather than n. Using the single sample t-test, for example, you may wish to test the null hypothesis that the mean of a set of values is not different from a specific value. You might wish to know, for example, whether the mean GFR of patients with renal stone disease is different from 60 ml/min (lower or greater than). The appropriate formula is

$$t = (\text{mean GFR} - 60) / \text{SE} \quad (6.4)$$

with n-1 degrees of freedom.

It is n-1 rather than n because you can imagine that the first GFR value in the sampled cohort could be either below or above 60. We then need to address the likelihood of which side of 60 the mean value lies. It is like the odds of having, say, four children of the same sex. The odds are 8 to 1, not 16 to 1, because the sex of the first child could be either male or female.

6.11 Significance of the Difference Between Two Groups of Patients (Unpaired T Test)

First, the pooled SD^2 based on all data from both groups is calculated, giving a value intermediate between the squared SDs of the two groups

$$\text{Pooled SD}^2 = \frac{SD_1^2.(n_1 - 1) + SD_2^2.(n_2 - 1)}{n_1 + n_2 - 2} \quad (6.5)$$

Multiplying the pooled SD by $(1/n_1 + 1/n_2)^{0.5}$ gives the pooled SE. The difference between the group means divided by the pooled SE gives a value of t with $n_1 + n_2$—2 degrees of freedom. The probability, that there is no difference between the two groups can then be derived from t and the number of degrees of freedom using the t-distribution table (or free internet programme).

When n_1 and n_2 are both large, pooled SE can be obtained more directly from

$$SE = \left(SD_1^2 / n_1 + SD_2^2 / n_2\right)^{0.5}$$
$$= \left(SE_1^2 + SE_2^2\right)^{0.5} \quad (6.6)$$

and

$$t = \text{difference between group means} / \text{SE} \quad (6.7)$$

For the t-test to be valid, it is a requirement that the values in both groups conform to a normal distribution. There are tests that give the probability that the distribution is not normally distributed. It is also a requirement that the variances of the two groups are similar; otherwise, it is necessary to establish the significance of the difference between the variances using the F test. Alternatively, non-parametric tests can be used that do not require a normal distribution, in which values are ranked, as described below.

6.12 Significance of the Difference Between Two Groups of Measurements in a Single Group of Patients (Paired T Test)

Frequently in medical research, we are interested in whether an intervention changes a quantitative attribute. Again, the SE, is the relevant measurement, being in this case the SE of the difference between the 'before and after' values. The value of t is then the mean difference divided by SE of the differences with n–1 degrees of freedom, n being the number of paired observations.

6.13 Testing the Null Hypothesis that There Is No Difference Between the Means of More than Two Groups (ANOVA)

When there are more than two groups of patients, it is not appropriate to perform multiple t-tests on pairs of the groups—three pairs for example when there are three groups—but instead to perform a single test that embraces all the groups simultaneously, called analysis of variance. ANOVA is based on the F-distribution and combines *within* group variance and *between* group variance to produce a ratio not unlike mean difference/SE. The higher the ratio, the smaller the ultimate p value. Take the following three-group data.

	Group 1	Group 2	Group 3	
	$n_1 = 3$	$n_2 = 5$	$n_3 = 4$	Total n = 12
	3 (1)	5 (4)	7 (4)	
	4 (0)	6 (1)	8 (1)	
	5 (1)	7 (0)	10 (1)	
		8 (1)	11 (4)	
		9 (4)		
Mean	4	7	9	

Each group has its mean value, namely 4, 7, and 9 for groups 1, 2 and 3. The overall mean embracing all 3 groups is 6.9 (i.e. 83/12), which for simplicity we will round off to 7.

To obtain the *within* group variance, each value is subtracted from the mean value of its group. The squared differences (shown in brackets in the table above) are all then summed to give in this example a total of 22.

To obtain the *between* group variance, the mean of each group is subtracted from the overall mean, squared and multiplied by n for the group. The three results are then summed,

$$\text{i.e. } n_1(4-7)^2 + n_2(7-7)^2 + n_3(9-7)^{2.}$$

$$\text{giving } 27+0+16=43.$$

The p value is obtained from the F-distribution. This carries degrees of freedom for this example of 2 for *between* (number of groups minus one) and 9 for *within* (total number of observations minus the number of groups). The degrees of freedom are divided into the summed values for *between* and *within* to give 43/2 (i.e. 21.5) and 22/9 (i.e. 2.44), respectively. The final test statistic is then 21.5/2.44, giving 8.81. In the F table, *between* is the numerator with 2 degrees of freedom and *within* is the denominator with 9 degrees of freedom, giving a p value of 0.008. The null hypothesis that there are no differences between the three groups in this example can therefore be rejected.

The principles are the same when there are more than three groups. *Between* and *within* are derived in the same way and have the appropriate degrees of freedom that depend respectively on the total number of groups (minus one) and the total number of individual values (minus the number of groups).

6.14 Strength of Correlation and Confidence Limits of Regression

Correlation measures the degree of association between two independent variables. It is given as the correlation coefficient (or Pearson's correlation coefficient), r, which is positive for a rising relationship and negative for one that is declining. Correlation analysis may test the relationship between two versions of the same variable, such as renal blood flow measured in two different ways, or between two different variables, such as GFR and age. The formula for calculating r is too complex for presentation here. The information given by r—in other words the strength of the association—is dependent on the number of observations, n, on which it is based, and this is reflected in the p value with which it is associated. As always, n is critical; thus, r may decrease as n increases, but p may still decrease. It is common to express r as r^2 to eliminate the negative sign when there is an inverse correlation.

In correlation, one variable is dependent on the other. Regression defines how the independent variable changes as a function of the dependent variable. For example, GFR declines with advancing age at the rate of about 1 ml/min per year. When the regression equation is known, it can be used to predict a y value from the corresponding x value. Indeed, for deciding the safety of prospective kidney transplant donation, normal ranges for GFR have been established for each age decade.

The regression gradient may pass through the origin of the graph (where y and x are both 0) or it may display an intercept. An intercept has both x and y values. When the x intercept is positive, the y intercept is negative, and vice versa. An SE can be calculated for an intercept and give a level of probability as to whether the intercept is significantly different from zero. Likewise, the regression gradient has an SE which can be used to derive the confidence limits of the gradient or whether a gradient differs significantly from the gradient in a separate cohort.

When x and y are different measures of the same variable (usually where x is the 'gold standard' and y a 'new method' for measuring the same thing), an alternative method to assess agreement can be used called Bland-Altman analysis, in which the difference between y and corresponding x is plotted against the average of y and corresponding x. The mean of the differences between x and y is called bias and the SD of the differences is called precision. These terms effectively replace correlation coefficient.

A major rule in correlation analysis is to ensure that x and y values are completely independent. If a variable is present in both axes, then the correlation will be invalid. Examples include correlating one tissue SUV in PET/CT with another in the same individual (an error that can readily be found in the literature) because both SUVs contain the individual's weight and the administered activity. If the weight is erroneously measured as low, for example, both SUVs will increase and increase the r value.

Extreme values also bias the association, and ideally both axes should be normally distributed. Figure 6.3 shows the effect of inclusion of an extreme value. Without the value, r^2 is 0.003, but with it, r^2 increases to 0.64. One solution to minimise the influence of the outlier is to take the reciprocals of the variable, which in Fig. 6.3 brings r^2 down to 0.185. This would be appropriate, for example if the variable, such as lung disappearance of an inhaled radiopharmaceutical, could be given either as a rate constant or half-time. Another is to use rank correlation, as described below, which is a non-parametric test, and for this relationship would give a Spearman rank correlation coefficient, r_s, of −0.38, similar to panel C of Fig. 6.3 ($r = -0.43$).

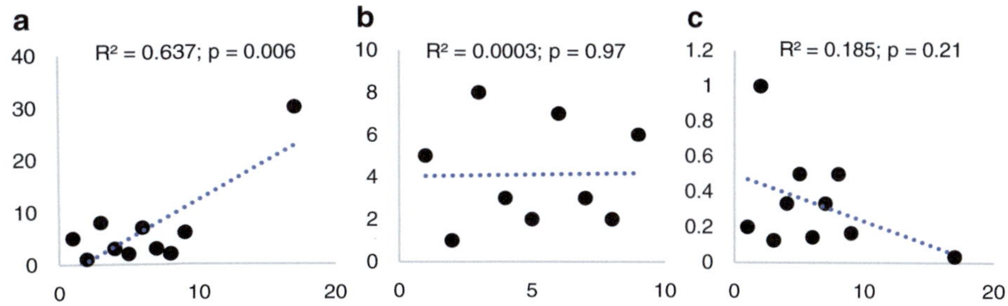

Fig. 6.3 Effect of an outlier on correlation analysis (**a**). Removing the outlier abolishes the correlation (**b**). Taking reciprocals of the y values partly restores it (**c**). Using, Spearman rank correlation, $r_s^2 = 0.144$

6.15 Interpretation of Correlation Coefficient and Regression

6.15.1 When the Correlation Coefficient Is of Greater Interest than the Regression

When, for example, it is suspected that a physiological variable predisposes an individual to cancer, a significant association between the variable and cancer risk is a crucial finding, even if r is low but nevertheless significant. The regression equation is less important, though still relevant. In such circumstances, the correlation coefficient may be quite low but still highly significant if the cohort is large.

6.15.2 When the Regression Is of Greater Interest than the Correlation Coefficient

Predicting a y value from a known association uses the regression equation. Establishing, for example, the normal range of GFR in the age group 60–70 requires not only knowledge of the regression equation of GFR on age but also its confidence limits. In Patlak-Rutland analysis (Chap. 3), the gradient of the regression is of predominant interest because it gives tissue tracer clearance. The correlation coefficient of the plot is nevertheless still relevant, as it portrays the confidence in the measured clearance value.

6.15.3 When Both Are Equally Important

An example of similar importance is the measurement of GFR with a filtration marker from the slope-intercept technique, as described in Chap. 11. Once a GFR marker has mixed throughout its distribution volume, the exponential decline in its plasma concentration (the regression) gives marker clearance per unit volume of distribution. It is routinely based, however, on only 3 samples, so the correlation coefficient needs to be at least 0.985, or the study is rejected.

Further Readings

1. Emami H, Singh P, MacNabb M, et al. Splenic metabolic activity predicts risk of future cardiovascular events: demonstration of a cardiosplenic axis in humans. JACC Cardiovasc Imaging. 2015;8:121–30.
2. Altman DG. Practical statistics for medical research. London: Chapman and Hall; 1991.

7 Non-parametric Statistics

When a dataset does not have a normal distribution, it is not appropriate to use parametric statistics. It may be possible, nevertheless, to convert a non-normal distribution to a normal one. For example, a distribution with a peak skewed to the left and a long tail to the right may be converted to a normal distribution by taking the logarithm of the x values—log transformation—giving a log-normal distribution. Tests are available to find whether a distribution is normal. A low p value in such tests rejects the null hypothesis that the distribution is not normal.

For comparing data from two groups, parametric statistical tests are only appropriate if the variances of the two groups are similar. The F test, which is based on the ratio of the variances, gives a p value which if low rejects the null hypothesis that the variances in the two cohorts are not similar. Non-parametric statistics should be used when parametric statistical tests are deemed inappropriate. Statistical significance in non-parametric tests is generally based on ranking the values in the datasets.

7.1 Significance of the Difference Between Two Groups of Patients (Equivalent to Unpaired T Test)

This is achieved with a test called the Mann-Whitney test, also known as the Wilcoxon rank test. Values are ranked irrespective of the group they are in. The total, Σ, of rank numbers (in brackets) in the smaller group (or either group if they have equal patient numbers) is then summed. For example,

Group 1 ($n_1 = 8$)	Group 2 ($n_2 = 7$)
19 (5)	25 (3)
38 (2)	10 (9)
12 (7)	7 (12)
11 (8)	9 (10)
21 (4)	4 (14)
8 (11)	3 (15)
14 (6)	6 (13)
63 (1)	
Σ (44)	(76)

The p value is obtained from Σ in the smaller group (76) using the Mann-Whitney p table. The range of values within which Σ is located widens as p decreases. Thus, the relevant line in the Mann-Whitney table for $n_1 = 8$ and $n_2 = 7$, is.

p	<0.1	0.05	0.02	0.01	0.001
	41–71	38–74	35–77	34–78	29–83

The last range, reading from left to right, within which 76 is not included is the range 38–74, so $p < 0.05$.

A. M. Peters, M. Vadrucci, *Introduction to Nuclear Medicine for Trainees in Imaging and Imaging Sciences*, https://doi.org/10.1007/978-3-032-18364-4_7

7.2 Significance of the Difference Between More than Two Groups of Patients (Equivalent to ANOVA)

When there are more than two groups and normal distributions cannot be assumed, a non-parametric test can be used, such as the Kruskal-Wallis test, which is based on the chi-squared distribution. Values are ranked irrespective of which group they are in. In this example (same data as above for ANOVA, above), overall rank numbers are shown in brackets.

	Group 1	Group 2	Group 3	
				Total
	$n_1 = 3$	$n_2 = 5$	$n_3 = 4$	n = 12
	3 (12)	5 (9.5)	7 (6.5)	
	4 (11)	6 (8)	8 (4.5)	
	5 (9.5)	7 (6.5)	10 (2)	
		8 (4.5)	11 (1)	
		9 (3)		
Rank Σ	32.5	31.5	14	
Rank Σ^2	1056.25	992.25	196	
Rank Σ^2/n	352	198	49	

The appropriate formula is

$$H = \frac{12}{\left[n(n+1)\right]} * \frac{\Sigma_1^2}{n_1} + \frac{\Sigma_2^2}{n_2} + \frac{\Sigma_3^2}{n_3} - 3(n+1) \tag{7.1}$$

$$\text{giving}\left[(12/156)*(352+198+49)\right]-39$$

$$= 7.12$$

(Note the term '12' does not refer to total n. It is a consistent term in the formula.)

The p value for 7.12, obtained from the chi-squared distribution, is 0.03, thereby rejecting the null hypothesis that there is no difference between the groups. Note the difference in p when this dataset is subjected to non-parametric statistics compared with parametric ANOVA, above, which gave a p value of 0.008.

7.3 Significance of the Difference Between Two Groups of Measurement in a Single Group of Patients (Equivalent to Paired T Test)

Significance is derived from the Wilcoxon matched pairs test. Non-zero differences between paired groups of measurements are ranked irrespective of whether they are positive or negative, *with ranking (in brackets) starting from the smallest difference*. For example

Positive differences	Negative differences
n = 10	n = 7
60 (13)	8 (3)
44 (11)	5 (2)
89 (16)	14 (5)
17 (6)	3 (1)
24 (9)	12 (4)
37 (10)	19 (7)
90 (17)	22 (8)
77 (15)	
53 (12)	
65 (14)	
Σ(123)	(30)

The p value is obtained from Σ in either group. As with Mann-Whitney, the range of values in the Wilcoxon table within which Σ is located widens as p decreases. Thus, the relevant line in the Wilcoxon table for n = 17, is

P	<0.2	0.1	0.05	0.02	0.01	0.001
	48–105	41–112	34–119	28–125	23–130	11–142

For 17 pairs of values, 123 and 30 are both located in the range 28–125, but not in the range 34–119, so there is a significant difference between paired values with $p < 0.02$.

7.4 Strength of Association (Equivalent to Pearson Correlation)

This is achieved with a test called Spearman rank correlation. The differences, d, between the ranks of paired values—ranked within their respective groups—are squared, thereby eliminating negative values, summed and inserted into the following equation to give the correlation coefficient, r_s.

$$r_s = 1 - \frac{\sum d^2 * 6}{n^3 - n} \tag{7.2}$$

where n is the number of pairs. Corresponding p values for r_s values can be looked up in published tables, as with r for Pearson correlation.

$$n^3 - n$$

For example, in the first pair, measurement 1 (12) is ranked eighth and measurement 2 (44) is ranked fifth, giving a squared difference between the two corresponding ranks of 9.

Measurement 1	Measurement 2	Rank difference	Squared
12 (8)	44 (5)	+3	9
26 (6)	39 (6)	0	0
14 (7)	7 (8)	−1	1
86 (2)	88 (2)	0	0
120 (1)	77 (3)	−2	4
65 (4)	93 (1)	+3	9
73 (3)	68 (4)	−1	1
43 (5)	25 (7)	−2	4
			Σ28

$$Rs = 1 - (168/504) = 0.67$$

$$P < 0.1$$

7.5 Diagnostic Accuracy

A diagnostic test to determine the presence or otherwise of disease may take the form of a numerical value or an image.

- *Test sensitivity* is the number of true test positives in a cohort of patients divided by the number of patients who have the disease.
- *Test specificity* is the number of true test negatives divided by the number of patients who do not have the disease.
- *Diagnostic accuracy* is the number of true positives plus the number of true negatives divided by the total number of patients in the cohort.
- *Positive predictive value* is true positives divided by all positives.
- *Negative predictive value* is true negatives divided by all negatives.

7.6 Receiver Operating Characteristic (ROC) Curve Analysis

ROC analysis is used to assess the diagnostic accuracy of an image or numerical measurement to determine whether a specific disease exists in a cohort of individuals. It enables selection of the optimum threshold or cut-off of a measurement above or below which an individual can be deemed to be normal or abnormal. Moreover, the diagnostic accuracies of two or more test measurements can be compared. ROC analysis is easier to understand with respect to a quantitative threshold rather than one based on image appearances.

The ROC curve plots sensitivity on the y-axis against 1-specificity on the x-axis and is therefore unitless. The area under the curve (AUC) is the endpoint and has a maximum value of one. In general, as cut-off values vary, sensitivity and specificity vary in opposite directions. Sensitivity therefore bears a positive relationship with 1—specificity. Take for example the diagnosis of renal artery stenosis (RAS) from reduced renal blood flow (RBF), the normal value of which is 10% of cardiac output. If 2% was taken as the cut-off point for RAS, many patients with RAS who have higher RBF values than 2% will be missed, giving a low sensitivity, but no one without RAS will be falsely diagnosed, giving a high specificity. Conversely, taking 9% as the threshold will result in false positives and low specificity. If sensitivity and specificity were both 50% at an RBF of say 6%, then the plot will be a straight

a

	sens	spec	1-spec	diag acc
	0	1.00	0	
●○●●	0.25	0.92	0.08	0.58
○●○●	0.42	0.75	0.25	0.58
●●○●	0.67	0.67	0.33	0.67
○●○○	0.75	0.42	0.58	0.67
●○●○	0.92	0.25	0.75	0.58
○○○●	1	0	1.00	0.50

b

	sens	spec	1-spec	diag acc
	0	1.00	0	
●●●●	0.33	1.00	0	0.67
○●●●	0.58	0.92	0.08	0.75
●●●○	0.83	0.83	0.17	0.83
○●○○	0.92	0.58	0.42	0.75
○○●○	1.00	0.33	0.67	0.67
○○○○	1.00	0	1.00	0.50

c

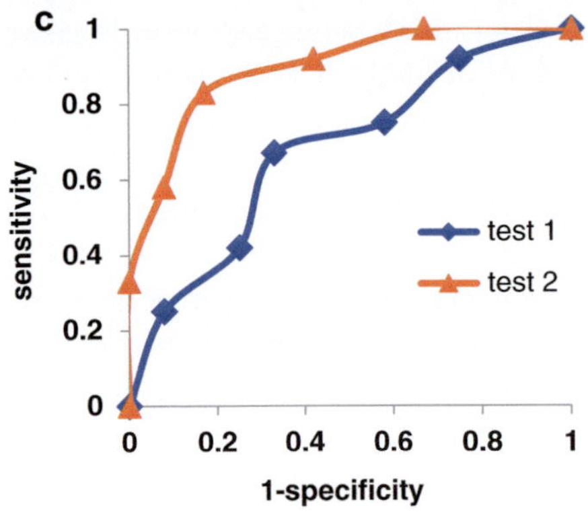

Fig. 7.1 ROC analysis for two different test measurements: A: Test 1, B: Test 2. Individuals with and without disease or disorder are shown as closed and open symbols, respectively (sens: sensitivity; spec: specificity; diag acc: diagnostic accuracy). Horizontal lines represent test measurement cut-off values. Note that the number of test measurement values, shown as equal here for the two tests, need not necessarily be equal. ROC curves are shown in C. AUC for test 1: ~0.7; AUC for test 2: ~0.9 (p = 0.09)

diagonal line from the origin to top right corner of the plot, indicating that the test has no value. On the other hand, high sensitivity *and* high specificity will place a point close to the top left corner of the plot and give a curve with an AUC close to unity.

The technique is illustrated in Fig. 7.1, which compares two test measurements. AUC is most easily determined by counting squares enclosed under the curve. In the two curves shown, AUC for the test measurement in A is ~0.7 (i.e., 70% of maximum area) and ~0.9 in B. The standard error of a curve depends on its AUC and the numbers of individuals with and without the disease (12 in both in Fig. 7.1). The significance of the difference between the two curves is based on their standard errors and can be calculated using an online calculator, which for these two curves gives a two-tailed p value of about 0.09.

ROC analysis requires the existence of a 'gold standard' to permit the derivation of sensitivity and specificity for a test measurement. A gold standard, however, may not always be available. Take disease of the basal ganglia, for example, which from I-123-ioflupane is quantified as a target-to-background ratio and expressed as a z score (Chaps. 6 and 24). ROC analysis has not been used to identify an optimum cut-off because confirming pathology in the basal ganglia can only be achieved post-mortem. So, instead, an age-dependent normal range has been derived and cut off based on the patient's z score.

Further Reading

1. Metz CE. Basic principles of ROC analysis. Semin Nuclear Med. 1978;8:283–98.

8 Interpretation of Statistical Significance

In general, you should not assume that the outcome of a study will be in the direction that you anticipate. Comparing two sets of unpaired data, for example, the mean of group A may turn out to be higher or lower than the mean of group B. This means that your test of significance needs to be two-tailed. If for some reason you are certain that the mean of group A cannot be higher than the mean of group B (or vice versa), the test can be one-tailed, which halves the p value for a corresponding t value and number of degrees of freedom. Similarly, in correlation, p for an r value should be two-tailed unless you are certain the correlation must be positive (or inverse).

The outcome of studies involving continuous data should not be regarded as positive or negative but as *probably* positive or *probably* negative, depending on how many samples are in the cohort and therefore on the p value. Sometimes one finds in publications the statement that the outcome in one group was significant because the p value was 0.045 and in another it was not significant because the p value was 0.061, so the two group outcomes are different. But, of course, this is an unjustified conclusion.

Positivity in outcome also carries publication bias. If an identical study, depending on precisely what it investigated, was performed in 20 different centres, one of them will end up with a p value of 0.05, increasing its likelihood of acceptance for publication over the 19 with negative outcomes.

Outliers are another problem, which often, as single values, determine whether a study has a positive or negative outcome, as shown in Fig 6.3. There are guidelines available as to whether and how outliers should be rejected, but they are difficult to understand for the relative novice. Strategies available to avoid discarding outliers are to take the logs of the values or their reciprocals or use non-parametric statistics. Alternatively, it is acceptable to present the results with and without the outlier and leave it to the discretion of the reviewers.

Acknowledgement Matthew Aldridge, King's College Hospital, London.

Further Reading

1. Altman DG. Statistics and ethics in medical research. BMJ. 1980;281:1.

A. M. Peters, M. Vadrucci, *Introduction to Nuclear Medicine for Trainees in Imaging and Imaging Sciences*, https://doi.org/10.1007/978-3-032-18364-4_8

Part III

Basic Sciences of Nuclear Medicine

Nuclear medicine is professionally highly diverse. In contrast to medicine and surgery, in which sub-specialisation has effectively led to the extinction of the general physician and general surgeon—and to general radiology now with numerous sub-specialities—nuclear medicine embraces all specialities and is supported by a diverse range of sciences including radiochemistry, radiopharmacy, clinical science and radiation physics.

9 Basic Sciences of NM

9.1 Radioactive Materials

Nuclear medicine is based on radioactive materials and detectors that record their emitted radiation. Radioactive materials range from single elements, such as radioactive iodine, through more complex radiopharmaceuticals that are chemically designed to target a tissue or system, to radiolabelled macromolecules, especially proteins, and radiolabelled blood cells. Some pharmaceuticals in nuclear medicine are the same as those used for drug therapy in general medicine, including bisphosphonates for osteoporosis, somatostatin analogues for neuroendocrine tumours and dihydroxyphenylalanine (DOPA) for idiopathic Parkinson's disease, but in infinitesimally smaller amounts for nuclear medicine.

9.2 Radionuclides

Radionuclides used for imaging emit gamma radiation generated in response to nuclear rearrangement in the atom—somewhat inappropriately called nuclear disintegration—in which a proton converts to a neutron or vice versa. Nuclei possess neutrons and protons in relative numbers to each other that give nuclear stability. In a nucleus that is unstable because of an excess of neutrons, a neutron may spontaneously convert to a proton. To maintain electrical neutrality, the conversion generates an electron, which is released from the nucleus as beta minus radiation. In contrast, a nucleus that is unstable because of an excess of protons may convert a proton to a neutron by capturing an electron from the inner orbiting shell of electrons. Proton-rich nuclei may also convert a proton to a neutron by emitting a positron, which almost immediately collides with an electron, resulting in annihilation of both. Some radionuclides decay by both beta minus emission and electron capture, such as K-40, which decays to Ca-40 (89%) and Ar-40 (11%).

As a result of these rearrangements, the nucleus is left in an 'excited' state with excess energy that is emitted as gamma radiation. An alternative process by which a nucleus may dissipate its excitement—internal conversion—is by transferring its energy to an orbiting electron, which is ejected as a high-energy electron, resulting in radioactive decay without gamma radiation.

A radionuclide therefore decays to a different element because its atomic number changes, but not its atomic mass. Most radionuclides decay directly to the ground state. Some, however, decay to a daughter with a nucleus that is still unstable and therefore continues to emit gamma radiation for periods ranging from a few seconds to several hours, or longer. Such radionuclides are called metastable and carry an 'm' in their notation. The best example is Tc-99m, the parent of which is Mo-99. This radionuclide decays by

A. M. Peters, M. Vadrucci, *Introduction to Nuclear Medicine for Trainees in Imaging and Imaging Sciences*, https://doi.org/10.1007/978-3-032-18364-4_9

beta minus emission with 12% of disintegrations leading directly to Tc-99 and 88% to Tc-99m, which then decays to Tc-99. The activity of a radionuclide is measured in MBq, where one Bq equates to gamma emission from a nuclear disintegration per second.

The relevant properties of radionuclides include half-life, energy of gamma radiation, and chemical properties that determine the ease with which they can be complexed to a given material. The science underpinning the attachment of radionuclides to pharmaceuticals and other materials, such as macromolecules and intact blood cells, is called radiochemistry. Radiopharmacy is the dispensation of radioactive materials for clinical use.

9.2.1 Half-Life ($t_{1/2}$)

Nuclear disintegration is random, so radionuclides decay exponentially with a rate constant of decay equal to ln $2/t_{1/2}$. Half-lives of medically useful radionuclides range from 13 s (Kr-81m) to 120 d (Se-75). Radiopharmaceuticals bearing ultra-short-lived radionuclides must obviously be administered continuously for the duration of image acquisition.

9.2.2 Emission

The emission relevant to nuclear medicine is gamma radiation, which, within the electromagnetic spectrum, has the highest photon energy, higher than X-rays. The emission energy of gamma photons—measured with a unit called an electron volt (ev)—determines their penetrability through materials, the most important of which are the tissues of the body and the detecting equipment. One can compare a radionuclide with a gun and think of the activity in MBq as the firing rate (bullets per second) and the energy in keV as the size of the bullets. If the energy is too low, I-125 for example, only photons from superficially located activity, such as in the skin, will escape from the body, whereas if the energy is high, such as from I-131, the photons are likely to go straight through the machine, detecting its presence. There is therefore an optimal energy for radioactive sources within the body, and this is in the region of 150 keV. Photons travelling in tissue have a distance value describing a 50% reduction in signal from attenuation—about 5 cm for Tc-99m. Attenuation means that the radioactive signals detected from the front of a patient who has received a radiopharmaceutical are different from those recorded from the back depending on the depth of the sources in the body.

9.3 Radiation Detectors

Detectors range from well counters, handheld probes, and whole-body counters—all of which simply detect a radiation signal—to gamma cameras and PET cameras, which provide an image of the distribution of the radiation sources within a patient. Detectors comprise three main components: crystal, collimator, and photomultiplier tube.

9.3.1 Crystal

This is a single crystal, which is completely transparent. When a photon is brought to a halt in the crystal, its energy is converted into a flash of light called a scintillation, hence the terms scintillation camera and scintigraphy. The scintillation is captured by a photoelectric cell in a photomultiplier tube (PMT) located immediately behind the crystal and converted and amplified to an electrical impulse (Fig. 9.1). The crystal in probes and gamma cameras is sodium iodide and in a PET camera generally LSO (lutetium oxyorthosilicate) or LYSO (lutetium yttrium oxyorthosilicate).

9.3.2 Collimator

The collimator in a probe is simply a lead cylinder that can be moved forwards or backwards over the probe to vary the angle of view. A

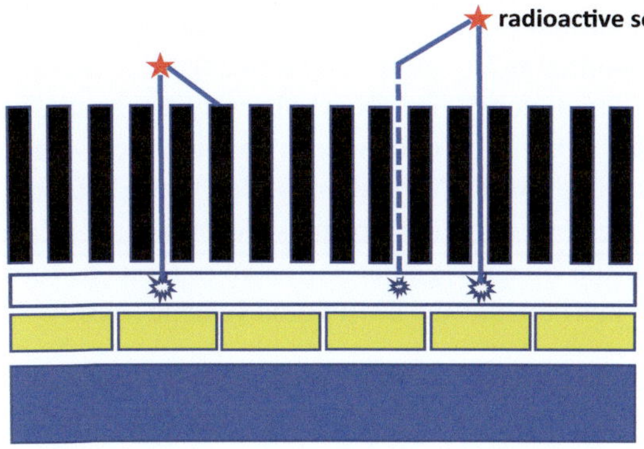

Fig. 9.1 Cartoon of structure of a gamma camera. Gamma photons from a radioactive source can only reach the transparent sodium iodide crystal if they are travelling perpendicular to the face of the collimator. If it stops in the crystal, a gamma photon converts its energy to a flash of light called a scintillation, which is detected by a photoelectric cell in the PMT and converted into an electric pulse. This will be highest in the PMT closest to the scintillation. The pulse is then amplified in the PMT. The computer accepts only those pulses arising from within a defined 'energy window'. Should a photon undergo deflection, it loses energy but may reach the crystal. However, its pulse will be rejected by the pulse height analyser. A deflected proton from a higher energy radionuclide, if present in the patient, may be recorded if its depleted energy level falls within the selected window and, as a result, degrade the image

collimator for a gamma camera is designed to form an image as described below.

9.3.3 Photomultiplier Tube

A PMT incorporates a photoelectric cell to convert the scintillation to an electrical impulse and an amplifier to amplify the pulse before sending it to the computer. Modern gamma cameras are switching to silicon photomultipliers (SiPMs), the physics of which are beyond this text.

Well counters measure activity in biological samples such as blood, urine, and sputum. The most common scenario is measurement of GFR from plasma samples. The sample in a container is inserted into a well of the counter, which has multiple wells for multiple samples, each well having its own scintillation detector. Handheld probes detect signals from parts of the body, such as when a surgeon searches for the sentinel node in the axilla of a patient with breast cancer who has received an injection into the breast a few hours earlier of a radiopharmaceutical that accumulates in axillary lymph nodes. Whole body counters are heavily shielded cubicles and contain multiple scintillation probes, making them highly sensitive to very small amounts of radioactivity. Although useful for research studies, such as counting whole body K-40 to measure whole body potassium, they are now sadly almost obsolete.

9.4 Image Formation

9.4.1 Gamma Camera

The gamma, or scintillation, camera was invented by an American engineer called Hal Anger and was previously known as an Anger camera. The collimator in a gamma camera is a sheet of lead approximately 40 cm in diameter when disc shaped or in length when rectangular. It has tens of thousands of small holes drilled through it. The septum is the lead between the holes. Septal thickness varies from small in a low-energy collimator suitable for a radionuclide like Tc-99m to large in a high energy collimator suitable for a radionuclide like I-131.

The crystal is located immediately behind the collimator and is of similar size in two dimensions to the collimator. Gamma photons emitted from a source of radioactivity within the camera's field of view will only reach the crystal if they are travelling in a direction that is perfectly parallel to the long dimension of the collimator's holes. Any at a slight angle will be absorbed in a septum. The PMT closest to the scintillation generates the greatest electrical impulse whereas PMTs remote to the scintillation generate lower impulses. The more PMTs, of which there are up to 100 in a modern camera, the better the image resolution. The system is highly inefficient, recording less than 1% of emissions.

Photons from the source collide with matter. Because this changes their direction of travel, they may enter distant irrelevant holes. This is called Compton scattering. Scattered photons lose energy and produce weaker scintillations if they reach the crystal. The system is therefore 'tuned' to select only those impulses within a specified energy range using a pulse height analyser. When there is another radionuclide present with a higher energy, the image may be degraded because the energy of scattered photons from this radionuclide may fall within the energy range or 'window' selected for the lower energy radionuclide. Many radionuclides emit gamma photons at several energies. In-111, for example, emits at 171 and 245 keV. Selecting both windows leads to a trade-off between more photons counted and degradation of the counts recorded in the lower window. Using techniques to correct such 'cross-talk', the gamma camera can simultaneously acquire separate images from two different radionuclides by selecting both their gamma energy windows—dual photon imaging.

After a scintillation probe or gamma camera records a scintillation, there is a very short time during which it is unresponsive, called deadtime. The time is so short that this is not generally a problem, but when confronted with a very active source, the detector will underestimate the number of incident photons and therefore the activity in the source, leading to errors in quantification. Photons arriving essentially simultaneously may be erroneously recorded as a single photon with double the energy and rejected by the pulse height analyser. Moreover, with very active sources, the energies of scattered photons may sum to be within the energy window.

Gamma cameras generally have two of the units shown in Fig. 9.1, called heads. For imaging the whole body, the heads—one posterior and one anterior to the patient—move together from the patient's head to toe, either continuously or in a 'step and shoot' mode, at a speed appropriate to gather sufficient photons to form an image, such as a whole-body bone scan.

9.4.2 PET Camera

A positron emitted from the nucleus of a radionuclide immediately collides with an electron and both undergo mutual annihilation. This gives rise to two photons of 511 keV that leave the annihilation site in exactly opposite directions. This is in addition to gamma emission from the nucleus that results from the excited state associated with the conversion of a photon to a neutron.

The two 511 keV photons are detected simultaneously by two scintillation detectors within a ring of multiple detectors surrounding the patient, and a 'line of response' is created. If one of the two photons fails to reach a detector, the system rejects the single photon that is recorded. The lines of response of photon pairs intersect at the site of the source, which can therefore be located. Alternatively, despite travelling at the speed of light, the difference in arrival times of the co-incident photons at their respective detectors can be measured and used to locate the source (time-of-flight PET). Identical flight times indicate that the source is in the centre of the ring (Fig. 9.2).

PET detectors mostly have LSO or LYSO crystals which are better suited to the high energy 511 KeV photons than sodium iodide. Each detector is furnished with several PMTs, typically 4, and modern PET cameras have multiple rings of detectors, enough even to enclose the entire patient from head-to-toe, thereby increasing sensitivity and reducing scan time. As with a gamma camera, a PET camera moves to cover the whole body, unless the camera encloses the whole body.

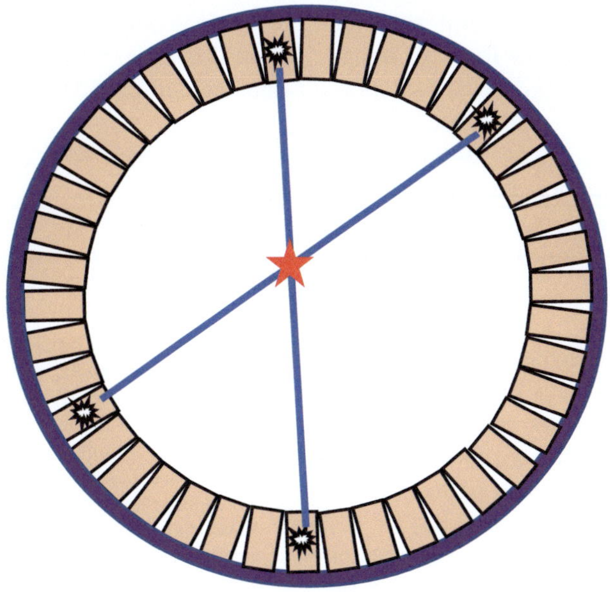

Fig. 9.2 Cartoon of a PET camera. A PET camera contains multiple rings of scintillation detectors that surround the patient. A positron emitted from the nucleus of an atom almost immediately encounters an electron with which it undergoes mutual annihilation. This results in the creation of two gamma photons of 511 KeV each, which leave the annihilation site in opposite directions from each other and are simultaneously recorded in scintillation detectors. Pairs of co-incidentally detected photons travel along lines of response that intersect at the site of the source (red star), thereby permitting location of the source. If one photon of a pair fails to reach a detector or goes through the ring without being stopped, then the scintillation from the other photon in the pair is rejected

9.4.3 Co-Registration

Nowadays, gamma and PET cameras can be combined with a CT machine to give hybrid cameras that provide images that combine the functional information of radionuclides and the anatomical information of CT. The functional and anatomical images—SPECT/CT and PET/CT—are acquired in sequence rather than simultaneously, so any patient movement in between may lead to slight degrees of misregistration. Frequently, a decision needs to be made immediately following completion of a study, usually a bone scan in which the location of a scintigraphic abnormality is not clear, whether to perform SPECT/CT. PET is essentially always acquired as PET/CT, although PET/MRI is becoming increasingly used.

9.5 Image (Data) Acquisition

For most nuclear medicine studies, the radioactive agent is injected intravenously. Other routes of administration are oral for gastrointestinal studies, inhalation for lung function, intradermal for imaging the lymphatic system, conjunctival sac for tear drainage, and, rarely, intra-arterial injection for blood flow measurement and intrathecal injection for CSF circulation.

Data acquisition may commence immediately following administration (dynamic imaging) or be delayed until the tissue of interest has accumulated sufficient radiopharmaceutical for imaging (static imaging). This may be 3 h for a bone scan, 24 h for an In-111 white blood cell scan or 7 days for a Se-75 scan. Ultra-short-lived radionuclides, such as Kr-81 m (13 s half-life), are administered continuously until sufficient counts have been acquired to form an image. Continuous infusion of longer-lived radiopharmaceuticals to achieve a steady state is rarely practiced. SPECT produces 3-dimensional images by rotating the camera around the patient and acquiring static images from multiple angles. SPECT cannot be performed during dynamic imaging. Image acquisition may be linked to a physiological event, such as in multiple gated cardiac acquisition in which a rapid sequence of images, usually 16 or 32, is obtained during a single cardiac cycle triggered by the p wave in the ECG, and the sequence is repeated a hundred-fold to generate an image of the beating heart (see Chap. 20).

Finally, in nuclear medicine, image orientation is as in regular photography. Thus, if the image is acquired from behind the patient, right is on the reader's right. So be careful not to get right and left mixed up!

Acknowledgement Ben Corcoran, Barts Health NHS Trust, London.

Further Reading

1. Surti S. Update on time-of-flight PET imaging. J Nucl Med. 2015;56:98–105.
2. Cherry SR, Jones T, Karp JS, Qi J, Moses WW, Badawi RD. Total-body PET: maximizing sensitivity to create new opportunities for clinical research and patient care. J Nucl Med. 2018;59:3–12.
3. Szczepura KR, Ruparelia P, Solanki CK, et al. Measuring whole-body neutrophil redistribution using a dedicated whole-body counter and ultra-low doses of ^{111}Indium. Eur J Clin Investig. 2011;41:77–83.

Part IV

Tc-99m Compounds

Tc-99m is the most frequently used radionuclide in nuclear medicine practice, either in the free state or complexed to a wide range of compounds and blood cells. Metastable radionuclides, of which Tc-99m is an example, are still excitable after nuclear disintegration of the parent and continue to emit gamma radiation until they reach the ground state. Mo-99 decays by beta minus emission to Tc-99 (12% of disintegrations) and Tc-99m (88%). Tc-99m decays to Tc-99 with a half-life of 6 h. A Mo-99 generator has a half-life of 2.75 days, which gives it a useful life span of 1 week and from which Tc-99m, as pertechnetate (Tc-99mO4), can be drawn daily.

10 Free Tc-99m (Pertechnetate; Tc-99mO$_4$; 161 Da; Half-Life 6 h)

Metastable radionuclides, of which Tc-99m is an example, are still excitable after nuclear disintegration of the parent and continue to emit gamma radiation until they reach the ground state. Mo-99, for example, decays by beta minus emission to Tc-99 (12% of disintegrations) and Tc-99m (88%). Tc-99m decays to Tc-99 with a half-life of 6 h. A Mo-99 generator has a half-life of 2.75 days, which gives it a useful life span of 1 week and from which Tc-99m, as pertechnetate (Tc-99mO$_4$), can be drawn daily.

Tc-99mO$_4$ is handled similarly to free iodide and accumulates in the thyroid (although, unlike iodide, not organified), gastric mucosa, and salivary glands after iv administration. It is therefore used to image firstly the thyroid and secondly ectopic gastric mucosa (usually in Meckel's diverticulum). Tc-99mO$_4$ is partly protein-bound in plasma, and some enters red cells. As a small hydrophilic molecule, the protein-free fraction exchanges across microvascular endothelium between plasma and interstitial space and undergoes glomerular filtration and urinary excretion.

10.1 Thyroid Scintigraphy

10.1.1 Thyroid Imaging in Adults

Thyroid scintigraphy in adults aims to distinguish between the 3 main causes of hyperthyroidism: thyroiditis, autonomous toxic nodule and Graves' disease. It may be used to determine whether a mediastinal mass is ectopic thyroid tissue (Fig. 10.1). Tracer accumulation in the thyroid is quantified as the percentage of administered activity in the thyroid at 20 min post-injection (normal range of 1–3%) or as the thyroid-to-surrounding tissue activity ratio, which is less favoured and has no clearly established normal range. Because TSH levels in blood are reduced in hyperthyroidism, each thyroid lobe should be separately quantified to evaluate 'suppression' of the lobe contralateral to an autonomous toxic nodule.

A. M. Peters, M. Vadrucci, *Introduction to Nuclear Medicine for Trainees in Imaging and Imaging Sciences*, https://doi.org/10.1007/978-3-032-18364-4_10

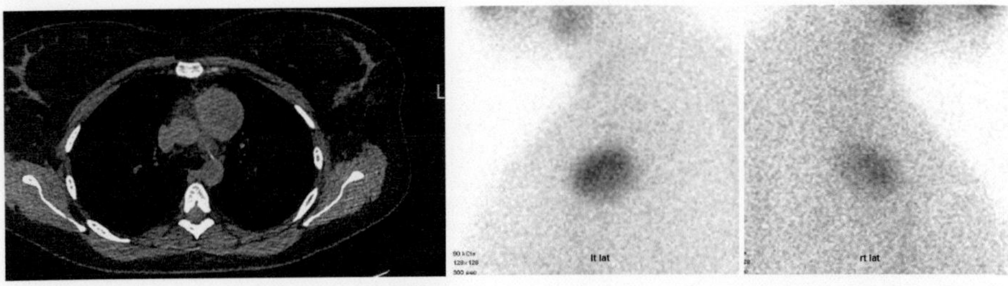

Fig. 10.1 Lateral planar Tc-99mO$_4$ scans and CT showing an ectopic thyroid in the chest

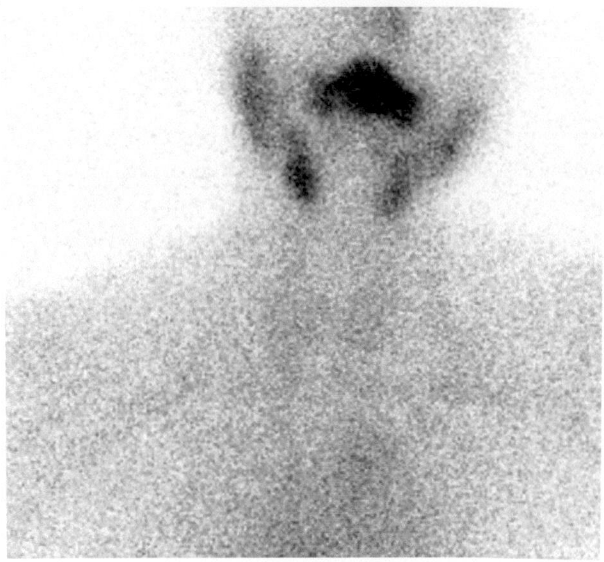

Fig. 10.2 Absent tracer accumulation in thyroid. Causes include thyroiditis, amiodarone therapy, recent contrast CT and iodine-containing medication or foods

10.1.1.1 Thyroiditis

In thyroiditis there is loss of cellular integrity of thyroidal cells resulting in the liberation of thyroxine into the circulation and thyrotoxicosis. The gland fails to accumulate Tc-99mO$_4$ and is not seen or only faintly seen on imaging (Fig. 10.2). The cause is usually a viral infection. Variants include the thyroiditis of pregnancy and thyroiditis induced by amiodarone therapy. Amiodarone also induces thyrotoxicosis in a thyroid with pre-existing abnormalities, such as multinodular goitre (Fig. 10.3). This is type 1 amiodarone-induced thyrotoxicosis, while type 2 is thyroiditis. Amiodarone is rich in iodine, and the thyroid is usually not seen in patients who have a recent history of amiodarone consumption because of competition with iodine. Types 1 and 2 amiodarone-induced thyrotoxicosis can be distinguished with Tc-99m-sestamibi (Chap. 16), which shows uptake in type 1, because the cells are intact, but not in type 2.

10.1.1.2 Autonomous Nodules

Thyroid nodules may escape TSH control, function autonomously, show increased Tc-99mO$_4$ accumulation, and give hyperthyroidism. Such nodules are solitary (Figs. 10.4 and 16.7) or multiple and may or may not be toxic (Fig. 10.5). Hyperthyroidism suppresses TSH secretion so that uninvolved thyroid tissue, for example, the contralateral lobe to a solitary toxic nodule, fails to accumulate Tc-99mO$_4$. A combination of autonomy and suppression explains the heterogeneity of Tc-99mO$_4$ accumulation in multinodular goitre. A dominant cold nodule (Fig. 10.6) raises a suspicion of thyroid cancer.

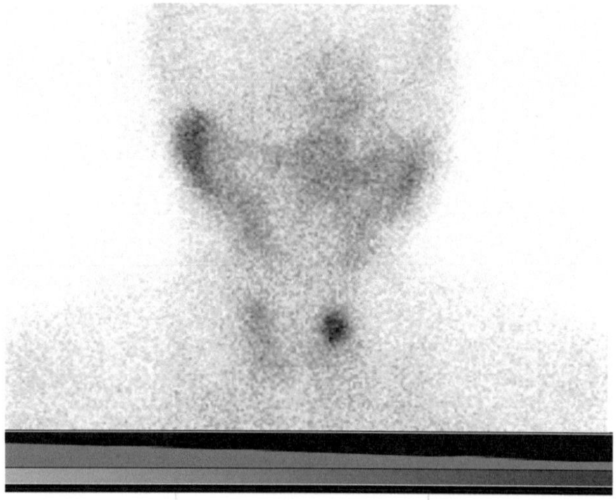

Thyroid	0.36 %	1.00 % - 3.00 %
Right Lobe	0.14 %	0.50 % - 1.50 %
Left Lobe	0.22 %	0.50 % - 1.50 %

Fig. 10.3 The patient was referred with suspected amiodarone-induced thyrotoxicosis. There is only faint tracer accumulation in the right lobe of the thyroid, but there is a focus of relatively increased uptake in the upper pole of the left lobe. Quantification is abnormally reduced at 0.36%. On a background of amiodarone suppression—on account of its high iodine content—the study suggests type 1 amiodarone-induced thyrotoxicosis, which generally occurs in thyroids with pre-existing disease. Type 2, a form of thyroiditis, would have shown no uptake

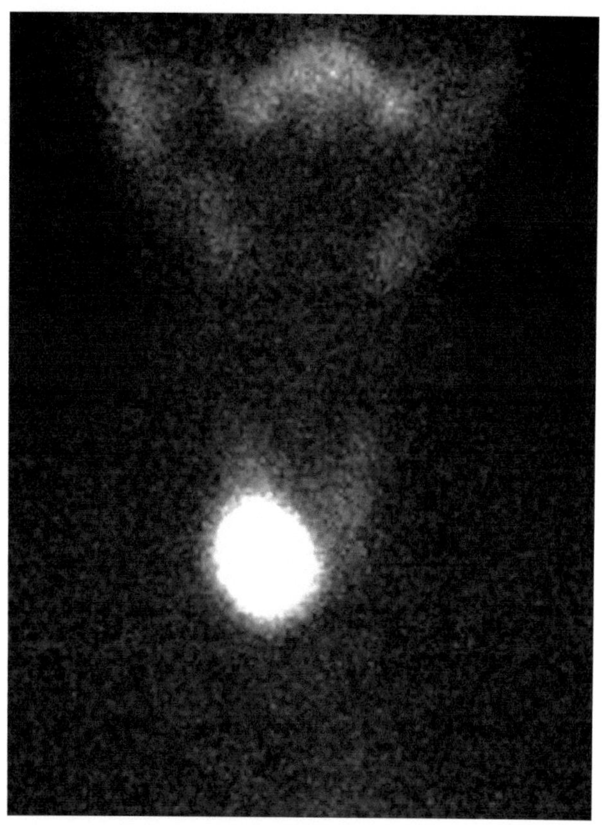

Fig. 10.4 Solitary autonomous toxic nodule in lower pole of right lobe of thyroid. The right lobe accumulated 3.7% of administered activity 20 min post-injection and the left lobe, 0.2% (normal range for whole gland is 1–3%). The upper pole of the right lobe and the left lobe show very little tracer uptake ('suppressed') because of low TSH levels

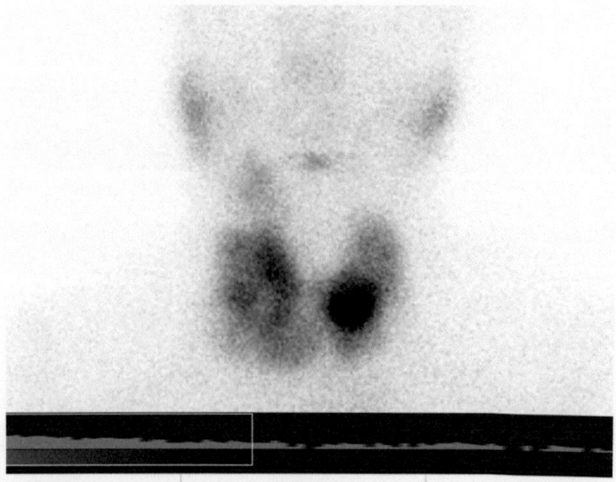

Thyroid	6.60 %	1.00 % - 3.00 %
Right Lobe	3.36 %	0.50 % - 1.50 %
Left Lobe	3.13 %	0.50 % - 1.50 %

Fig. 10.5 Toxic multinodular goitre showing heterogenous overall increased tracer accumulation throughout the thyroid. Quantification of tracer accumulation as a percentage of administered activity at 20 min post-injection is abnormally increased at 6.6% (normal range 1–3%). Note absent uptake in left submandibular gland

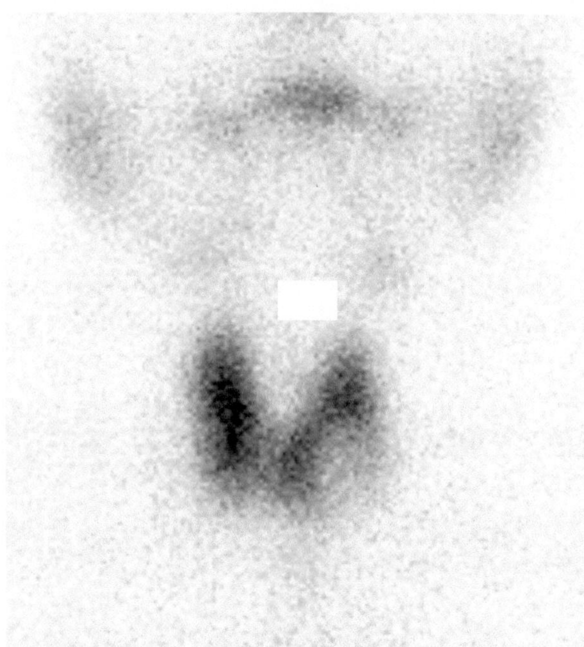

Fig. 10.6 Dominant cold nodule in left lower pole in a Tc-99mO_4 thyroid scan

10.1.1.3 Graves' Disease

Graves' disease is caused by antibody-mediated stimulation of the thyroid via its TSH receptors. The thyroid may or may not be enlarged and typically shows symmetrical and prominent homogeneous Tc-99mO_4 accumulation amounting to >3% of the administered activity at 20 min post-injection. The pyramidal lobe is often visualised and supports a diagnosis of Graves' disease (Fig. 10.7). An uptake value within the normal range does not exclude the diagnosis and may be reduced if the patient is receiving carbimazole. Rarely, uptake values are subnormal because the patient has self-medicated with iodine-containing substances or eaten fish containing iodine, and patients should be questioned accordingly. Patients who have been given radiological contrast medium must wait 6 months before thyroid scintigraphy because of the iodine content of the medium (Fig. 10.8). This period is similar to that required for amiodarone escape.

Graves' disease may occur in a pre-existing nodular gland and resemble toxic multinodular goitre. A nodule may not be responsive to the anti-thyroid antibody causing the disease and remain 'cold' because TSH levels are suppressed, giving rise to a dominant cold nodule. When the patient is treated with anti-thyroid medication and the TSH levels return to normal, the nodule may become visible, an event referred to as Marine-Lenhart syndrome.

10.1.1.4 Reporting an Adult Tc-99mO_4 Thyroid Scan

Most patients have biochemical thyrotoxicosis, and it is not the purpose of the scan or the quantification to diagnose thyrotoxicosis but instead to establish its cause. Always compare with thyroid ultrasonography if available. Note the size and position of the gland, whether there is retrosternal extension, and whether the pyramidal lobe is visible. Note whether the patient is receiving carbimazole, which reduces thyroid Tc-99mO_4 accumulation, or self-medicating with iodine-rich substances.

Homogeneous and symmetrical tracer accumulation points to Graves' disease. Prominent heterogenous uptake points to toxic multinodular goitre but may also be seen in Graves' disease involving a multinodular gland. A visible pyramidal lobe clinches Graves'. Note the presence or otherwise of a dominant cold nodule. Solitary autonomous nodules result in suppression of extra-nodular thyroid tissue. Absent or negligible tracer accumulation throughout the gland points to thyroiditis, provided the patient has not consumed iodine or been given radiological contrast within 6 months.

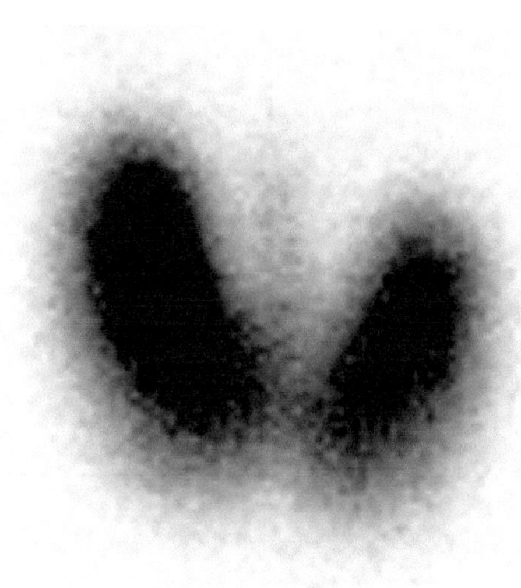

Fig. 10.7 Visualisation of a midline pyramidal lobe confirming Graves' disease

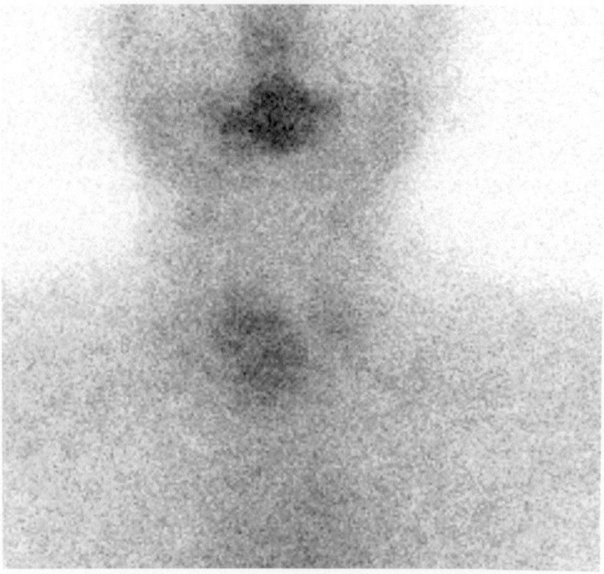

Fig. 10.8 Thyroid scan in a hyperthyroid patient with a multinodular goitre who 2 months previously had CTPA. Uptake at 20 min post-injection was 0.37%

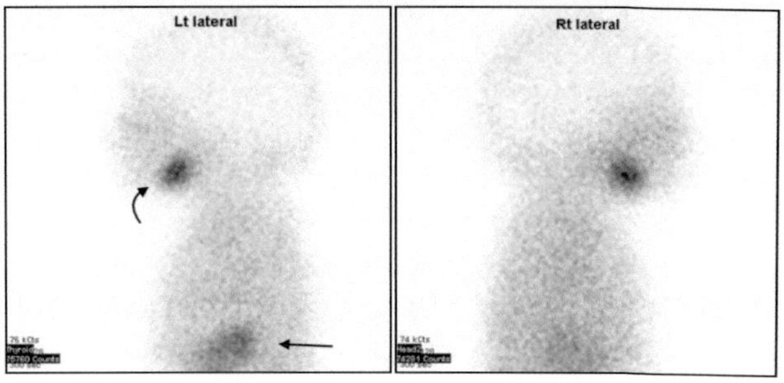

Fig. 10.9 Sublingual thyroid (curved arrow) in a neonate with congenital hypothyroidism. Note gastric activity (straight arrow). No normal range exists for quantification in this age group

10.1.2 Paediatric Thyroid Imaging

In contrast to scintigraphy in adult thyroid disease, which generally aims to identify the cause of hyperthyroidism, children (usually young infants) are routinely referred with hypothyroidism (usually from birth), the causes of which include thyroid agenesis, thyroid hypoplasia, ectopic thyroid and dyshormonogenesis. In dyshormonogenesis, there is an inborn error of metabolism in which the thyroid is unable to organify iodine and produce thyroxine. In a hypothyroid infant, Tc-99mO_4 uptake is reduced in aplastic or ectopic thyroid (Fig. 10.9), while in dyshormonogenesis it is increased or at least shows a level of uptake incompatible with thyroid hypofunction, because although the thyroid cannot manufacture thyroxine, it is still able to respond to raised TSH levels and concentrate iodine and Tc-99mO_4 (Fig. 10.10). There is no normal range for thyroid accumulation in children.

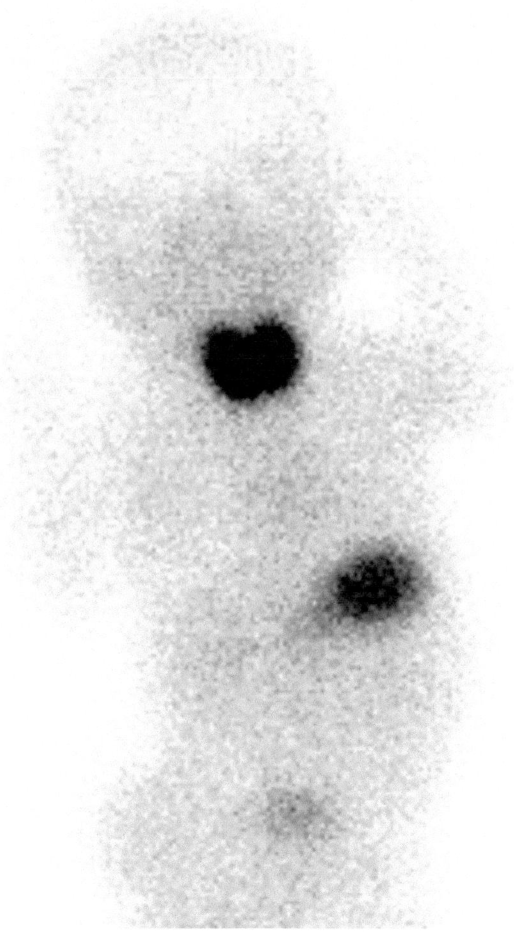

Fig. 10.10 Dyshormonogenesis in a 4-week-old infant. Thyroid accumulation of tracer in thyroid is markedly increased because of high TSH level in blood

10.2 Ectopic Gastric Mucosa

Ectopic gastric mucosa may ulcerate and bleed, giving rise to the typical presentation of painless melaena, most often in a child. The contained gastric mucosa accumulates Tc-99mO_4 with a time course that parallels physiological accumulation in the stomach. A Meckel's diverticulum, present in the appendix, is the commonest site for ectopic gastric mucosa and on Tc-99m0_4 scanning is usually seen as a focus of activity in the right iliac fossa (Fig. 10.11). Or it may move to different locations in the abdomen—'wandering' Meckel's (Fig. 10.12). Duodenal reduplication cysts may also contain gastric mucosa and be seen in the right upper quadrant. Although referrals for 'Meckel's scans' are numerous, positive scans identifying gastric mucosa are rare—you will see fewer than four or five in your career.

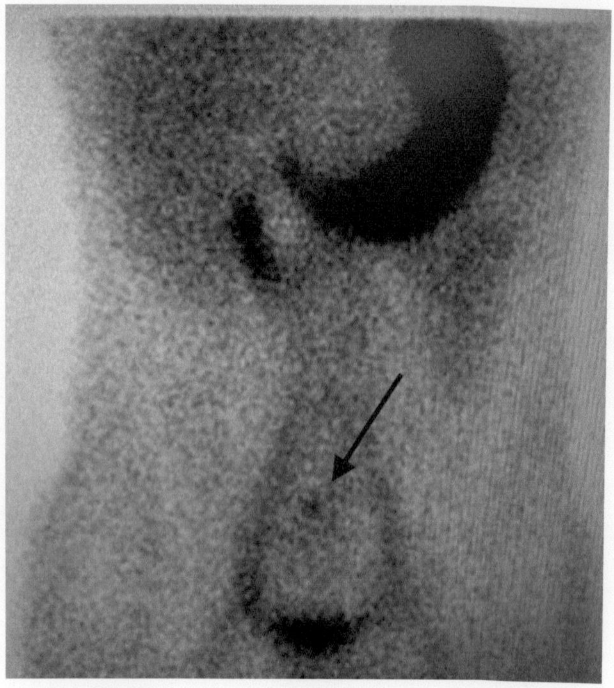

Fig. 10.11 Positive scan for ectopic gastric mucosa in a Meckel's diverticulum

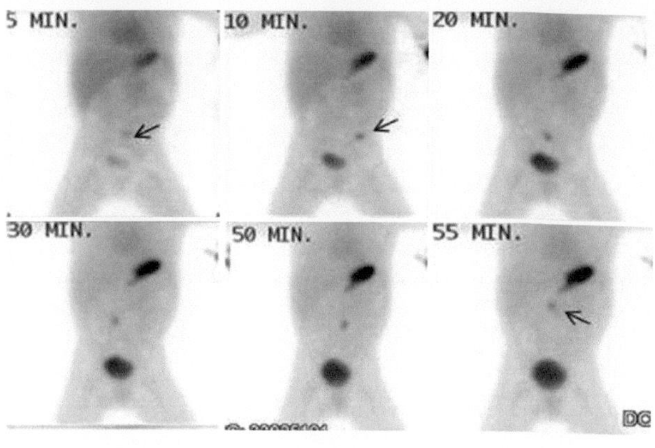

Fig. 10.12 'Wandering' Meckel's diverticulum. Small bowel is mobile so a focus of increased uptake in a Meckel's diverticulum may move over time

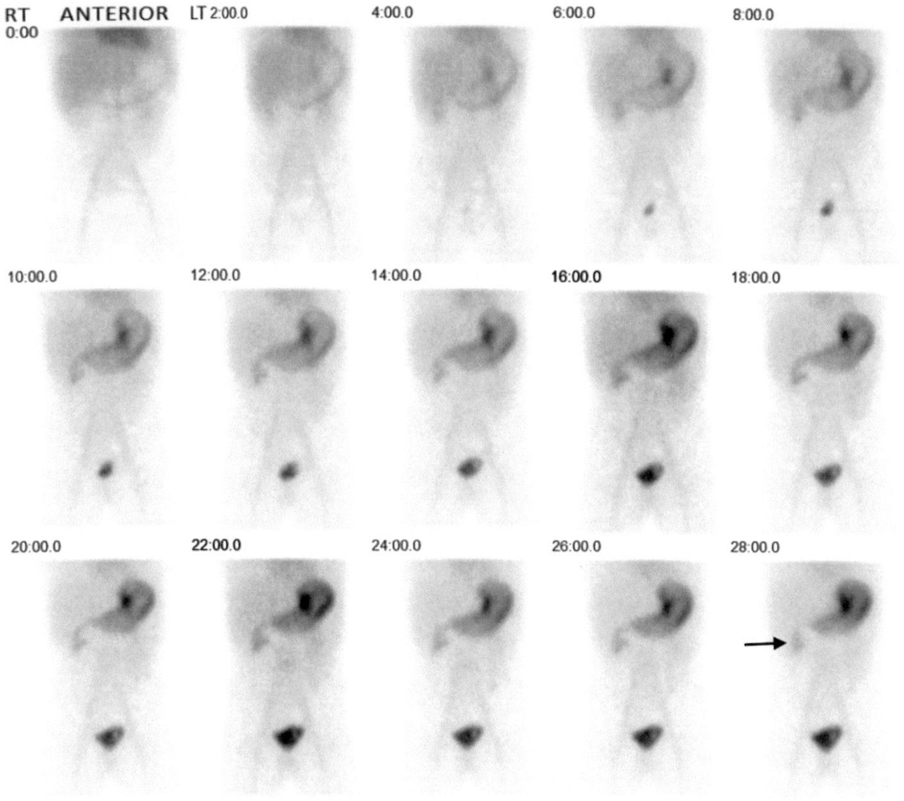

Fig. 10.13 Tc-99mO$_4$ scan in a patient with rectal bleeding. In the stomach, the activity remains confined to gastric mucosa, indicating good suppression of acid secretion following premedication with cimetidine. No abnormal focus seen. Avoid confusion with renal activity (arrow)

Because the gastric mucosal secretion of Tc-99mO$_4$ is linked to acid secretion, it is important to premedicate patients with an acid blocker, such as cimetidine or proton pump inhibitor; otherwise, Tc-99mO$_4$ will leave the stomach, enter small bowel and confuse the picture (Figs. 10.13 and 10.14). Equally important, premedication also inhibits secretion of Tc-99mO$_4$ from ectopic gastric mucosa, thereby 'locking' the activity within it and avoiding a false-negative result.

The usual imaging protocol is 30 min of dynamic acquisition followed by anterior and posterior static imaging. Lateral static imaging is widely practised but usually unhelpful. False positives arise from urinary activity in a ureter or renal pelvis, or accumulation of tracer in a loop of inflamed bowel (Fig. 10.15). The latter occurs because of the expanded interstitial fluid space and increased endothelial permeability associated with inflammation. Blood pool activity, which may appear focal in major vessels, is usually obvious and declines over time rather than increases.

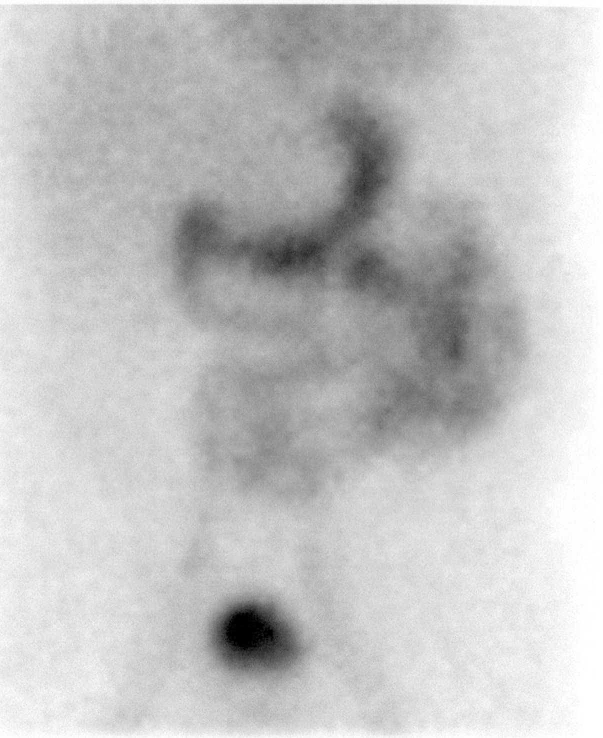

Fig. 10.14 There is abundant intestinal activity in this scan for a Meckel's diverticulum, indicating inadequate pre-medication. Not only will this result in secretion of tracer from gastric mucosa but also from ectopic mucosa in the diverticulum

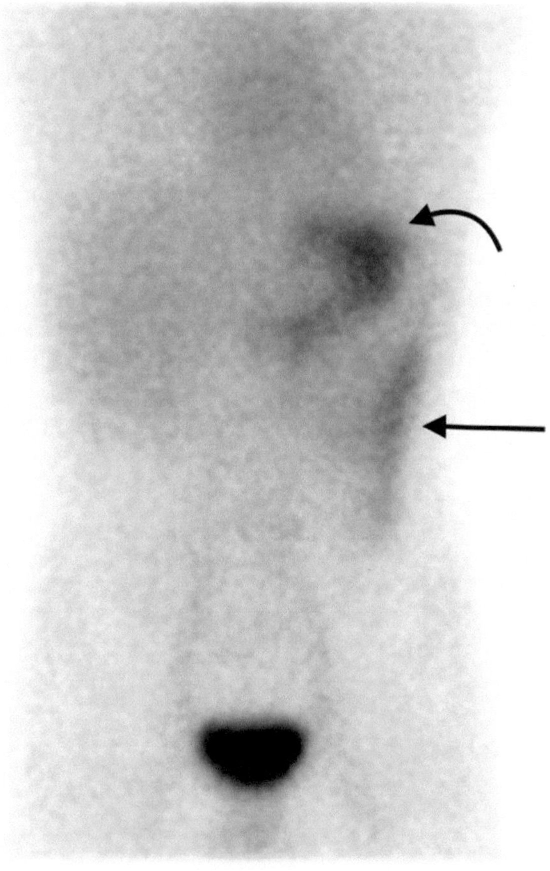

Fig. 10.15 Tc-99mO$_4$ is a small molecule that diffuses from plasma to interstitial fluid throughout the body. Endothelial permeability and interstitial space are increased in inflammation. Inflammatory bowel disease, therefore, is a potential cause of a false positive scan for ectopic gastric mucosa, as seen in this patient in whom the tracer can be seen in splenic flexure and proximal descending colon (straight arrow). The study is negative for ectopic gastric mucosa. Stomach shown by curved arrow

Further Reading

1. Tsujioka Y, Yamada Y, Hasegawa T, Hashimoto M, Jinzaki M. Imaging findings of thyroid diseases in children. Clin Pediatr Endocrinol. 2025;34:89–104. https://doi.org/10.1297/cpe.2024-0082.

11 Tc-99m-Diethyltriaminepentaacetic Acid (DTPA; MW 650 Da)

DTPA is a chelating agent that chelates Tc-99mO_4. Tc-99m-DTPA does not bind to plasma protein, is essentially biologically inert and is the nuclear medicine equivalent of radiological contrast medium. As a small hydrophilic molecule, it diffuses across capillary endothelium and enters the interstitial fluid space of the whole body, except the brain. Being hydrophilic, however, it does not enter the whole-body intracellular space. Its distribution volume is therefore the extracellular fluid volume (ECV). Like contrast, it is unable to cross the blood-brain barrier unless the latter is damaged. It is freely filtered at the glomerulus and passes into urine without tubular secretion or reabsorption. It therefore belongs to a family of substances called filtration markers that have identical plasma, renal and urinary clearances. The classical member of the family is inulin. Another member is Cr-51-EDTA, which, until recently in Europe, was routinely used to measure GFR but has now been withdrawn and replaced by Tc-99m-DTPA. The family also includes iohexol and I-125-iothalamate.

11.1 Measuring Glomerular Filtration Rate (GFR) with a Filtration Marker

GFR is routinely measured by taking 3 or 4 blood samples between 2 h and 4 h following iv injection of a filtration marker such as Tc-99m-DTPA. Plasma concentration initially falls rapidly because of tracer diffusion into the whole-body interstitial fluid space. After the tracer has mixed between plasma and interstitial fluid, plasma concentration declines at a slower rate determined by GFR. The plasma concentration-time curve is therefore a double exponential, becoming a single exponential from about 2 h post-injection when mixing of tracer between plasma and interstitial space is complete (Fig. 11.1). The rate constant, α_2, of the second exponential is almost equal to the ratio of GFR to ECV. Tracer concentration at zero-time is estimated from extrapolation of the second exponential and divided by α_2 to give the area under the time-concentration curve (AUC). As explained in

A. M. Peters, M. Vadrucci, *Introduction to Nuclear Medicine for Trainees in Imaging and Imaging Sciences*, https://doi.org/10.1007/978-3-032-18364-4_11

Chap. 3, tracer clearance is administered activity divided by AUC (Eq. 3.6).

Taking samples 2 h after tracer injection rather than immediately simplifies the procedure but ignores the area under the first exponential, thereby underestimating AUC and overestimating GFR. This overestimation is corrected to give 'true' GFR using a second-order polynomial formula described in 1972 by Jens Brochner-Mortensen (Fig. 11.1).

To scale for body size, GFR is conventionally scaled to a body surface area of 1.73 m^2. In healthy young adults, GFR is 80–120 ml/min/1.73 m^2. It declines normally from about age 35 at a rate of about 1 ml/min/1.73 m^2 per year (Fig. 11.2), so a value of 50 ml/min/1.73 m^2 is regarded as normal in a person of 80. It declines slightly faster in women (Fig. 11.3).

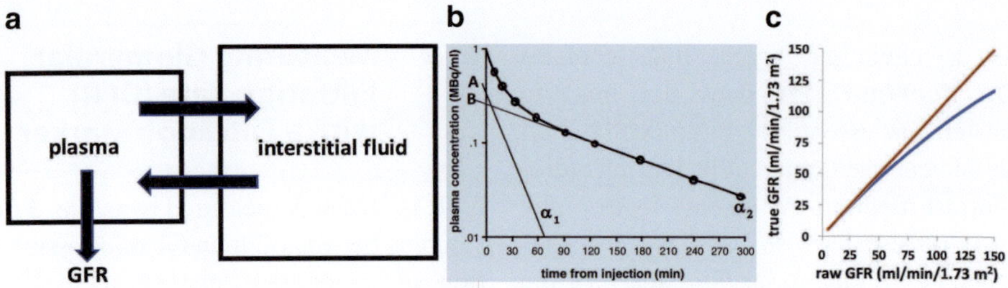

Fig. 11.1 Model depicting distribution of Tc-99m-DTPA following intravenous injection (**a**). Tracer exchanges between plasma and interstitial space whilst undergoing glomerular filtration, yielding a double exponential decline in plasma Tc-99m-DTPA concentration (**b**). Plasma clearance is equal to administered amount (dose) divided by area under plasma time-concentration curve to infinite time. Therefore, GFR = dose/[(A/α_1) + (B/α_2)], where A and B are the zero-time intercepts and α_1 and α_2 are the corresponding rate constants of the two exponentials. In most departments, 3 samples are taken at 2, 3 and 4 h, and GFR is approximated to dose/(B/α_2). This, the 'raw' GFR, is therefore overestimated and requires correction. This is conventionally done with a polynomial equation that relates 'true' GFR to 'raw' GFR: true = raw—raw^2*0.00146 (**c**; blue line: polynomial relationship between true and raw; red line: identity). The correction factor is 0.85 at raw GFR of 100 ml/min/1.73 m^2. The factor declines to zero as α_2 approaches zero at low values of GFR

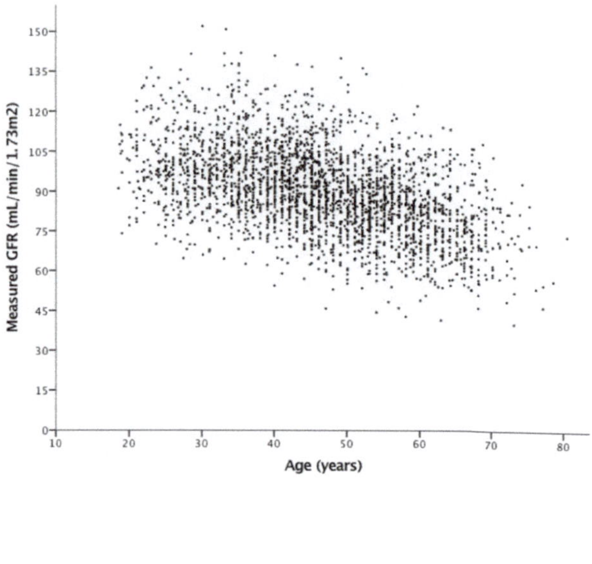

Fig. 11.2 GFR declines with advancing age from about 35 at a rate of slightly less than 1 ml/min/1.73 m^2, as shown in this population of 2974 healthy potential renal transplant donors from multiple centres in the UK. (From Fenton et al. [1])

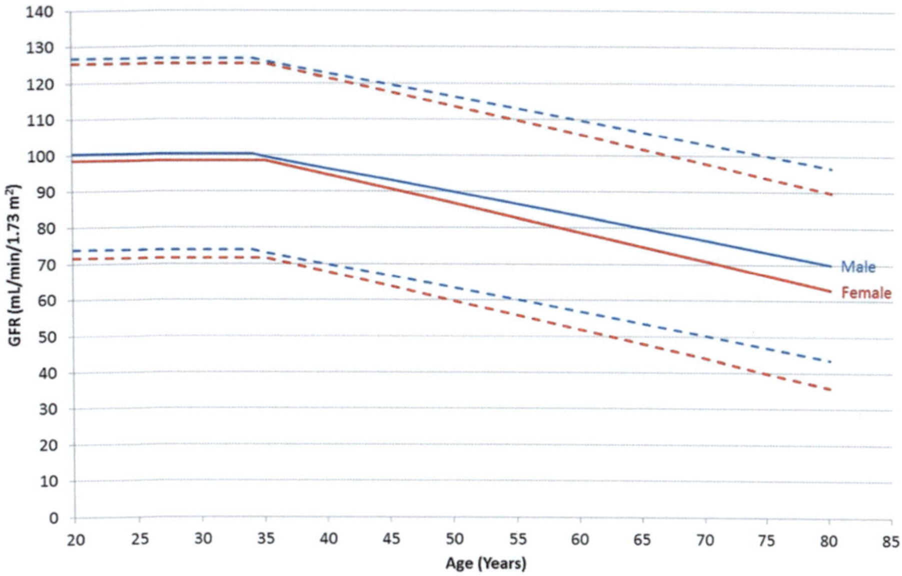

Fig. 11.3 GFR declines slightly more rapidly with advancing age in women compared with men. Continuous lines are means from Fig. 11.2, and dashed lines are two standard deviations from mean. (From Fenton et al. [1])

11.2 Tc-99m-DTPA Renography

Tc-99-DTPA may be used for renography. As it is filtered at the glomerulus, dynamic images of the kidney can be recorded as the tracer progresses through the renal tubules to the collecting system. The time course of activity in the kidney captured by a region of interest (ROI) over the kidney is displayed as a time-activity curve, called a renogram. The ROI includes non-renal tissue, the signal from which is subtracted as background. The renogram has 3 phases. The first lasts about one minute and portrays the kidney's blood flow. The second is the rising phase, which reflects the rate of glomerular filtration of the tracer. It terminates at the peak of the renogram which is normally at about 2.5 min post-injection when the amount of tracer arriving in the kidney from plasma is equal to the amount leaving the kidney and entering the ureter, or more precisely, leaving the ROI drawn over the kidney. The renogram then progressively declines—phase 3—reflecting urinary drainage.

The main indication for renography is to exclude outflow tract obstruction in patients with a dilated collecting system. It is seldom performed in acute obstruction because such patients generally present to the A and E department with renal colic. More often the patient has longish-standing, non-total obstruction or simply a dilated upper renal tract with no obstruction.

Intravenous furosemide is routinely administered to distinguish between obstructed and non-obstructed dilated tracts. It may be given 15 min before (F-15), at the same time as (F0) or 20 min after (F + 20) administration of tracer. Urine flow rate increases up to 10-fold in a healthy kidney in response to furosemide but less in a diseased kidney. Furosemide is a loop diuretic that induces diuresis by inhibiting the transporter in the ascending loop of Henle called the NKCC2 cotransporter, which functions to absorb sodium against its concentration gradient, along with potassium and chloride. Water transport in the tubule takes place through protein channels called aquaporins. Critically, there are no aquaporins in the ascending limb, so water cannot accompany the absorbed sodium. Instead, the sodium enters the vasa recta. Blood flow in the vasa recta travels in the opposite direction to urinary flow in the loop, thereby carrying the sodium deep into the medulla and creating the concentration gradient that controls urine osmolarity. Meanwhile, water is flushed out of the medulla by entering the ascending limb of the vasa recta. Following i.v. injection, furosemide is secreted into the proximal tubule and exerts its action from within the lumen of the ascending limb of the loop of Henle. Its effectiveness as a diuretic therefore depends on the ability of the proximal tubule to secrete it and therefore on renal function.

Differential or split function is measured from renography. With Tc-99m-DTPA this is specifically differential GFR and is equal to the differential gradients of the second phase of the renogram following background subtraction. Background includes the non-renal tissue in the ROI and the non-filtered tracer in the kidney, which is mostly intravascular.

Renogram analysis and interpretation will be described below under Tc-99m-MAG3, which has largely replaced Tc-99 m-DTPA for renography.

11.3 Imaging the Distribution of Pulmonary Ventilation

Tc-99m-DTPA is used to image the distribution of ventilation in V/Q lung scanning (Chap. 23). The tracer, in aqueous solution, is nebulised and converted to an aerosol which the patient inhales. The main drawback is the tendency for the aerosol to deposit in main airways because of turbulent air flow, frequently encountered in obstructive lung disease. Because of the dynamics of aerosol propulsion, the distribution of activity in the lungs is not always strictly the same as the distribution of ventilation, and, in this respect, aerosols are inferior to a radioactive gas, such as Kr-81m (Chap. 23).

11.4 Imaging the Integrity of the Lung Blood-Gas Barrier

During the HIV epidemic of the 1980s, the clearance rate from the lungs of inhaled Tc-99 m-DTPA across the blood-gas barrier was used to assess the severity of acute pulmonary interstitial disease. In normal subjects, inhaled Tc-99m-DTPA clears from the lungs via this route exponentially with a half-time of about 80 min (Fig. 11.4). This falls to less than 20 min in severe inflammatory lung disease. The technique fell out of use because healthy cigarette smokers also have markedly reduced clearance half-times of about 20 min. Interestingly, non-smoking people who live with smokers also have a reduced half-time, around 40–50 min. Although Tc-99m-DTPA for this application is essentially obsolete, it is nevertheless important to appreciate the physiology because in ventilation lung scanning, lung counts may decline quite rapidly in heavy smokers, leading to the appearance of activity in the kidney (Fig. 11.4). This finding may lead to the serendipitous detection of interstitial lung disease if the patient is a non-smoker.

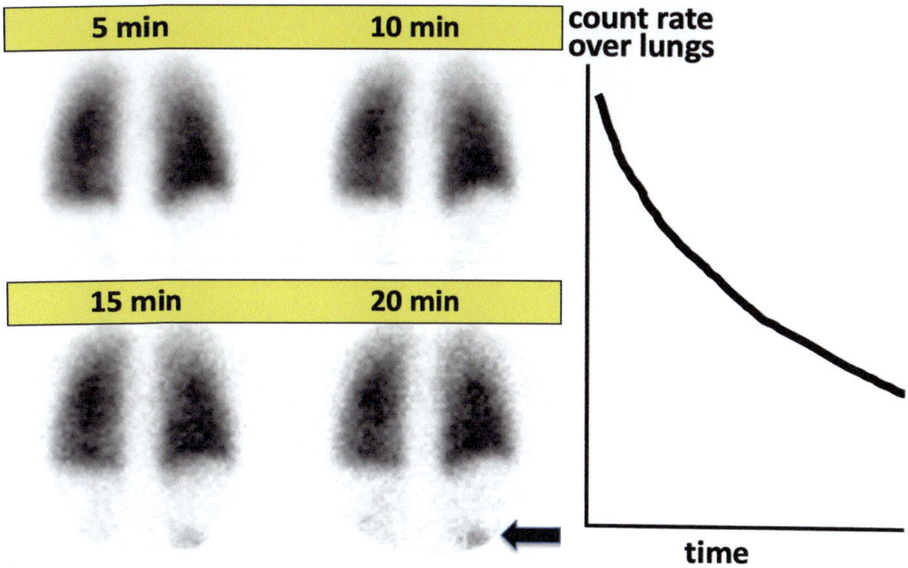

Fig. 11.4 Testing the integrity of the lung blood-gas barrier by measuring the rate of disappearance of inhaled Tc-99m-DTPA aerosol from the lungs. This results from diffusion of tracer into pulmonary arterial blood, is exponential and can be expressed as a rate constant or half-time. The arrival of activity in blood can be appreciated from the accumulation of tracer in the renal collecting systems (arrow)

Further Reading

1. Fenton A, Montgomery E, Nightingale P, Peters AM, Sheerin N, Wroe AC, et al. Glomerular filtration rate: new age- and gender-specific reference ranges and thresholds for living kidney donation. BMC Nephrol. 2018;19:336. https://doi.org/10.1186/s12882-018-1126-8.

12 Tc-99m-Mercaptoacetyltriglycine (MAG3) (MW 417 Da)

Tc-99m-MAG3 is the preferred tracer for renography for most indications and has largely replaced Tc-99m-DTPA for two reasons. Firstly, it is heavily protein-bound in plasma (~95%) giving it a smaller volume of distribution than Tc-99m-DTPA, which, instead, diffuses unopposed into interstitial fluid. Secondly, it has a higher renal extraction efficiency (~50%) than Tc-99m DTPA, the extraction efficiency of which is the filtration fraction (20%). Tc-99m-MAG3 is secreted in the proximal tubule and not reabsorbed, so features relating to subsequent tubular transit are essentially the same as those of Tc-99m-DTPA.

Tc-99m-MAG3, as with many other substances including furosemide, is extracted from peritubular blood at the base of the tubular cell by a family of proteins called organic anion transporters (OATs), and then transported across the apical surface of the tubular cell into the tubular lumen by another protein family called ABC transporters, also known as multiple drug resistance (MDR) proteins. This family, the most prevalent member of which is P-glycoprotein, functions to prevent the entry of xenobiotics into the body or to mediate their exclusion. OATs and MDRs are also active in the liver, explaining why Tc-99m-MAG3 may be seen in the gallbladder (Fig. 12.1).

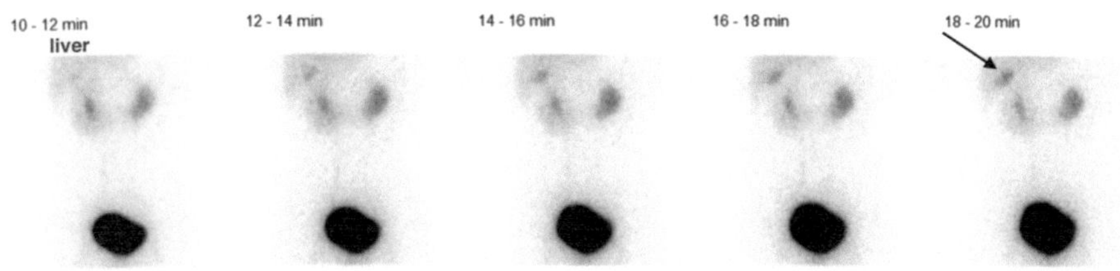

Fig. 12.1 Gallbladder activity (arrow) can be seen in this Tc-99m-MAG3 renogram (anterior projection), illustrating hepatic tracer accumulation, which can be explained by the liver and kidney sharing similar organic anion transporters (OATs) and multiple drug resistance (MDR) proteins. Note the horseshoe kidney

A. M. Peters, M. Vadrucci, *Introduction to Nuclear Medicine for Trainees in Imaging and Imaging Sciences*, https://doi.org/10.1007/978-3-032-18364-4_12

12.1 Renography

Most departments give furosemide 15 min before the tracer (F-15) for adults and at the same time as tracer (F0) for children, thereby establishing an enhanced urine flow rate before or shortly after tracer injection. Alternatively, it can be given 20 min after the tracer (F + 20) when, in the absence of obstruction, pelvic tracer is flushed out by the induced diuresis.

12.1.1 Reporting a Tc-99m-MAG3 Renogram

For F-15 and F0 protocols, do not use the phrase 'renography was performed under maximal urinary flow', because it pre-supposes no obstruction. The report is based on the 3 phases of the renogram, as described under Tc-99m-DTPA (Fig. 12.2). There is no need to comment on renal blood flow (RBF) in native kidneys, and so the

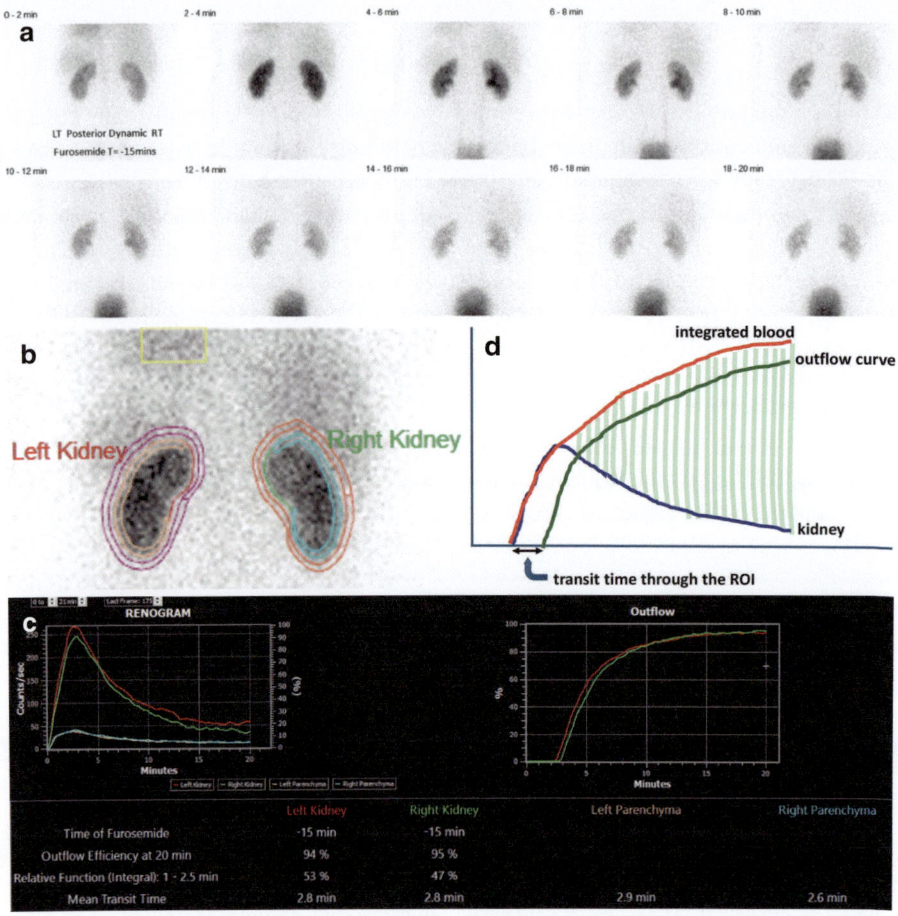

Fig. 12.2 (**a**) Normal Tc-99m-MAG3 renogram. (**b**) Regions of interest (ROIs) from which the curves are generated. Taking the left kidney, the whole kidney curve is derived from the inner of the two purple ROIs. The area between the two purple ROIs gives background activity. The contained counts in background are scaled according to the respective pixel numbers in kidney and background ROIs and subtracted from the whole kidney curve to give the background-corrected curves displayed in (**c**). The orange ROI is placed over parenchyma, avoiding the collecting system to give the parenchymal curves. Mean parenchymal transit time is calculated from the impulse response function (IRF) derived using the ROI (yellow) over the heart (see Fig. 3.8). The ratio of the area of the IRF to its initial amplitude gives mean parenchymal transit time. The heart ROI is also used to derive the outflow curve, the time course of which portrays tracer leaving the kidney (or, more precisely, the whole kidney ROI). It is derived (**d**) as the difference (green curve) between activity arriving in the kidney (red curve) and activity remaining within it (the renogram; blue curve)

first phase can generally be ignored. Do not use phrases such as 'perfusion is delayed' or 'the kidney is well perfused', because they are meaningless in the context of renography. The best way to comment on perfusion in the native kidney—if felt necessary—is by comparing it with the spleen, assuming the latter is normal (Fig. 12.3), because normal renal perfusion is greater than splenic perfusion. If the spleen is more prominent than the kidney in the perfusion phase, then RBF is reduced. RBF in the transplanted kidney, however, is important, and various indices have been described to semi-quantify it.

The second phase of the renogram portrays activity accumulating within the renal parenchyma and the time it takes to reach the collecting system. This is the parenchymal transit time (PTT), which is important because in obstruction it is prolonged. A comment may be made about the kidney's size and position and the gross appearance of the parenchyma, which, although not as well defined as in a Tc-99 m-DMSA scan, should nevertheless be described if clearly abnormal. Thus, is it hydronephrotic, small or large, duplex, horseshoe (Fig. 12.1) or ectopic (Fig. 12.4): and are there any obvious focal defects that may indicate scarring, cysts, infarcts or tumour?

Split function (which is differential Tc-99m-MAG3 renal clearance) can be measured from the relative gradients of the 2nd phase (slope method) or from the relative areas under the renogram curves between two time points prior to the peak (integral method). If the renograms 'take off' at slightly different times, the integral method is subject to error (Fig. 12.5). Ideally, split function should be measured using Patlak-Rutland graphical analysis, as described in Chap. 3. If split function is the principal question in the referral, and there is no issue with drainage, the appropriate tracer is Tc-99m-DMSA, not Tc-99m-MAG3. Tc-99m-DMSA gives a more accurate estimate of split function because firstly, it is based on a delayed static image with no limit to scan duration, in contrast to Tc-99m-MAG3 which gives less than 2 min (i.e., the duration of the second phase); and secondly, it is based on the geometric mean (square root of product) of

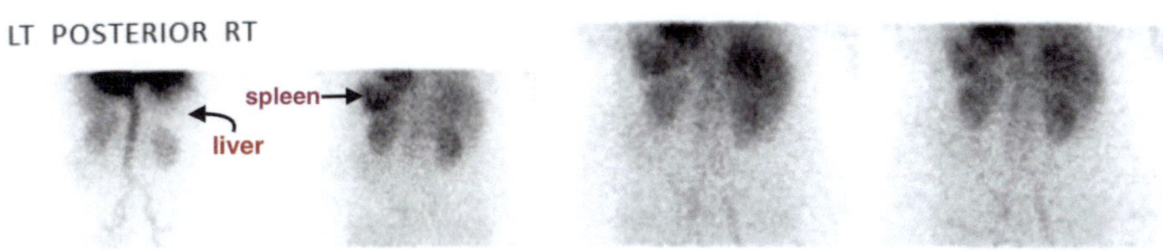

Fig. 12.3 There is limited value in commenting on renal blood flow when reporting a renogram unless it is a transplant renogram for which perfusion is important and should be quantified. For native kidneys, perfusion can be assessed from the count density over the kidney during the first pass of tracer compared with the spleen. Renal perfusion normally exceeds splenic perfusion, so in this example it can be concluded that renal perfusion is reduced. Note the paucity of hepatic activity in the first frame (curved arrow). This is because on first pass most hepatic activity arrives later via the portal vein (75% of hepatic blood flow)

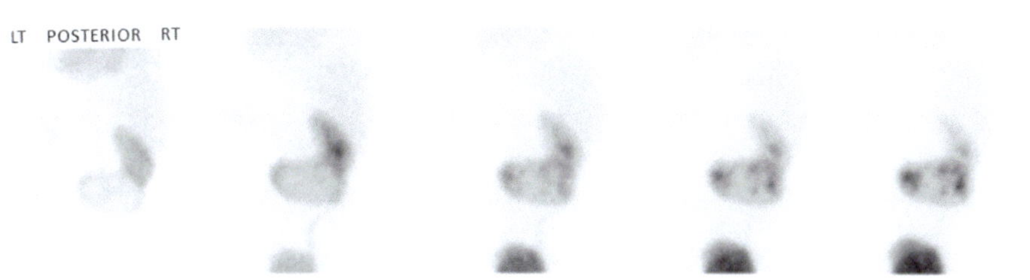

Fig. 12.4 Tc-99m-MAG3 renogram in a patient with crossed fused ectopia. The ectopic left kidney is dilated and shows prolonged parenchymal transit time and poor drainage. The ureter, visible from the 2nd frame of the dynamic, is draining the non-ectopic kidney

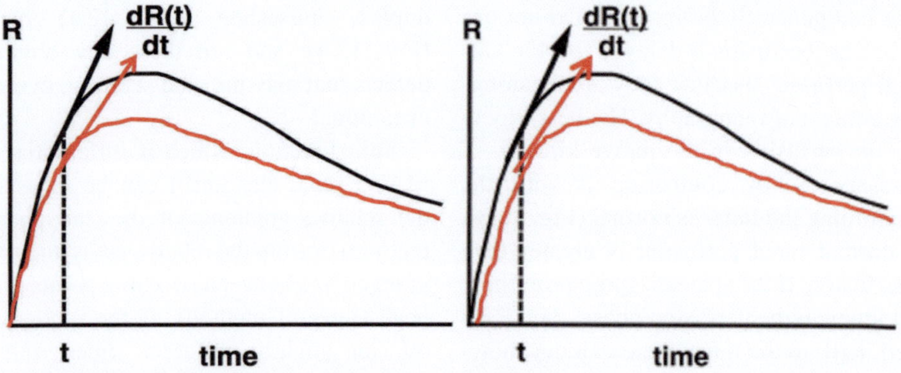

Fig. 12.5 Measurement of split function using slope and integral methods. Upper panel: split function is the relative gradients of the upslopes (dR(t)/dt). Lower panel: split function is the relative areas under the upslopes between t and an earlier value of t. If the renograms 'take off' at different times, there will be an error in split function using this method

anterior and posterior images, which corrects for any difference in depth in the abdomen between the two kidneys. In renography, split function is routinely based only on the posterior projection. If CT is available, kidney depth should be checked. Tc-99m-MAG3 split function can be derived from the geometric mean if an anterior dynamic sequence has also been acquired.

When the 2nd phase in a Tc-99m-MAG3 renogram fails to progress to the 3rd phase, and instead the renogram continues to rise or remains flat, the principal objective is to distinguish between outflow tract obstruction and collecting system dilatation without obstruction. Given that obstruction influences collecting system pressure and urinary flow rate, this distinction is challenging because renography gives no information concerning either. Instead, it provides information only on tracer transit time, which is approximately equal to the ratio of volume to urinary flow rate. Normal pelvic volume is about 10 ml. For a single kidney with a urine flow rate of 1 ml/min, mean pelvic transit time would be 10 min, decreasing to 2 min if, after furosemide, there was a 5-fold increase in flow rate. A pelvic volume of say 100 ml, however, would give a mean post-furosemide transit time of 20 min. Mean pelvic transit time in a malfunctioning kidney will be longer if urinary flow rate shows a poor physiological response to furosemide. This makes it difficult to diagnose obstruction in poorly functioning and dilated kidneys.

These pathophysiological considerations need to be borne in mind when interpreting the renogram, especially for F-15 and F0 protocols. For F + 20 renography, washout of tracer in response to furosemide can be quantified from the decline in activity (Fig.12.8), such as the half-time, but again remember that this is influenced as much by pelvic volume as urine flow rate. Delayed

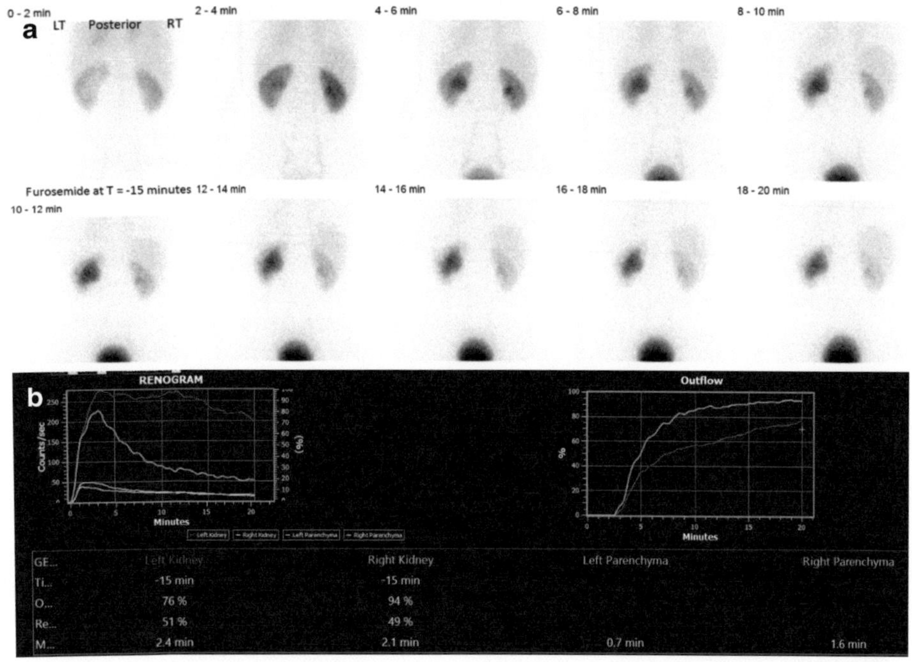

Fig. 12.6 Tc-99m-MAG3 renogram (F-15) showing a hydronephrotic but non-obstructed left kidney (**a**). Parenchymal transit time is normal, and function is symmetrical (**b**)

static pre- and post-micturition imaging, which is routinely performed about 30 min post-injection for F-15 and F0 protocols, may help decide whether there is obstruction, but there is almost always considerable activity present in the collecting system of a hydronephrotic kidney simply because of long transit time through its high volume.

In patients with poor global renal function, background activity remains high during the renogram because the plasma tracer clearance is reduced, resulting in a renogram that remains relatively flat. This does not indicate poor drainage—it is because of a tracer input that is slow to fall (Fig. 12.7). The renogram in a heathy subject in contrast falls in parallel with the plasma tracer concentration and should approach baseline by 20 min post-injection. The renogram peaks early in global kidney disease because of osmotic diuresis.

An important marker of obstruction is parenchymal transit time (PTT). This is measured using a technique called deconvolution analysis that uses ROIs over the cortex of the kidney (excluding collecting system) and blood pool (over the chest) to generate a curve, called an

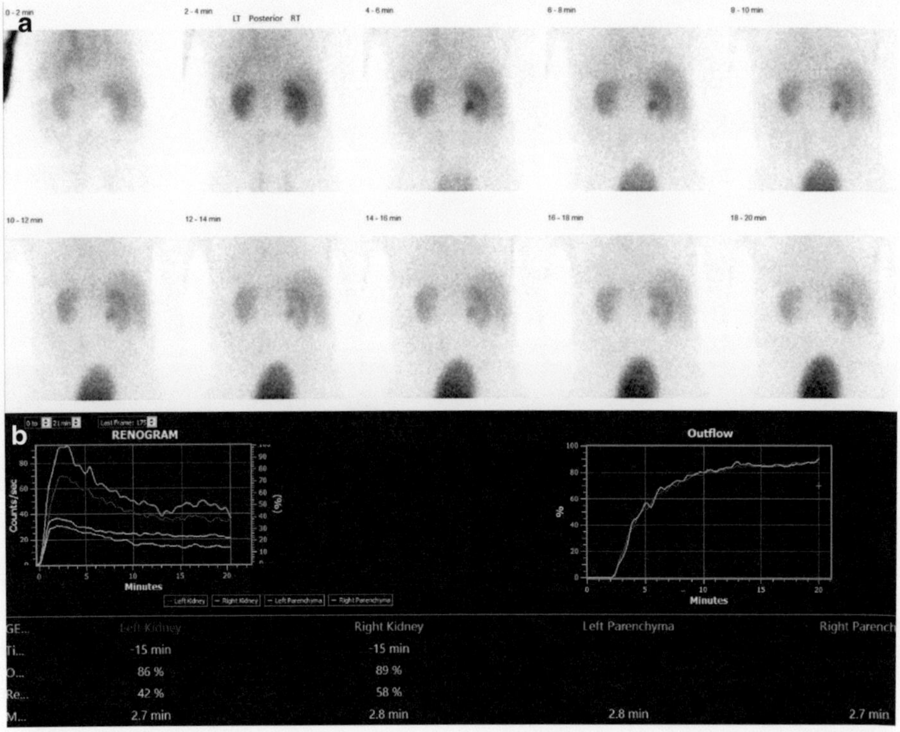

Fig. 12.7 Impaired renal function. There is increased background activity in the later frames of the renogram (**a**). The curves (**b**) remain symmetrically flat because of slow plasma tracer clearance. When function is normal, the renograms approach baseline by 20 min (Fig. 12.2), by which time incoming tracer is minimal. Early renogram peaks are another feature of renal impairment because of osmotic diuresis

impulse response function (IRF), that would be recorded if the tracer was to arrive as a bolus in the kidney and not recirculate (Fig. 3.8). PTT is then equal to the area divided by the initial height of the IRF. This technique is not robust, so PTT should also be judged by eye from inspection of the dynamic sequence of images, comparing the two kidneys.

Patients are commonly referred for renography with a provisional diagnosis of PUJ obstruction following the incidental discovery of hydronephrosis without ureteric dilatation. The majority show no evidence of obstruction on renography and drain in response to diuretic (Fig. 12.6). It is easier to exclude outflow tract obstruction than to diagnose it. The three critical

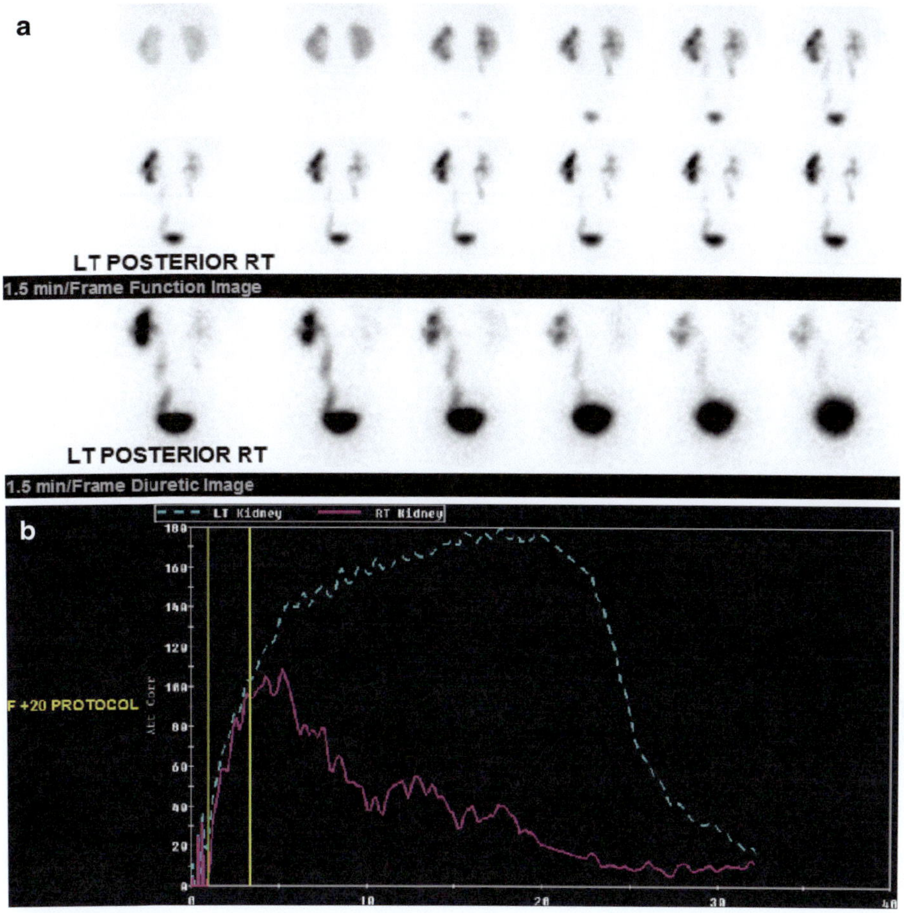

Fig. 12.8 Dilated left upper tract (**a**). Brisk washout in response to furosemide administered 20 min post-tracer injection excludes obstruction (**b**)

features of PUJ obstruction are (1) prolonged PTT, (2) a progressively rising renogram, and (3) impaired function (Fig. 12.9). No ureteric activity is seen and there is no washout with the F+20 protocol. A nephrostomy tube should be clamped (before the diuretic) until completion of the study when it should be opened, and the drainage response recorded (Fig. 12.10). Regarding patients having sequential studies, stable split function argues strongly against obstruction unless it is intermittent. Recent obstruction may also leave split function normal. A full bladder may delay drainage so renography protocols routinely include pre- and post-void static imaging (Fig. 12.11).

The phrase partial obstruction is best avoided because obstruction is virtually always partial. Complete obstruction (Fig. 12.12) is rarely seen

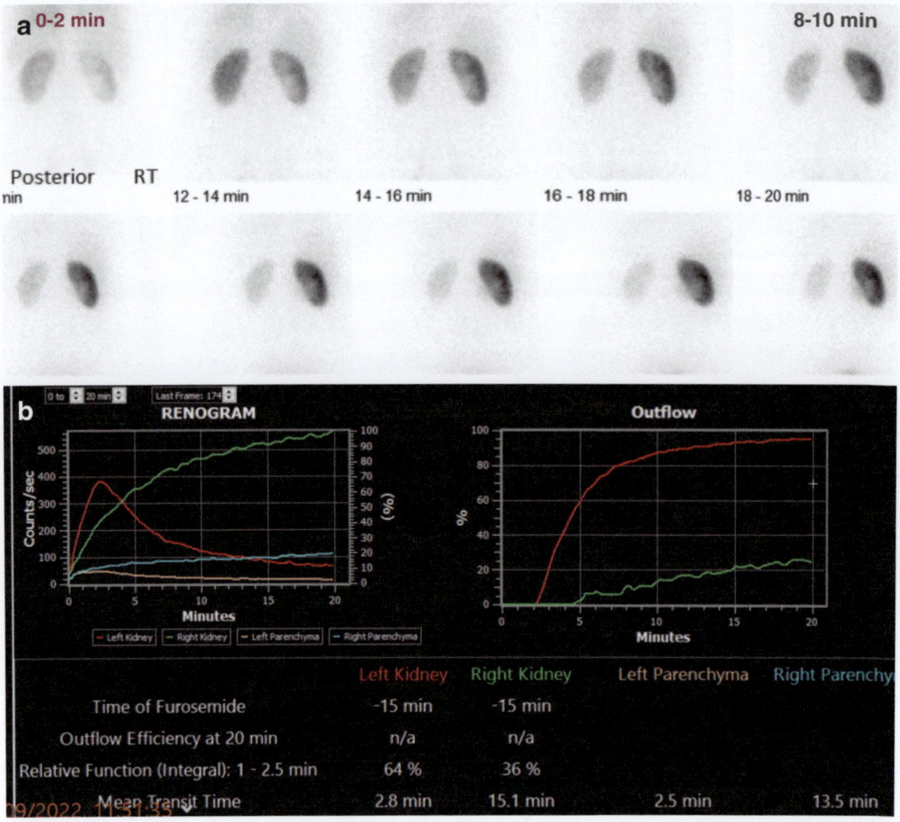

Fig. 12.9 Tc-99 m-MAG3 renogram (F-15). Obstructed right kidney showing increased parenchymal transit time (**a**), progressively rising renogram, and impaired function (**b**)

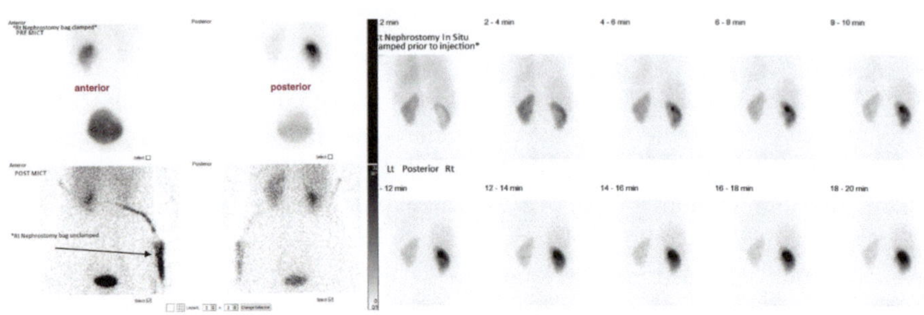

Fig. 12.10 A nephrostomy tube should be clamped during renography before diuretic is administered. The hydronephrotic right kidney shows a prolonged parenchymal transit time and poor drainage (right panel), in keeping with obstruction. It drained after the nephrostomy tube was unclamped, confirming obstruction (left panel). The left kidney looks normal

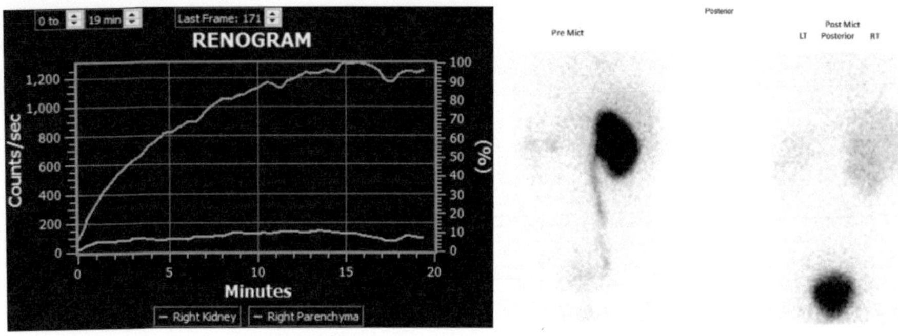

Fig. 12.11 This hydronephrotic kidney looks obstructed, generating a progressively rising renogram, but drained briskly following voiding, excluding obstruction

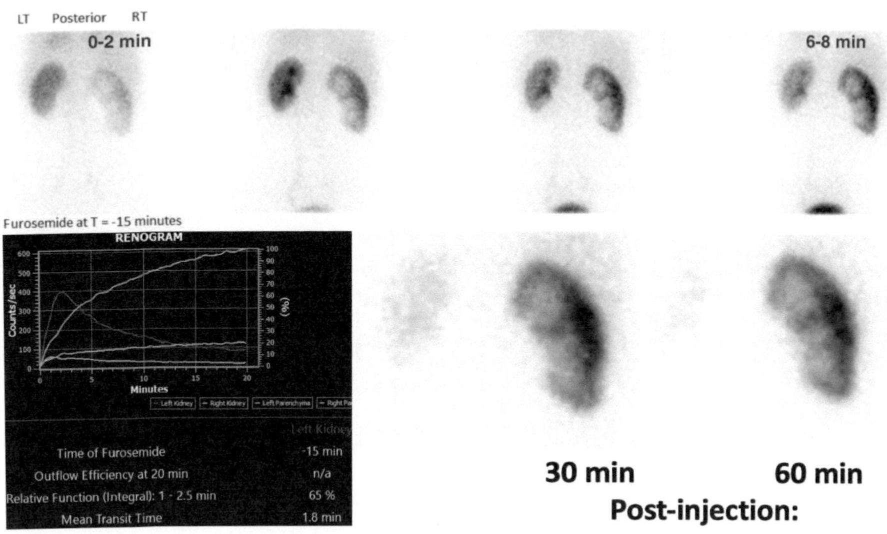

Fig. 12.12 No activity can be seen in the right collecting system even at 60 min post tracer injection, in keeping with complete obstruction

because the patient is likely to attend the A and E rather than the nuclear medicine department. Low-grade or high-grade obstruction are better terms.

Antenatally diagnosed hydronephrosis (ANH) is a common indication for renography in young infants (Fig. 12.13). Again, despite prominent pelvic dilatation, clear renographic evidence of obstruction is often lacking, and the kidney shows no loss of function compared with the contralateral kidney. Indeed, the hydronephrotic kidney in ANH is noted, not infrequently, for showing greater function—for unexplained reasons. Such children may undergo repeat renography until they are several years old, each time showing persisting dilatation but no loss of function.

Obstruction at the vesicoureteric junction (VUJ) leads to dilatation of ureter as well as the pelvis. It is encountered less often in practice than PUJ obstruction and is more difficult to diagnose because of its distal location in the upper tract. Conditions such as endometriosis, colorectal tumours or fibroid uterus (Fig. 12.14) may cause obstruction at a mid-ureteric level. With regard to duplex kidneys, the upper moiety tends to be obstructed at the VUJ, while the lower moiety tends to be associated with vesicoureteric reflux (VUR), which typically gives rise to a dilated and tortuous ureter. Bilateral upper tract dilatation in young males is a feature of posterior urethral valves.

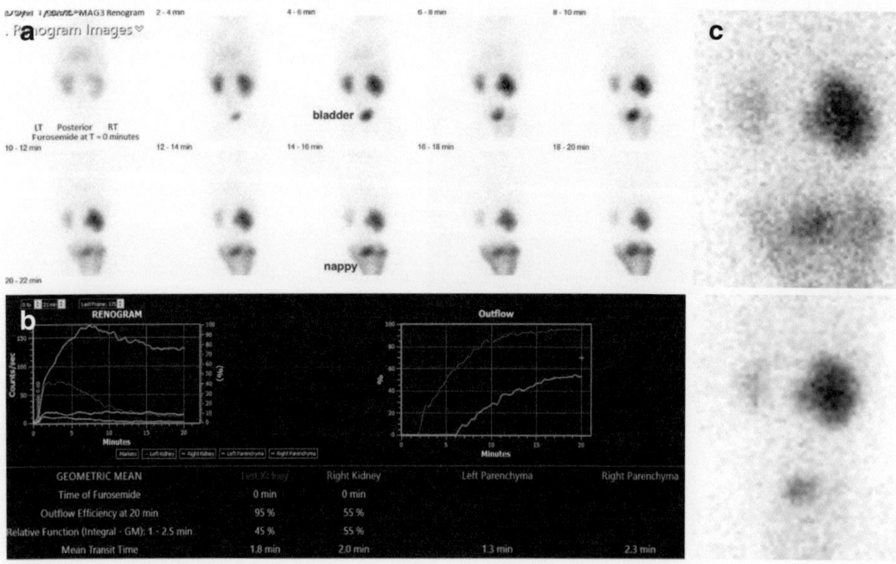

Fig. 12.13 Antenatally diagnosed hydronephrosis in an infant. There is prominent pelvic dilatation on the right (**a**) but the renogram declines from 7 min post-injection and there is no loss of function compared with the left kidney (**b**). Delayed pre- and post-void imaging (**c**) shows a pelvis full of activity but as transit time is the ratio of volume-to-flow, this is not surprising and does not indicate obstruction. Note that the child voided into his nappy at 10 min into the renogram. Sometimes in small children this provides an opportunity to see vesicoureteric reflux, but not here

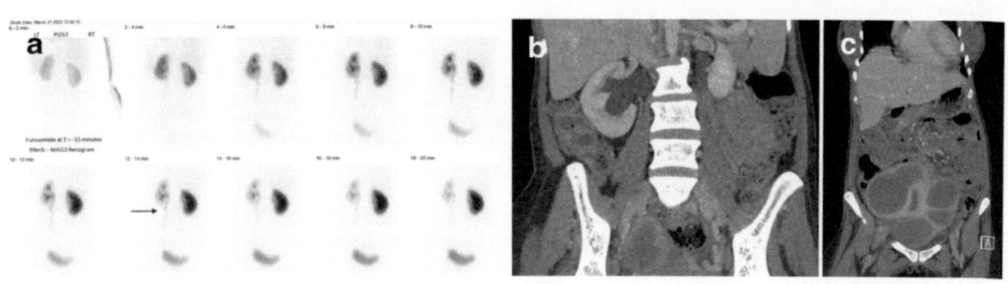

Fig. 12.14 Fibroid uterus causing obstruction to the right kidney. The Tc-99m-MAG3 renogram (**a**) shows a markedly prolonged parenchymal transit in a hydronephrotic right kidney (**b**). The left ureter (arrow) is slightly dilated but only in its upper half. This is because of a large fibroid uterus (**c**) causing obstruction on the right but not yet on the left

A rather poorly recognised cause of prolonged PTT in the native kidney is tubular injury. The proximal tubule actively reabsorbs about two-thirds of the glomerular filtrate but otherwise presents a tight barrier to solutes. Damage to the barrier allows indiscriminate solute and water reabsorption, thereby reducing water flow along the tubular lumen and increasing PTT. This is seen at its extreme in acute tubular necrosis (ATN), especially in renal transplants. In ATN, perfusion is typically maintained at near-normal levels, but the renogram progressively rises as Tc-99m-MAG3 accumulates in the tubular cell and is unable to enter the lumen against the flow of water coming in the opposite direction. Less severe degrees of tubular injury manifest as increased PTT, typically bilateral in native kidneys, giving rise to symmetrically rising renograms and a risk of misdiagnosis of bilateral obstruction (Fig. 12.15). Unlike Tc-99m-MAG3, Tc-99m-DTPA can distinguish between tubular injury and obstruction. Thus, the renogram pro-

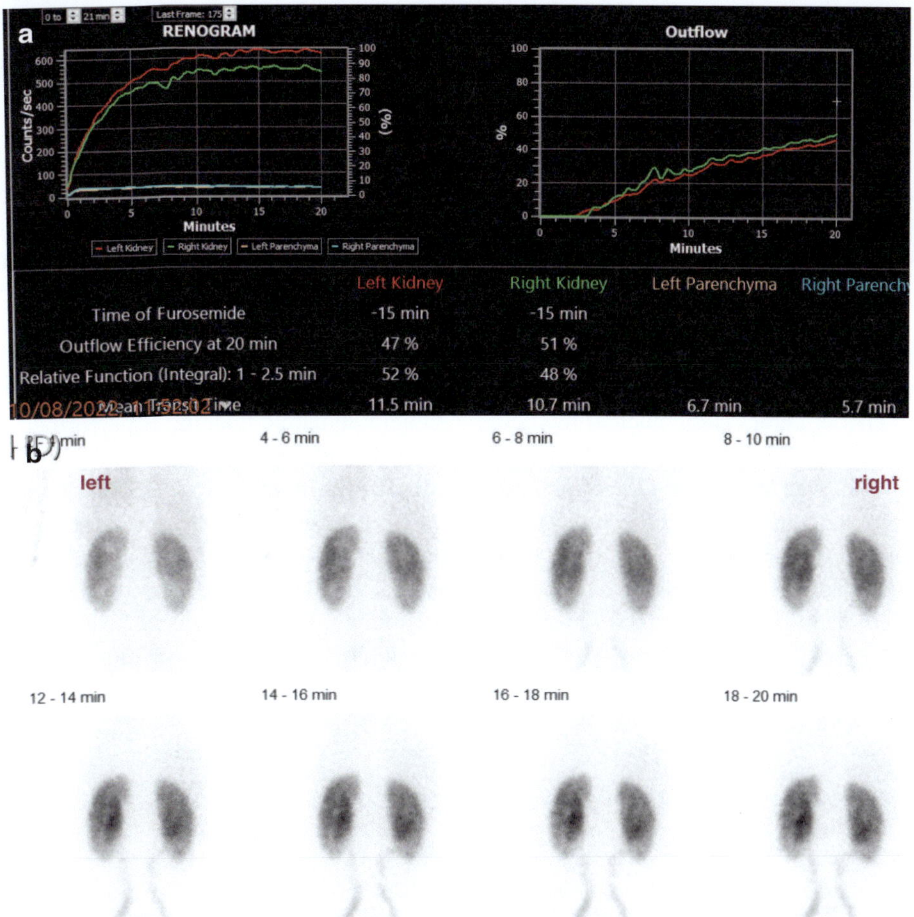

Fig. 12.15 The Tc-99m-MAG3 renograms (**a**) in this patient with systemic lupus erythematosus rise in an almost perfect symmetrical fashion and the images (**b**) show retention of activity in the parenchyma of both kidneys, in keeping with impaired tubular function, in which the ability of the proximal tubular cell to secrete tracer is impaired

gressively rises in obstruction but displays no second phase in tubular injury because the tracer diffuses back from lumen into the tubular cell and then capillary blood. Current chemotherapy is also associated with increased PTT because it may block the MDR proteins that mediate Tc-99m-MAG3 transport from proximal tubule into the tubular lumen. A similar phenomenon related to anti-rejection medication may be responsible for the commonly seen 'flat' renogram of the renal transplant.

Another cause of prolonged PTT is functionally significant renal artery stenosis (RAS). When renal blood flow is reduced from RAS, renin is secreted by the granular cells of the juxtaglomerular apparatus in the efferent (post-glomerular) arteriole and acts locally on circulating angiotensinogen to produce angiotensin 1. This is then converted to angiotensin 2 (A-ll) by angiotensin-converting enzyme (ACE), located in the endothelial cells of the efferent arteriole. A-ll constricts the efferent arteriole, thereby raising glomerular pressure and maintaining GFR at the expense of a further reduction in RBF. An ACE inhibitor, such as captopril, abolishes this response, and the GFR of the kidney falls. Captopril renography was popular in the 80 s and 90 s but is less frequently performed nowadays.

We suspect that this is another unwelcome result of moving from Tc-99m-DTPA to Tc-99m-MAG3 for renography. Thus, as a filtration agent, Tc-99m-DTPA directly portrays the reduction in GFR, but, as a tubular agent, Tc-99m-MAG3 relies instead on detecting a prolonged PTT resulting from the fall in GFR.

12.2 Radionuclide Cystography

Radionuclide cystography may be direct (DRC) or indirect (IRC). Direct is the nuclear medicine equivalent of MCUG but rarely performed. Its only advantage over MCUG is a lower radiation exposure. To perform IRC, which is more physiological than either MCUG or DRC, one simply waits for the bladder to fill with radioactive urine following iv injection of Tc-99m-MAG3. IRC is therefore an extension of renography.

Furosemide should not be administered otherwise micturition may be premature, especially in young children, and the urine too dilute. The patient should have an empty bladder at the time of tracer administration to maximise subsequent urinary tracer concentration. Routine renography is performed followed by static imaging to ensure adequate bladder filling. Withholding furosemide may result in significant retention of tracer in the renal pelvis with the potential to obscure any VUR. It is at this point that furosemide should be considered to drain the upper tracts. With back to camera, dynamic imaging is performed while the patient voids, and time-activity curves are constructed for both kidneys and the bladder.

To diagnose VUR, activity reaching the renal pelvis must be recorded (Fig. 12.16). In other words, the ROIs for IRC are over the kidneys, not the ureters. VUR may occur prior to voiding, so inspect the data prior to voiding. Beware of sta-

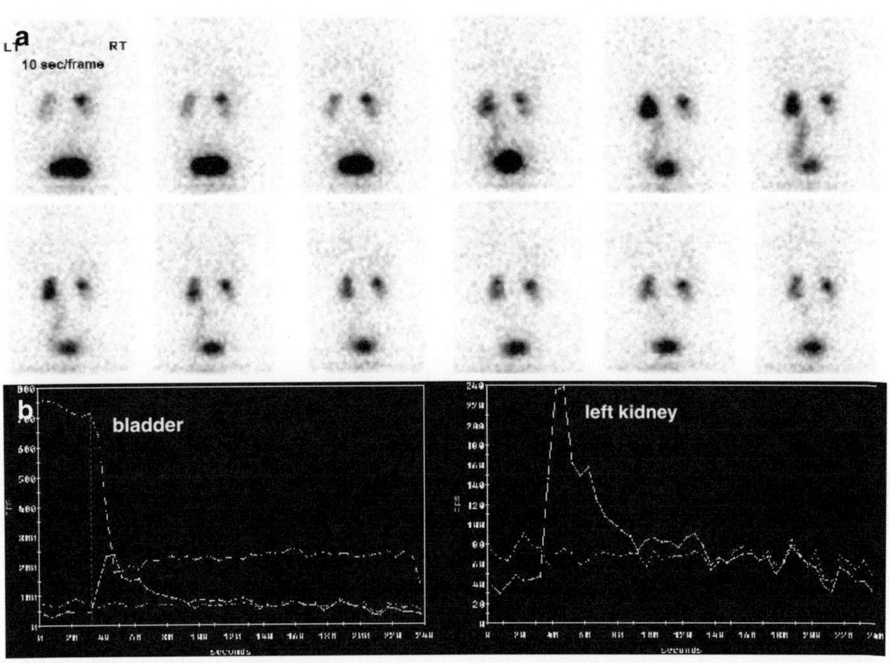

Fig. 12.16 Vesicoureteric reflux. Tc-99m-MAG3 renography has been completed, and the bladder is adequately filled with radioactive urine (**a**). The patient then voids with back to gamma camera. The dilated left ureter drains the lower moiety of a duplex kidney, and the tract has drained well prior to voiding. There is, however, retention of urine in the upper moiety of the right kidney which is also duplex but there is no ureteric dilatation. During voiding, there is reflux on the left but not the right. The left panel of curves (**b**) includes bladder and both kidney curves. The right panel shows only the kidney curves. This case illustrates the general rule that in a duplex kidney, the upper moiety tends to be obstructed while the lower moiety tends to reflux

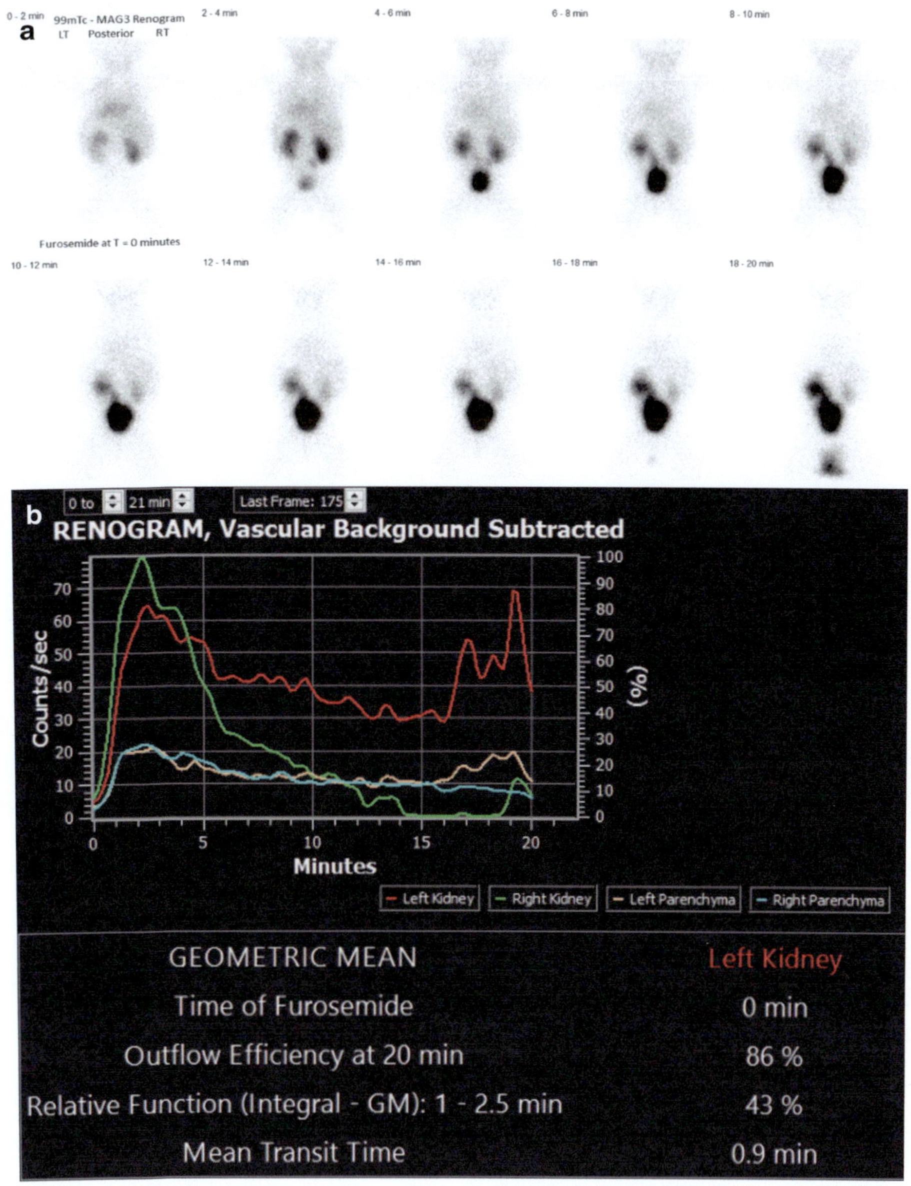

Fig. 12.17 For an elective vesicoureteric reflux study, a child must be potty trained to void on request. In young infants who are not potty-trained, however, reflux may be seen during renography if the patient spontaneously voids. This baby with bilateral ureteric dilatation—especially on the left—voided towards the end of the renogram (**a**), producing a clear 'spike' on the left in the recorded curves (**b**)

tistical noise in the time-activity curves—VUR cannot occur once the bladder is empty! The bladder does, however, refill following VUR. A child needs to be potty-trained for IRC so that voluntary voiding can be recorded during dynamic imaging. Reflux, nevertheless, may occasionally be recorded during renography if the patient spontaneously voids (Fig. 12.17).

Further Reading

1. Cherney DZI, Perkins BA, Soleymanlou N, Maione M, Lai V, Lee A, et al. Renal hemodynamic effect of sodium-glucose cotransporter 2 inhibition in patients with type 1 diabetes mellitus. Circulation. 2014;129:587–97.
2. Gilmer GG, Deshpande VG, Chou C-L, Knepper M. Flow resistance along the rat renal tubule. Am J Physiol Renal Physiol. 2018;315:F1398–405.
3. Shikano N, Kanai Y, Kawai K, Ishikawa N, Endou H. Transport of ^{99m}Tc-MAG3 via rat renal organic anion transporter-1. J Nucl Med. 2004;45:80–5.
4. Upsdell SM, Leeson SM, Brooman PJ, O'Reilly PH. Diuretic-induced urinary flow rates at varying clearances and their relevance to the performance and interpretation of diuresis renography. Br J Urol. 1988;61:14–8.

13 Tc-99m-Dimercaptosuccinic Acid (DMSA) (MW 182 Da)

Tc-99m-DMSA circulates in blood bound to alpha-1-microglobulin (MW 30KDa). Because of its molecular size, the complex undergoes glomerular filtration at a slower rate than Tc-99m-DTPA with a renal extraction efficiency of about 5%. Filtered complex is reabsorbed intact into the proximal tubule where the DMSA component forms disulphide bridges with cortical proteins. Unabsorbed complex passes into the urine, which even in healthy subjects, always contains activity.

Static imaging is performed 3 h after injection but can be later if there is renal impairment and renal tracer clearance is reduced. Plasma clearance is greater than renal clearance because the tracer accumulates in tissues other than the kidney, although this only becomes clearly visible when there is renal impairment. In normal kidneys, the cortico-medullary junction should be visible (Fig. 13.1), so in your report do not describe accumulation in a healthy kidney as homogeneous. If it really is, it may be abnormal. Each kidney accumulates about 30% of the administered activity by 3 h post-injection, with 30% of extrarenal activity distributed throughout the body and 10% excreted in urine. If the patient has global renal impairment, extrarenal (background) activity is conspicuous and should be mentioned in the report (Fig. 13.2).

Split function is the relative accumulated activity in regions of interest over the kidneys and measures relative, not absolute, function. It is measured as the geometric mean (square root of the product) from posterior and anterior projections to account for potential differences in depth in the abdomen between the two kidneys (Fig. 13.3). The normal range for the split function is 56/44%, which is slightly narrower than with Tc-99 m-MAG3 because it is more accurately measured. Posterior-only split function should also be recorded in case comparison is to be made with split function from renography—previous or prospective—which is routinely based only on the posterior image. When available, CT should be used to check renal depths.

The main indication for Tc-99m-DMSA is suspected focal renal pathology. When split renal function is the principal question, it should be measured with Tc-9m-DMSA rather than Tc-99m-MAG3. Focal defects seen on Tc-99m-DMSA include scars, cysts, infarcts (typically wedge-shaped), tumours and lobar nephronia (Figs. 13.4, 13.5, 13.6, 13.7, and 13.8). The last-mentioned is pyelonephritis localised to a lobe and resembles an infarct. Generalised reduction in tracer accumulation with loss of the cortico-medullary boundary is seen in current pyelonephritis, in which the kidney may be enlarged (Fig. 13.9), in reflux nephropathy and in renal artery stenosis.

Split function is usually abnormal in unilateral renal disease but may be normal in bilateral disease. Abnormal split function in the absence of abnormal scintigraphic features in either kidney,

A. M. Peters, M. Vadrucci, *Introduction to Nuclear Medicine for Trainees in Imaging and Imaging Sciences*, https://doi.org/10.1007/978-3-032-18364-4_13

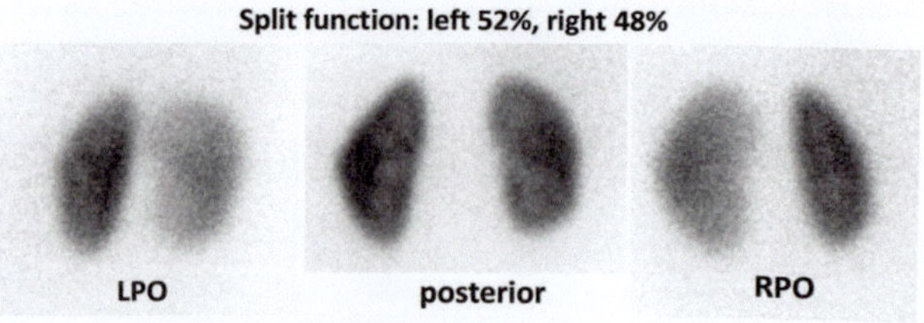

Fig. 13.1 Normal Tc-99m-DMSA scan. Note the presence of a corticomedullary distinction. LPO left posterior oblique; RPO right posterior oblique

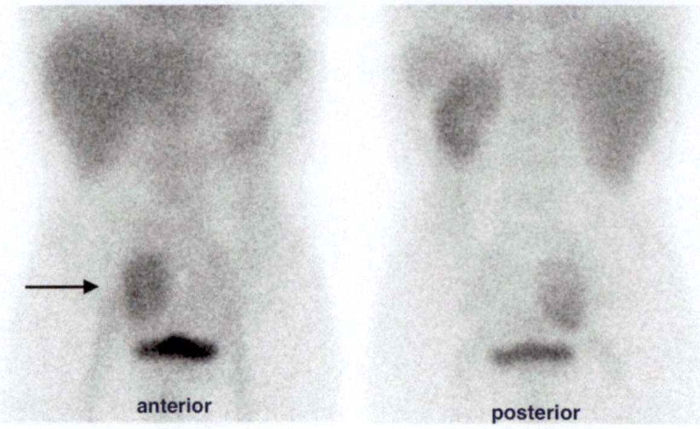

Fig. 13.2 Tc-99m-DMSA scan in patient with globally impaired renal function showing increased blood pool activity. Hepatic and splenic activities are a combination of cleared tracer and blood pool and background activity. Relatively high urinary activity in bladder likely reflects impaired tubular reabsorption of filtered tracer-protein complex. Note that the right kidney is in the pelvis (arrow)

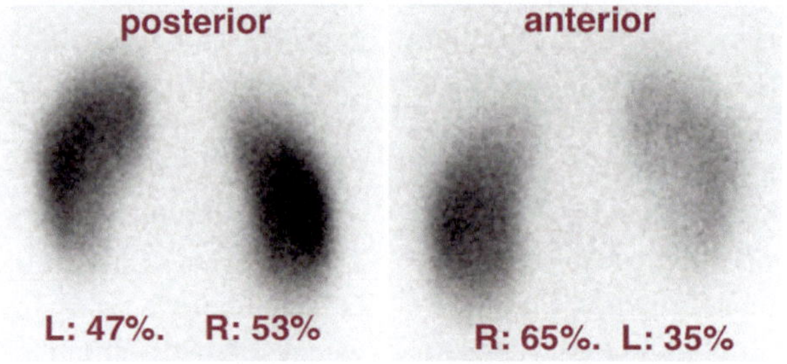

Fig. 13.3 In this Tc-99m-DMSA scan, the left kidney contributes 47% of overall renal function on the posterior view (**a**) but only 35% on the anterior view (**b**). This is because the right kidney is more anterior in the abdomen than the left kidney. Taking the geometric mean of anterior and posterior counts, i.e., square root of product: $(47*35)^{0.5} = 41$, corrects for the difference in renal depths and gives the correct split function. Note that this scan shows movement artefact, a common problem in paediatrics

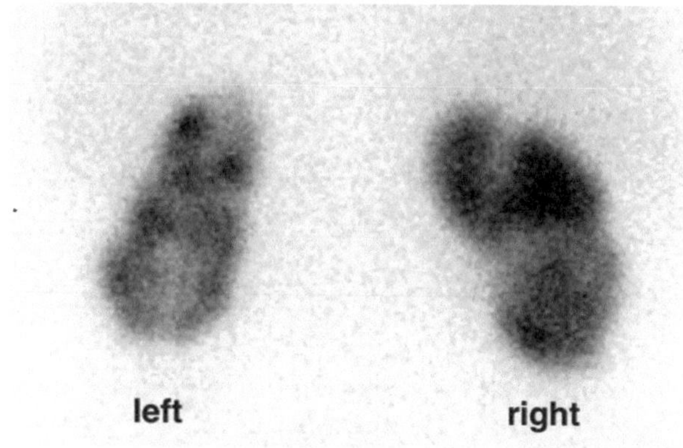

Fig. 13.4 Bilateral renal scarring shown in the posterior projection of a Tc-99m-DMSA scan with split function of left 36%, right 64%

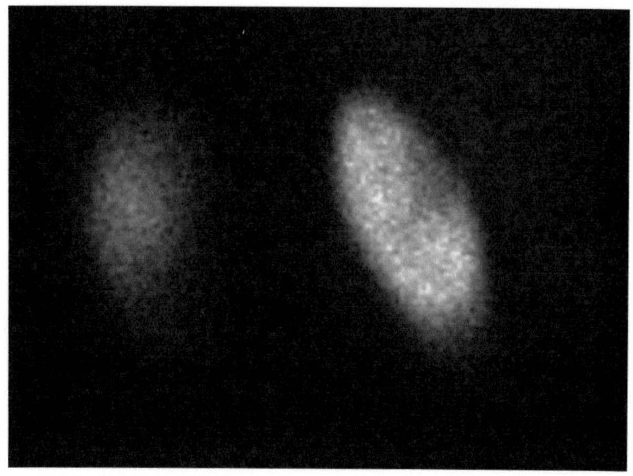

Fig. 13.5 Tc-99m-DMSA scan showing lobar nephronia, a focal infection restricted to a lobe of the kidney. The focus is typically wedge-shaped and may therefore be confused with a renal infarct

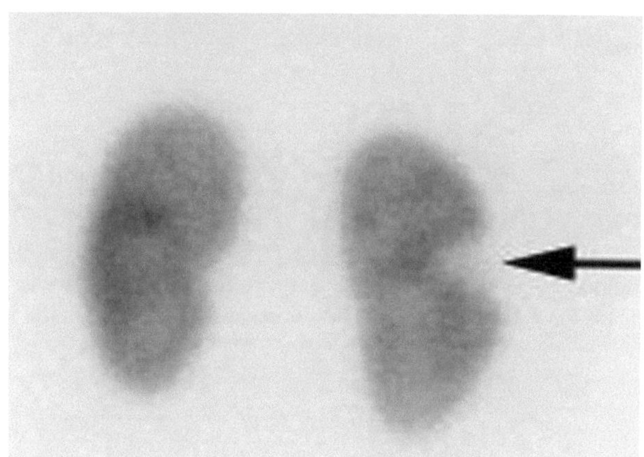

Fig. 13.6 Renal infarct showing as a wedge-shaped parenchymal defect

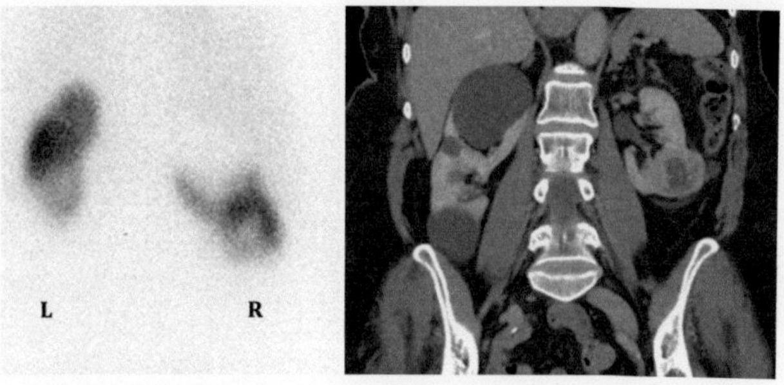

Fig. 13.7 Bilateral renal cysts

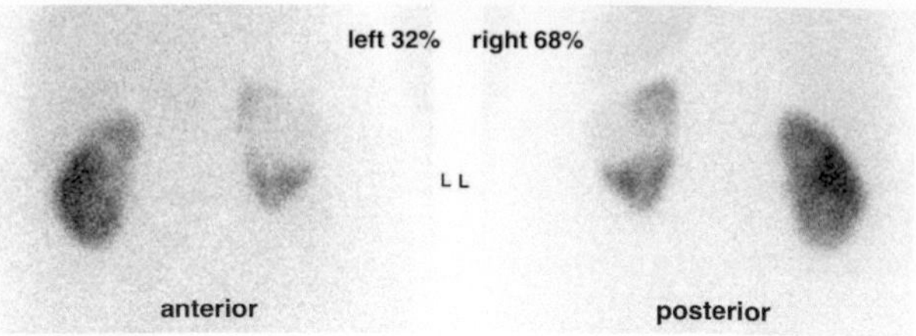

Fig. 13.8 Renal tumour in the left kidney. The purpose of Tc-99m-DMSA is to provide split function to aid surgical management

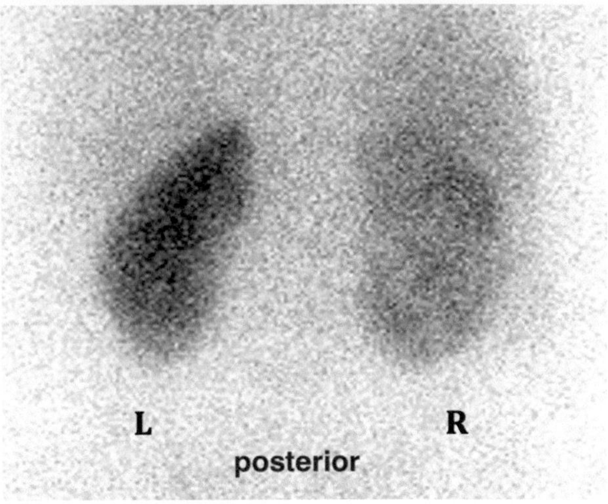

Fig. 13.9 Current pyelonephritis. Both kidneys are abnormal with overall reduced tracer accumulation and no definition of the corticomedullary junction. The right kidney is swollen. Tc-99m-DMSA scintigraphy in urinary tract infection is usually delayed by several months with the aim of identifying residual scarring but occasionally requested to make a diagnosis of acute pyelonephritis

but one is larger than the other, raises a suspicion of an intact unilateral duplex (Fig. 13.10). The contribution of the duplex is in the region of 60–65% as there are effectively two kidneys on one side and one kidney on the other. Failure to recognise a healthy unilateral duplex may result in the contralateral simplex kidney being misdiagnosed as damaged.

Variants in Tc-99m-DMSA imaging, in addition to duplex, include dromedary hump, splenic impression, pelvic kidneys, foetal lobulation, crossed fused ectopia and horseshoe kidneys (Figs. 13.11, 13.12, 13.13, and 13.14). In the presence of severe unilateral disease, the healthy contralateral kidney is likely to be hypertrophied. Horseshoe kidneys are usually fused at the lower poles but may rarely fuse at the upper pole (Fig. 13.15). The dromedary hump, also known as a hypertrophied column of Bertin, is a normal variant but may be misinterpreted as tumour with other imaging techniques.

Paediatric diseases referred for Tc-99m-DMSA include renal scarring from recurrent urinary tract infections, multicystic dysplastic kidney (showing no tracer accumulation), unexplained hypertension, and the complications of a duplex kidney in which a damaged upper moiety is usually from obstruction (Fig. 13.16) and a damaged lower moiety from VUR.

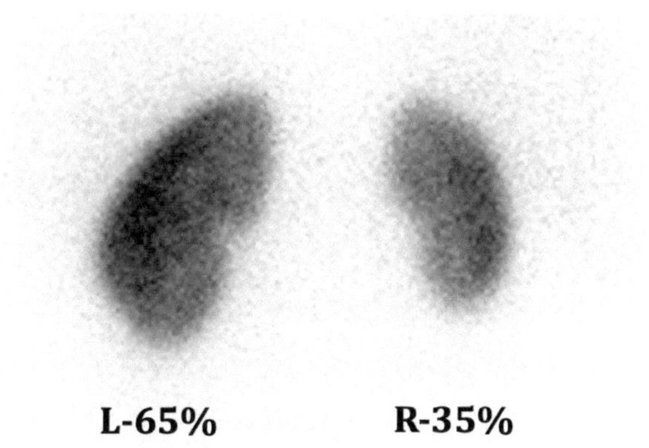

Fig. 13.10 Normal kidneys. Left is duplex. The split function is outside normal limits because there are effectively three kidneys, of which two are on one side and one is on the other side. In a Tc-99m-MAG3 or Tc-99m-DMSA scan always suspect an intact unilateral duplex when one kidney is smaller than the other, contributes only 30–40% of overall function but otherwise looks normal

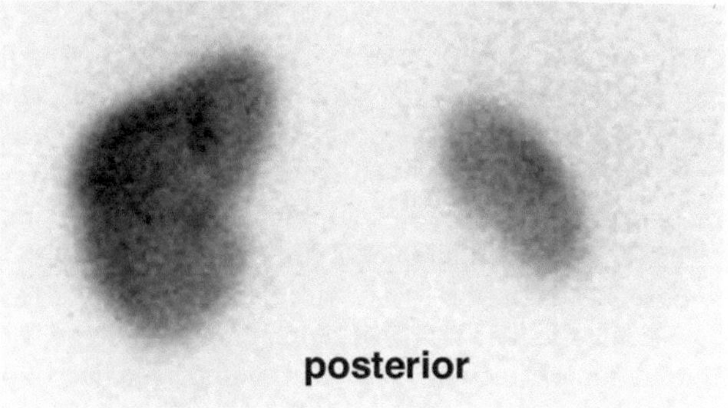

Fig. 13.11 Tc-99m-DMSA scan showing a dromedary hump (hypertrophied column of Bertin). This is a normal variant but on CT may be mistaken for a mass. The right kidney is atrophic

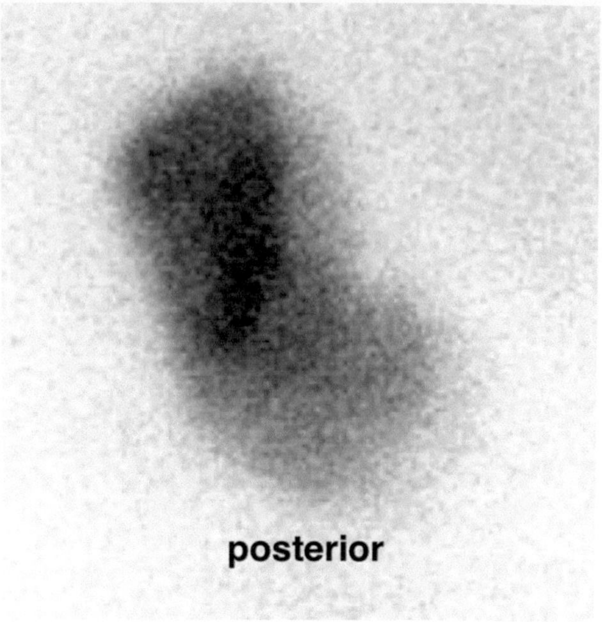

Fig. 13.12 Crossed fused ectopia. The right kidney is the ectopic one

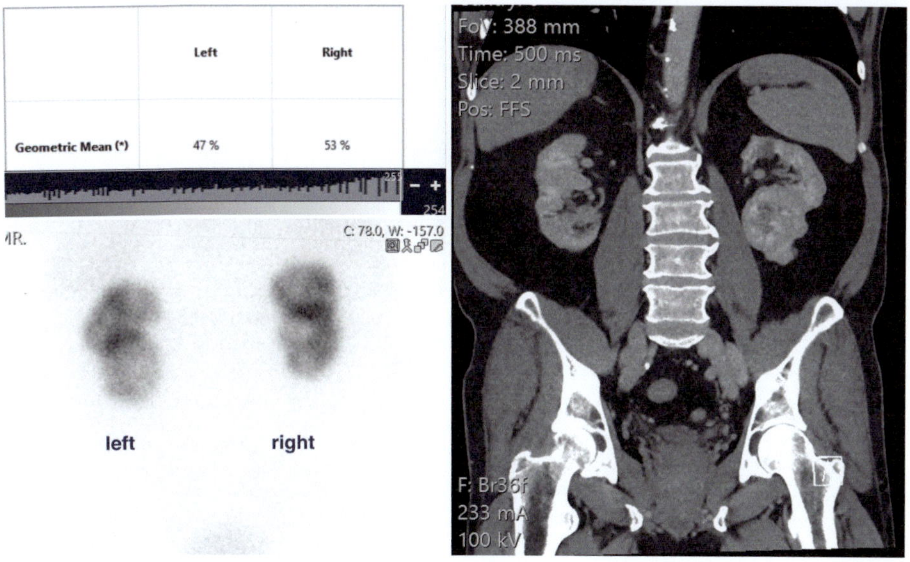

Fig. 13.13 Tc-99m-DMSA scan showing bilateral, symmetrical irregular cortical outlines, with a differential of foetal lobulation, which is a normal variant, and multiple bilateral scars

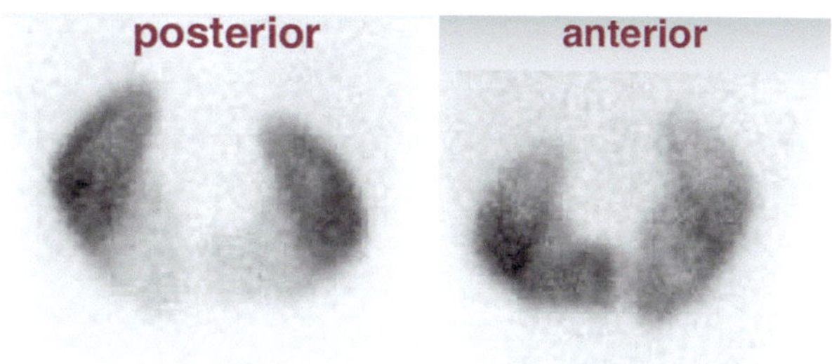

Fig. 13.14 Horseshoe kidney with lower pole fusion

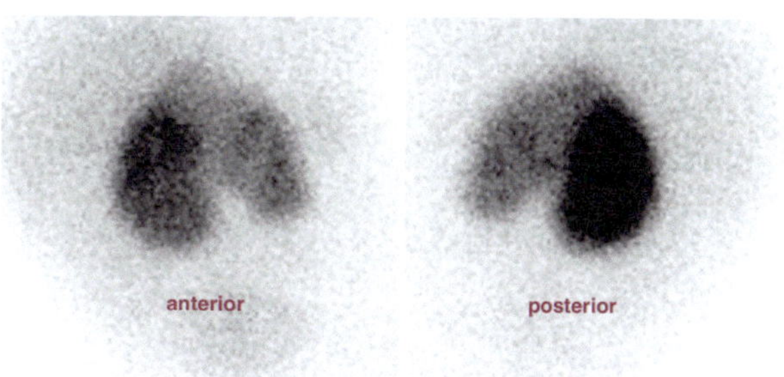

Fig. 13.15 Horseshoe kidneys usually fuse at the lower poles but may fuse at the upper poles as shown in this Tc-99m-DMSA scan

	Left	Right
Geometric Mean (*)	61 %	39 %

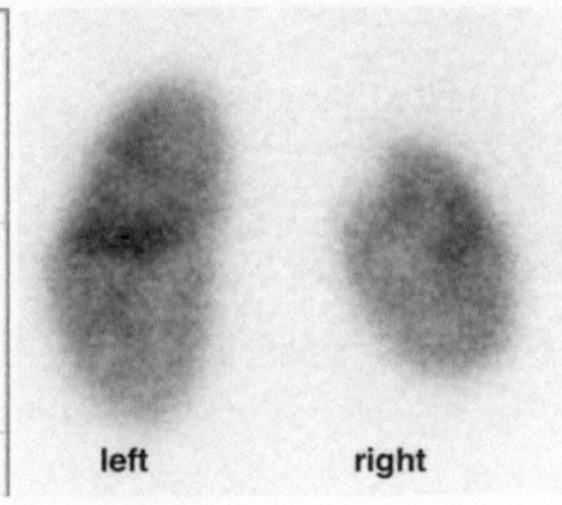

Fig. 13.16 Bilateral duplex kidneys. Left is intact but the right is scarred in the upper moiety. A feature of a duplex kidney, displayed on the left, is the impression of a 'band' of activity extending across the midzone

Further Reading

1. Weyer K, Nielsen R, Petersen SV, Christensen EI, Rehling M, Birn H. Renal uptake of 99mTc-dimercaptosuccinic acid is dependent on normal proximal tubule receptor–mediated endocytosis. J Nucl Med. 2013;54:159–65.

14 Tc-99m-Iminodiacetic Acid (HIDA) (MW 177 Da)

Tc-99m-HIDA is an organic anion that, along with other organic anions, including indocyanine green, bromsulphthalein, rose Bengal and Evans blue, accumulates in hepatocytes with an extraction efficiency approaching 100%. Organic anions are secreted into the bile canaliculi and excreted in bile. Their physiological analogue is bilirubin. Like the transfer of Tc-99m-MAG3 from plasma to tubular lumen, the transfer of Tc-99m-HIDA from plasma to hepatocyte and then from hepatocyte to bile canaliculus is mediated respectively by a family of proteins called organic anion transporters (OATs) and by multiple drug resistance (MDR) proteins. Tc-99m-HIDA is bound to plasma protein in the circulation and only enters urine when there is severe conjugated hyperbilirubinaemia.

Tc-99m-HIDA is used to image the hepatobiliary system. Imaging protocol is dynamic acquisition over 30–60 min followed either by delayed static imaging at 1–3 h, or a second dynamic, after consumption of food. Hepatic time activity curves are constructed for both dynamics, plus a blood time-activity curve over the cardiac chambers for the first dynamic. Like conjugated bilirubin, Tc-99m-HIDA undergoes bidirectional transfer between plasma and hepatocytes (Fig. 14.1).

The relative likelihoods of a HIDA molecule returning to plasma (k_2) or entering bile (k_3) are about 2:1. The blood pool curve declines as a double exponential, the first representing tracer exchange between sinusoids and hepatocytes, and the second reflecting tracer movement into bile canaliculus following mixing between blood and hepatocytes. The liver curve (the hepatogram), which rises to a peak and then declines, is the difference of the same two exponentials that comprise the blood time-concentration curve (Figs. 1.7 and 1.8).

A. M. Peters, M. Vadrucci, *Introduction to Nuclear Medicine for Trainees in Imaging and Imaging Sciences*, https://doi.org/10.1007/978-3-032-18364-4_14

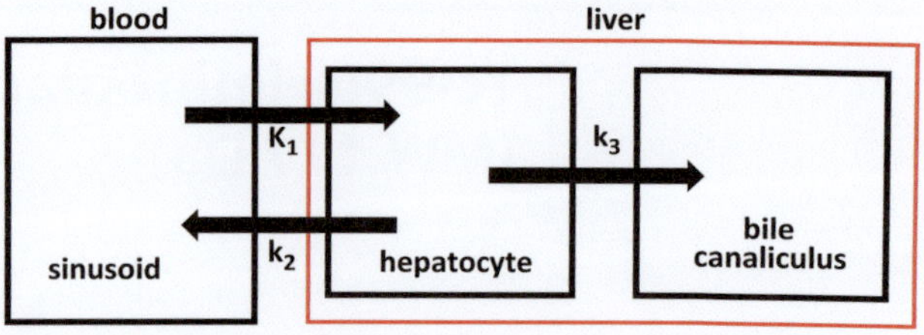

Fig. 14.1 Kinetics of Tc-99m-HIDA in the liver. Kinetics of bilirubin are similar and account for the conjugated hyperbilirubinaemia of jaundice

A pathological model in which transfer to the biliary system cannot occur is biliary atresia in which the liver has no communication with the extrahepatic biliary tree. In this condition, there is dynamic exchange of Tc-99m-HIDA between hepatocytes and blood, with equilibrium between the two compartments reached within 30 min of injection (Fig. 1.9).

In severe drug-induced hepatic cholestasis, MDR is overwhelmed by the drug, and negligible activity enters bile canaliculi from the hepatocytes. As in biliary atresia, equilibrium of Tc-99m-HIDA between hepatocytes and blood is established within 30 min, with negligible activity moving into bile canaliculi. The jaundice of pregnancy probably has a similar cause, where the MDR substrate is oestrogen, which is present in excess. Cholangitis also causes severe cholestasis.

The indications for Tc-99m-HIDA scintigraphy are biliary obstruction, biliary dyskinesia, cholangitis, biliary atresia, neonatal hepatitis, progress of piggyback transplantation for acute hepatic failure, drug-induced cholestasis, choledochal and other cysts, intrahepatic bile reflux or obstruction in a blind Roux loop, biliary leak and cholecystitis. In hospitals with specialist liver units, many referrals for a Tc-99m-HIDA scan come from the transplant surgeons querying drainage through surgical reconstructions. Otherwise, the most frequent referrals in general hospitals are for suspected biliary dyskinesia.

14.1 Reporting a Tc-99m-HIDA Scan

For biliary dyskinesia, check the patient has fasted, otherwise, the gallbladder will have contracted and will not fill with activity. For post-cholecystectomy sphincter of Oddi dysfunction (SOD), it makes sense to give a meal before tracer administration, because, in SOD, the sphincter inappropriately contracts in response to cholecystokinin. Gross hepatic morphology should first be commented on if there is anything of significance, such as bile duct dilatation, as in Caroli disease (Fig. 14.2). The excretion half-time, measured from the gradient of the downslope of the hepatogram (Fig. 14.3), describes intrahepatic transport of the tracer and has a normal upper limit of 30 min. The report should then focus, as in renography, on tracer drainage and gallbladder response to a meal.

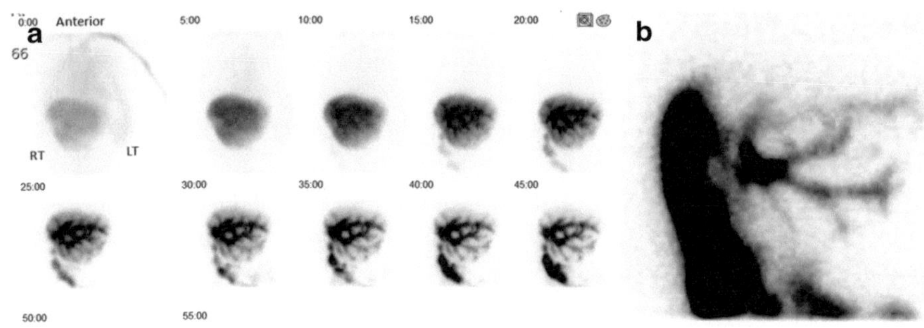

Fig. 14.2 Gross dilatation of intrahepatic biliary tree. Activity is visible in bile ducts from 5–10 min post-injection (**a**), so obstruction can be excluded. Confirmation is provided by delayed static image at 2 h post-injection (**b**). Tc-99m-HIDA and Tc-99m-MAG3 scintigraphy are similar in that parenchymal transit time is prolonged in outflow obstruction

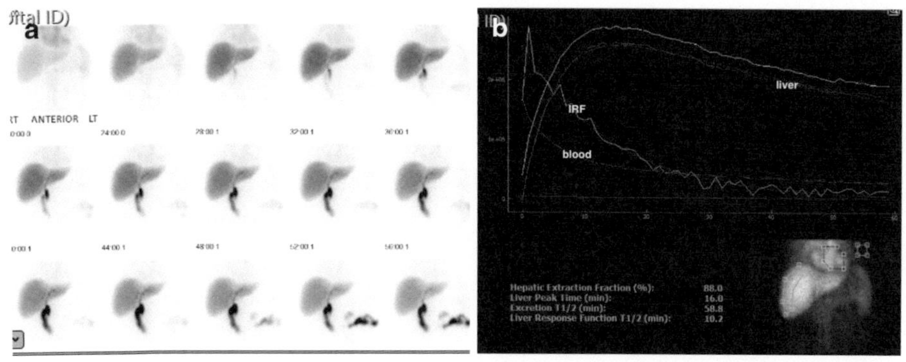

Fig. 14.3 (**a**) There is no biliary obstruction as shown by early appearance of activity in common bile duct (timing not shown for first 5 frames) but the parenchyma is slow to clear with an excretion halftime of 59 min (upper limit of normal 30 min), indicating cholestasis. (**b**) Time activity curves for liver (with and without background correction) and cardiac blood pool. IRF is the impulse response function, the rate constant of which is equal to $k_2 + k_3$ (see Figs. 14.1 and 3.8). It us used to calculate hepatic tracer extraction efficiency (K_1 in Fig. 14.1 divided by hepatic blood flow), normally 100%

14.2 Biliary Dyskinesia

There are three biliary dyskinesia syndromes: cystic duct syndrome (CDS), sphincter of Oddi dysfunction (SOD) and hyperkinetic gallbladder (HGB). Normally, during fasting, the cystic duct is open, and bile enters the gallbladder for storage. It is not unusual, therefore, to see no activity entering the duodenum up to 60 min post-injection because the sphincter of Oddi is appropriately closed. In response to cholecystokinin (CCK), secreted into the circulation from enterocytes when food enters the duodenum, the gallbladder contracts, and the sphincter of Oddi opens, releasing bile into the duodenum. In CDS, the cystic duct inappropriately constricts in response to CCK and the gallbladder fails to eject bile (Fig. 14.4). In SOD, the sphincter fails to open in response to CCK, limited bile enters the duodenum (Fig. 14.5), and instead may reflux into the intrahepatic biliary tree. In HGB, the gallbladder shows an exaggerated response to CCK and ejects more than 80% of its contents, usually rapidly (Fig. 14.6). Duodeno-gastric reflux (Fig. 14.7) may contribute to symptoms of biliary dyskinesia.

The lower normal limit of gallbladder ejection fraction is conventionally taken as 35% at 30 min post-stimulation. This, however, was established when intravenous CCK was used as the stimulant instead of food, and the protocol was reasonably rigid. The lower limit following a meal, however, is now less certain and made even less certain by protocol variations, such as (a) meal composition (*Calogen* is a standardised meal), (b) static imaging before and after the meal versus dynamic imaging after the meal, and (c) 30 min versus 60 min for dynamic imaging. Moreover, the CCK response to food may be delayed if stomach emptying is slow, potentially giving a false-positive result for CDS. We believe 60 min dynamic imaging is essential to fully document gallbladder

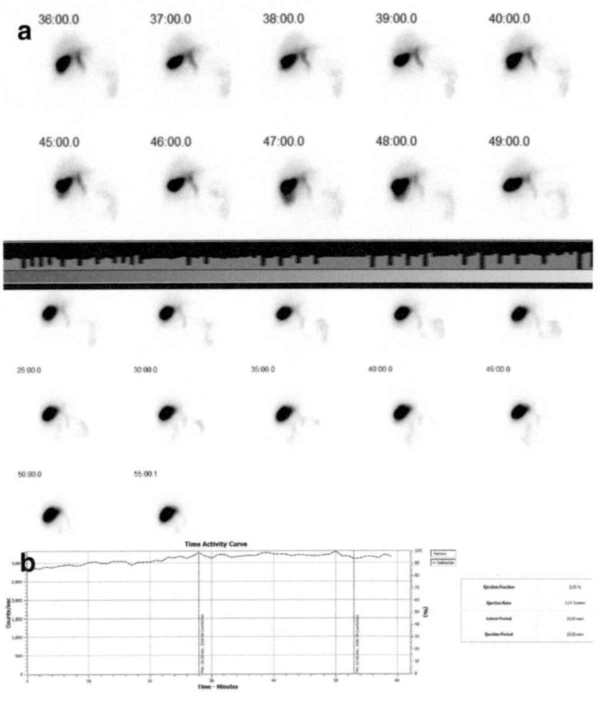

Fig. 14.4 Cystic duct syndrome is a variant of biliary dyskinesia, the other variants being sphincter of Oddi dysfunction and hyper-responsive (or hyperkinetic) gallbladder. In CDS, the gallbladder fills normally (**a**, upper panel) but fails to respond to cholecystokinin released from enterocytes in response to *Calogen* (**a**, lower panel). The gallbladder ejection fraction is essentially zero (**b**). Severely delayed gastric emptying resulting in impaired cholecystokinin release may produce a false positive result

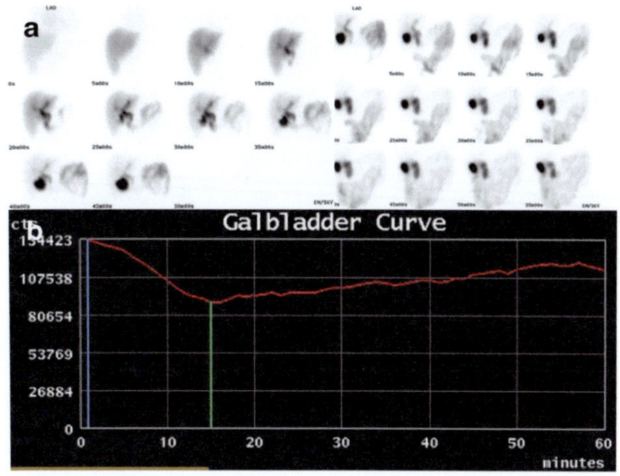

Fig. 14.5 Scoring systems for the diagnosis of SOD have been published based on several features of the dynamic scan such as hepatic excretion halftime in relation to counts over the CBD. But these systems have focussed on post-cholecystectomy SOD, in which the study should be performed after a standard meal, despite the absence of a gallbladder. SOD, like CDS, is a functional disorder in which instead of the sphincter opening in response to cholecystokinin it undergoes contraction. In this case, which is not post-cholecystectomy, SOD can be diagnosed because although activity is visible in jejunum prior to the meal (**a**, left panel), the sphincter appears to undergo contraction after the meal (**a**, right panel), leading to build up of activity in the CBD and re-filling of the gallbladder (**b**)

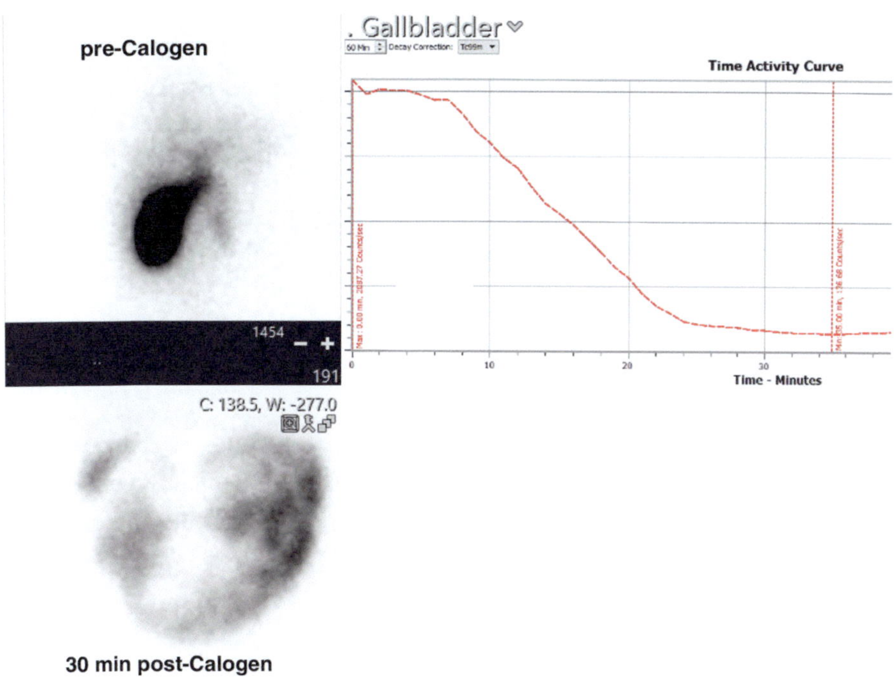

Fig. 14.6 Hyperkinetic (hyper-responsive) gallbladder is a less well recognised cause of biliary dyskinesia. Nevertheless, symptoms to which it is ascribed have been shown to be abolished by cholecystectomy. Ejection fraction is in the region of 90% over 30 min post-meal, as shown in this case

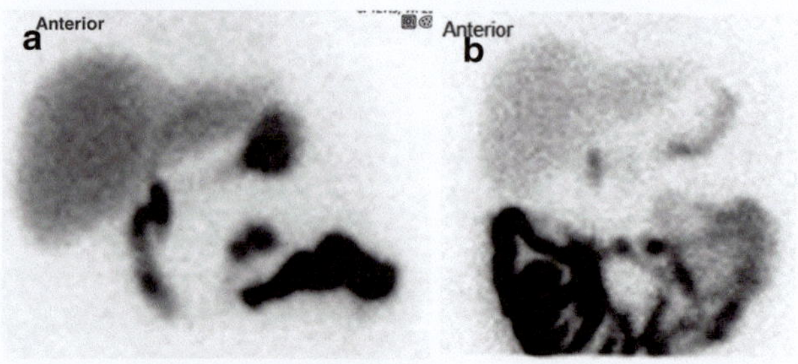

Fig. 14.7 Duodeno-gastric reflux in a Tc-99m-HIDA scan. Static images obtained 1 (**a**) and 2 h (**b**) post-injection are shown

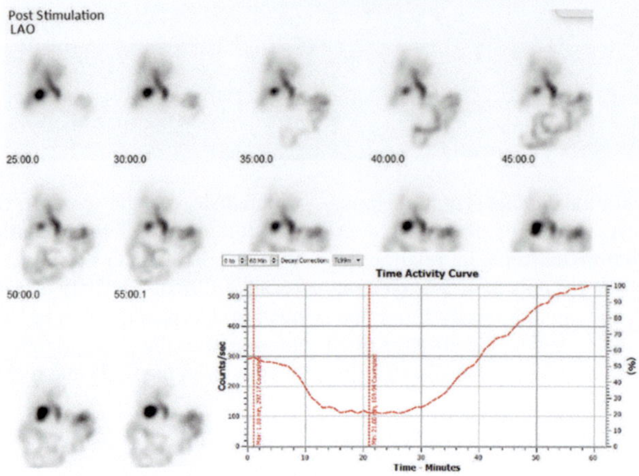

Fig. 14.8 Unusual re-filling of the gallbladder following a brisk response to a standard *Calogen* meal with an initial ejection fraction of 63%. This illustrates the importance of dynamic imaging up to 60 min after a meal for a full assessment of biliary malfunction, as opposed to the wide practice of static imaging post-meal, often at 30 min post-meal

kinetics, as shown for example when a gallbladder refills (Fig. 14.8). For post-cholecystectomy biliary dyskinesia (i.e., SOD), food should be given before the tracer to increase bile flow and to induce (inappropriate) sphincter contraction. The effect on bile flow, however, is minimal, with a flow increment of less than 1.5-fold (compared with five to tenfold in urine flow in a healthy kidney following furosemide).

14.3 Localising a Bile Leak

Bile leaks usually arise from the cut surface of the liver after surgery (Fig. 14.9) or from a punctured extrahepatic bile duct (Fig. 14.10). SPECT/CT is routinely performed immediately after the initial 60 min dynamic imaging sequence but can be delayed, allowing physiological activity in the intestine to move distally and out of the field of

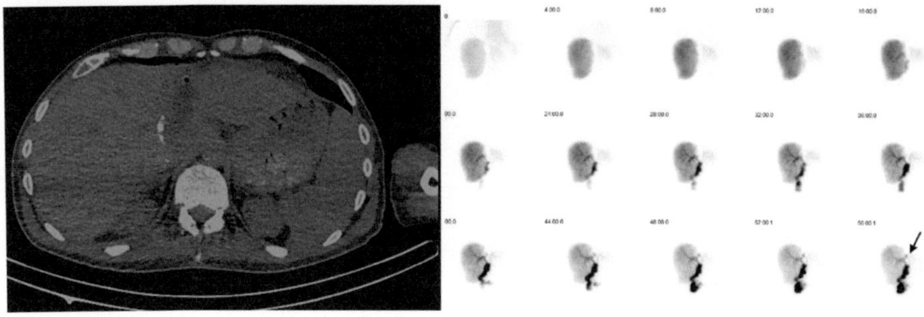

Fig. 14.9 Bile leaks mostly occur at two typical sites. Firstly, involving small intrahepatic bile ducts at the surface of the liver following surgical procedures that involve cutting the liver, shown here (arrow), and secondly leaks involving larger extrahepatic bile ducts that often lead to intra-abdominal collections

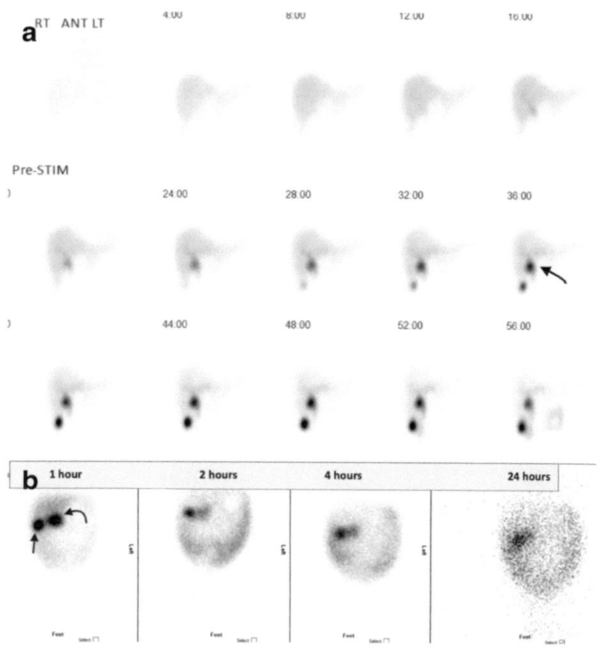

Fig. 14.10 Leaking common bile duct in a young infant. There is a choledochal cyst (curved arrow) in which tracer accumulated before entering the gallbladder (straight arrow) (**a**). No activity is visible in bowel but instead is seen throughout the abdomen in ascitic fluid (**b**), placing the leak in the CBD

interest. Delayed planar imaging is useful to capture activity if it is trapped at the site of the leak. The leak may form a collection, hence the importance of SPECT/CT. Delayed imaging of drainage bags is also important.

14.4 Biliary Atresia and Neonatal Hepatitis

In biliary atresia there is no anatomical connection between the intrahepatic and extrahepatic bile ducts, and bile is unable to access the duodenum. Blood pool and hepatic activities decrease and increase, respectively, with identical exponential rate constants and remain in equilibration over many hours (Fig. 14.11). Imaging at 24 h shows liver activity but no gut activity. Some activity, however, enters urine, which should not be confused with intestinal activity, especially if it is in a nappy over the infant's abdomen. Appearances may be similar in neonatal hepatitis (Fig. 14.12) or cholangitis (Fig. 14.13) when there is slow entry of tracer into duodenum. Any activity entering the intestine excludes biliary atresia.

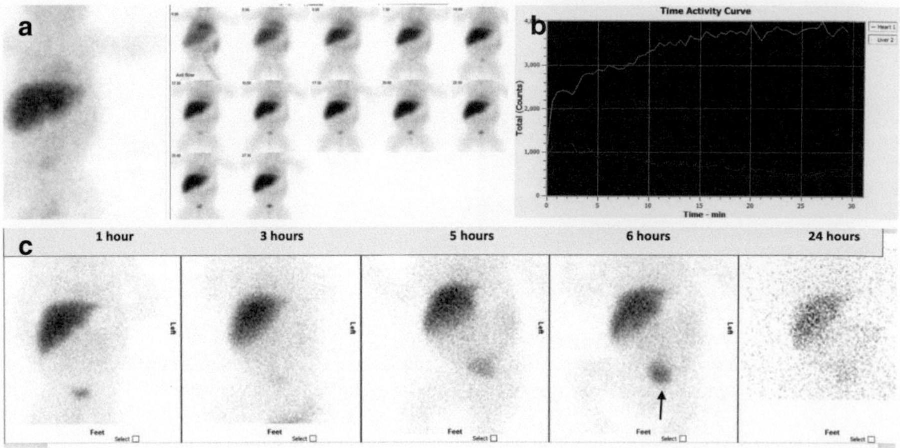

Fig. 14.11 In biliary atresia, there is no anatomical connection between liver and gut and no means for bile to drain from liver. Tc-99m-HIDA accumulates in hepatocytes (**a**) and re-enters plasma giving time activity curves over cardiac blood pool and liver that respectively decline and rise with identical rate constants (**b**). Delayed imaging up to 24 h post-injection shows no bowel activity (**c**). Note urinary activity (arrow)

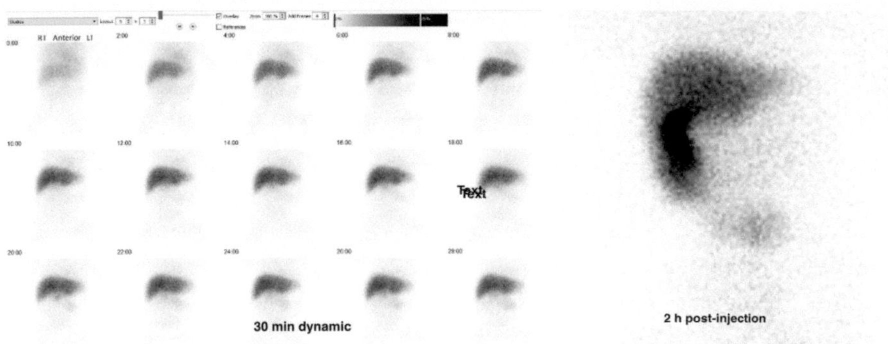

Fig. 14.12 Because of severe intrahepatic cholestasis, neonatal hepatitis, shown here, may be confused with biliary atresia (left panel), but the latter is excluded by the appearance of activity in bowel (right panel). Despite its name, neonatal hepatitis may be encountered in infants up to at least 8 weeks of age

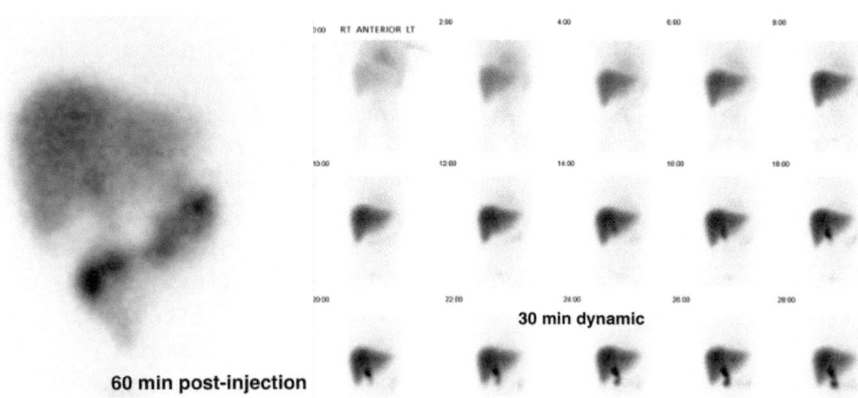

Fig. 14.13 Cholangitis in an infant. Note similar appearances to neonatal hepatitis

14.5 Choledochal Cyst

Choledochal cysts are focal dilatations of the biliary tree and therefore visible on Tc-99m-HIDA scintigraphy (Fig. 14.14). There are 5 anatomical variants, the commonest of which is type 1, which involves the extrahepatic tree. Biliary obstruction and malignant change are the prime reasons for resection of a choledochal cyst. Tc-99m-HIDA scintigraphy may be used to exclude biliary communication with a cyst that is not suspected to be a choledochal cyst (Fig. 14.15).

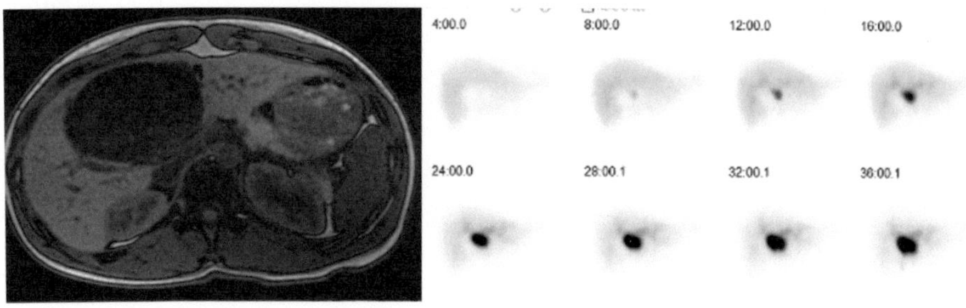

Fig. 14.14 Choledochal cyst involving the common hepatic duct

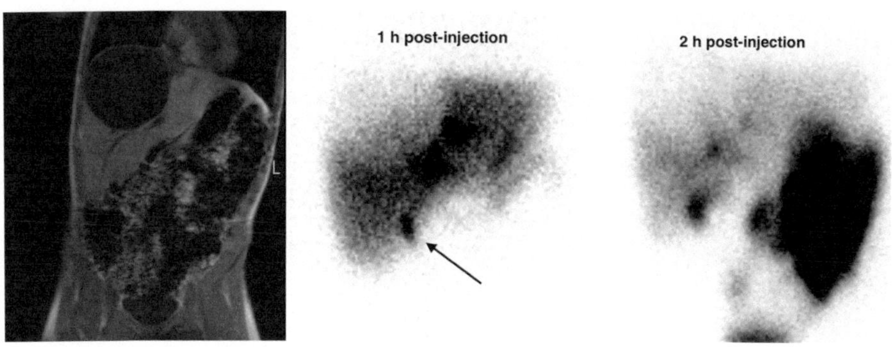

Fig. 14.15 A large intrahepatic cyst that does not communicate with the biliary tree and is therefore not a choledochal cyst. Left panel: MRI; middle panel: 1 h post-injection; right panel: 2 h post-injection. Arrow: gallbladder

14.6 Biliary Obstruction

Biliary obstruction may be intra- or extrahepatic. If it is intrahepatic within a lobe, it may be missed because tracer can escape from hepatocytes as a result of bidirectional tracer transfer between blood and liver (Fig. 14.1). Anastomotic strictures may be post-surgical, such as following hepaticojejunostomy. Obstruction gives a prolonged parenchymal phase—as in renography—followed by delayed appearance of activity in a dilated biliary tree (Fig. 14.16). Excretion halftime is prolonged, and delayed static imaging shows tracer retention in the intrahepatic biliary tree. Partial obstruction may occur in the second or third part of the duodenum (Fig. 14.17), one cause of which is superior mesenteric artery syndrome that results from entrapment of duodenum between the artery and the aorta, generally diagnosed, at least scintigraphically, from a gastric emptying study, rather than Tc-99m-HIDA.

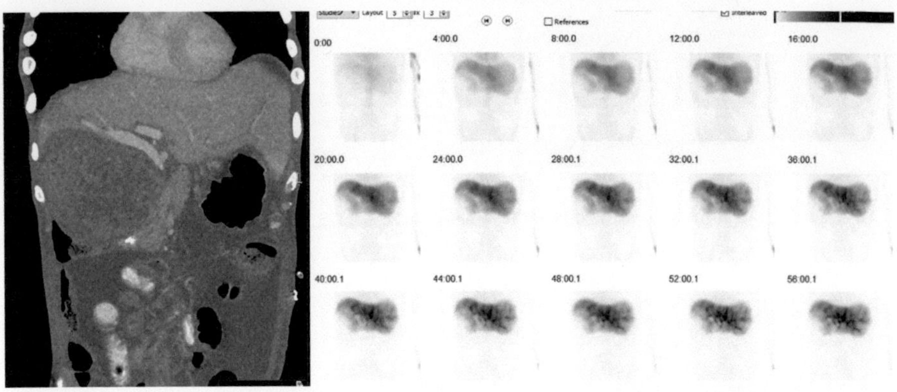

Fig. 14.16 Renal cell carcinoma causing biliary obstruction. Activity slowly accumulates in the intrahepatic biliary tree which is dilated. No activity seen in bowel over the initial 60 min dynamic image acquisition

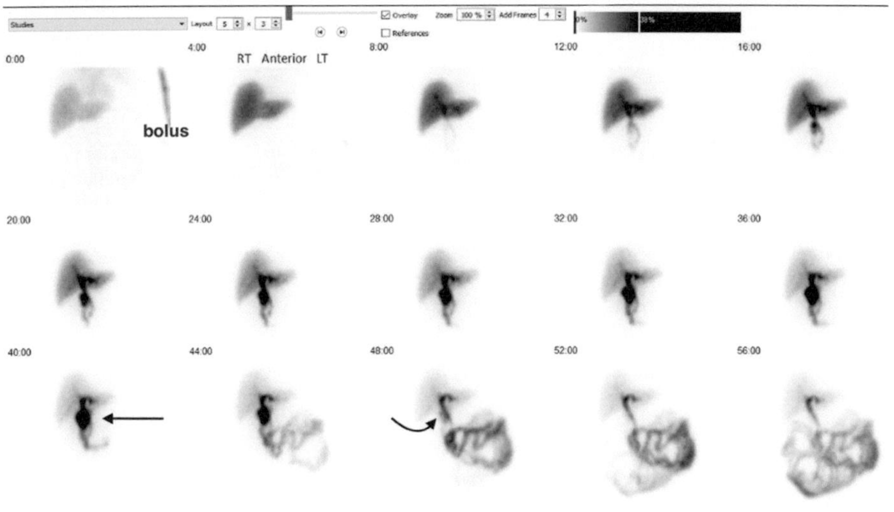

Fig. 14.17 Hold-up of Tc-99m-HIDA in the second part of the duodenum (straight arrow), which may have contributed to this patient's right upper quadrant pain. Note the rapidity of intestinal transit once the tracer passes the duodenum (curved arrow). Gallbladder is not visualised

14.7 Cholecystitis

Acute cholecystitis is not frequently encountered in nuclear medicine departments because of the availability of alternative imaging techniques. Delayed gallbladder filling of Tc-99m-HIDA, however, may be seen in patients with suspected biliary dyskinesia and suggests chronic cholecystitis (Fig. 14.18).

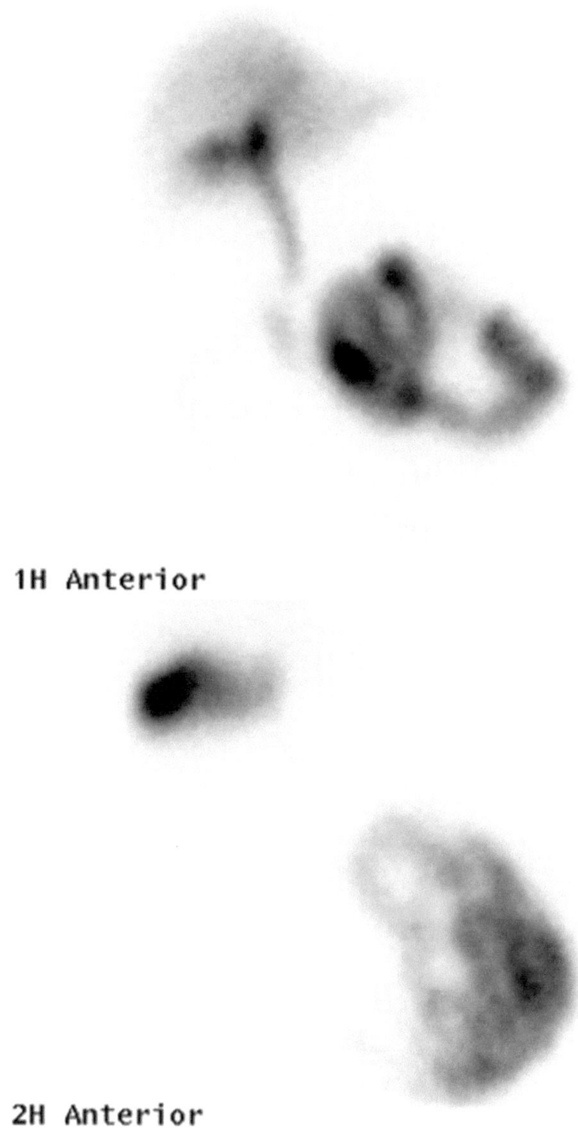

Fig. 14.18 Delayed filling of the gallbladder suggesting chronic cholecystitis. Make sure the patient has fasted!

14.8 Focal Nodular Hyperplasia (FNH)

FNH is an important scintigraphic diagnosis because, like a hypertrophied column of Bertin, it may be misdiagnosed as a tumour in morphological imaging. FNH is readily diagnosed with Tc-99m-labelled colloid because it contains Kupffer cells (Chap. 22). FNH, however, contains functioning hepatocytes as well as Kupffer cells and accumulates Tc-99m-HIDA (Fig. 14.19). The uptake becomes more prominent as a result of ongoing biliary drainage in normal liver.

14.9 Auxiliary Transplant

Acute liver failure, from paracetamol overdose for example, may be treated by transplanting an auxiliary liver which functions alongside the native liver while the latter recovers. The progress of the native liver compared with the auxiliary is monitored with sequential Tc-99m-HIDA scintigraphy with measurement of split function. As the native liver recovers, immunosuppression is tailed off and function in the auxiliary transplant declines (Fig. 14.20). As with renography, split function gives no indication of absolute function.

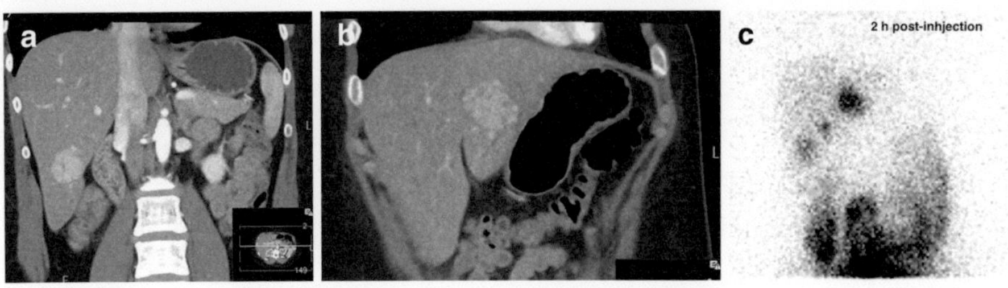

Fig. 14.19 Focal nodular hyperplasia (FNH). Tc-99m-colloid is recommended for the identification of FNH but the condition is also evident with Tc-99m-HIDA. In this case, CT scans (**a** and **b**) show two of the 3 lesions seen on the HIDA scan (**c**). The lesions contain functioning hepatocytes but no draining bile ducts—hence their gradual appearance on delayed static images as tracer clears into bile

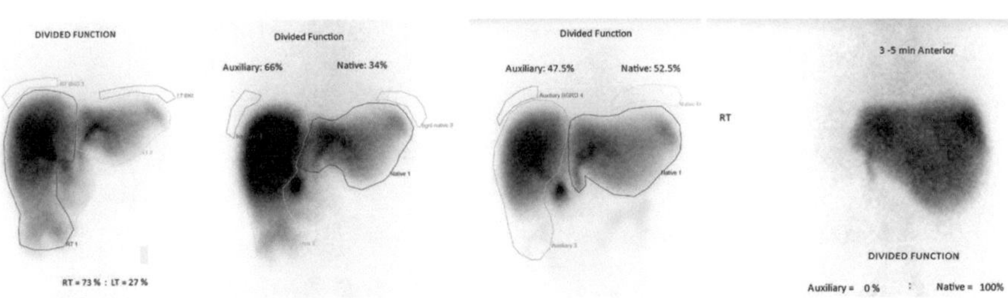

Fig. 14.20 Declining function, captured in split function in the 3–5 min time frame, in an auxiliary liver transplant given for acute liver failure. As the native liver recovers, in this case from 27%, through 34%, 52%, to 100% of overall function, immuno-suppression can be tailed off so that the auxiliary liver finally becomes non-functional. As in renal split function, no information is given on absolute function

Further Reading

1. Krishnamurthy GT, Brown PH. Comparison of fatty meal and intravenous cholecystokinin infusion for gallbladder ejection fraction. J Nucl Med. 2002;43:1603–10.
2. Saurabh S, Green B. Is hyperkinetic gallbladder an indication for cholecystectomy? Surg Endosc. 2019;33:1613–7. https://doi.org/10.1007/s00464-018-6435-2.
3. Sostre S, Kalloo AN, Spiegler EJ, Camargo EE, Wagner HN. A noninvasive test of sphincter of Oddi dysfunction in postcholecystectomy patients: the scintigraphic score. J Nucl Med. 1992;33:1216–22.

15 Tc-99m-Labelled Diphosphonates (MW ~300 Da)

A range of diphosphonates are labelled with Tc-99m for imaging the skeleton, including Tc-99m-MDP (methylene diphosphonate), Tc-99m-HDP (hydroxy-diphosphonate) and Tc-99m-DPD (diphosphono-propanodicarboxylic acid). A diphosphonate is an example of a pharmaceutical in therapeutic use (e.g., for osteoporosis) complexed with a radionuclide to produce a radiopharmaceutical. Tc-99m-diphosphonates accumulate in the osteoid seam of osteoblastic bone. They therefore portray osteoblastic activity in bones without accumulating in osteoblasts or osteoclasts.

Tc-99m-MDP is hydrophilic and therefore distributes, like Tc-99m-DTPA, throughout the ECF space. It is filtered at the glomerulus and excreted in urine with minimal tubular reabsorption. Plasma clearance of Tc-99m-MDP is about 200 ml/min of which about half is into the skeleton and half into the urine. Imaging is undertaken 3 h following injection (Fig. 15.1). In many patients, usually with musculoskeletal disease, dynamic imaging is performed immediately after injection to assess blood flow to the area of interest, followed immediately by static imaging completed within 5 min of injection to reinforce information on vascularity. This sequence constitutes a 3-phase bone scan. Phases 1 and 2 give essentially the same information about blood flow (Fig. 15.2).

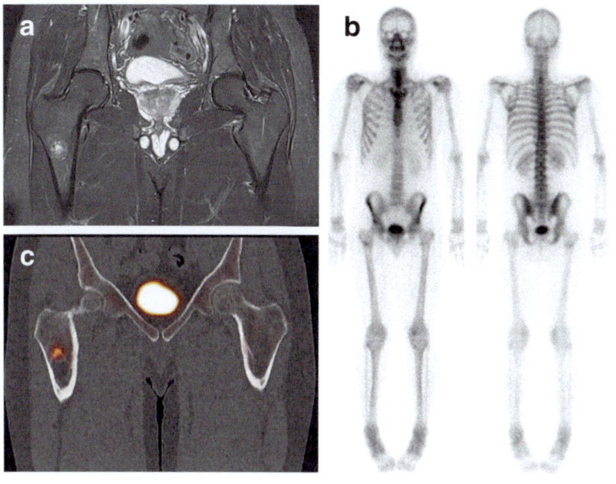

Fig. 15.1 Isolated benign bone tumour in the proximal right femur (**a**) in a young man with an otherwise normal whole body bone scan (**b**). Variation in bone tracer uptake broadly depends on weight-bearing stress and muscle traction. The bone scan can be co-registered with low-dose CT (**c**) for accurate anatomical localisation

A. M. Peters, M. Vadrucci, *Introduction to Nuclear Medicine for Trainees in Imaging and Imaging Sciences*, https://doi.org/10.1007/978-3-032-18364-4_15

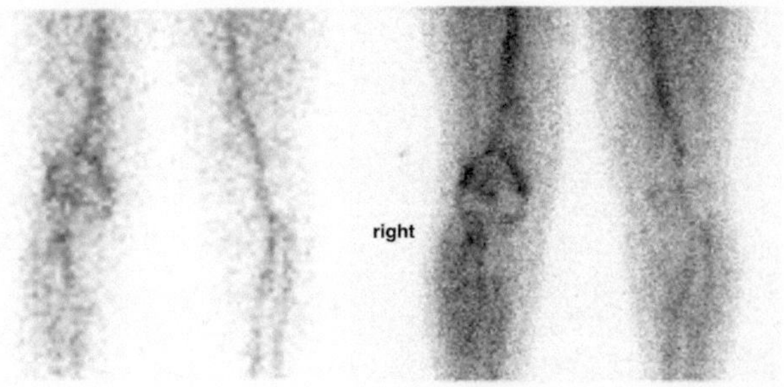

Fig. 15.2 Phases 1 (left panel) and 2 (right panel) give similar information about vascularity in a 3-phase bone scan. This patient with a painful right total knee replacement has synovial hypervascularity indicating synovitis

Fig. 15.3 Whole body bone scan showing increased soft tissue activity in a patient with impaired renal function. Left panel: posterior blood pool image (phase 2) showing poor tracer concentration in the kidneys. Right panel: anterior 3 h image showing prominent soft tissue activity.The skull looks prominent because in overweight individuals there is less overlying soft tissue to attenuate the emitted photons. Note hypervascularity and increased uptake in left wrist and soft tissue uptake in the right breast

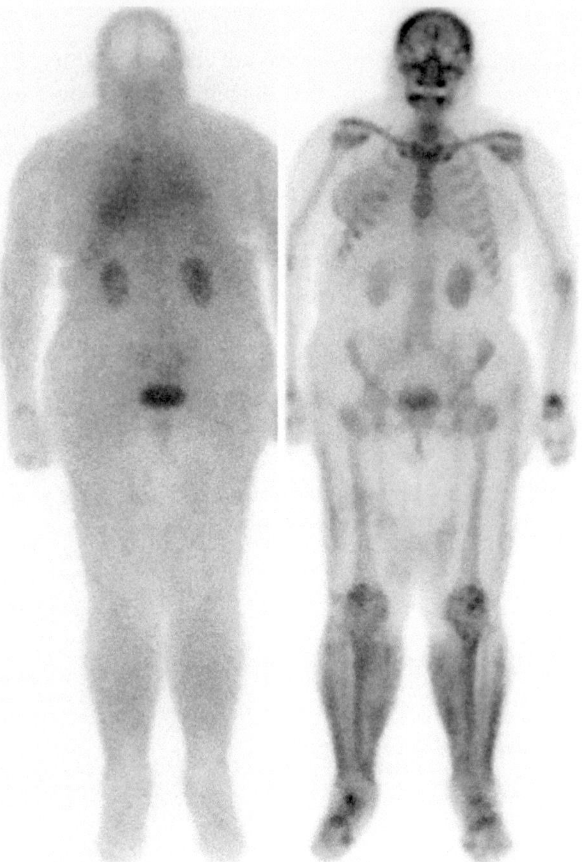

In patients with poor renal function, reduced renal clearance leaves more activity in the ECF at 3 h. Even if there is normal clearance into the skeleton, the increased background activity results in what is perceived as a poor-quality bone scan (Fig. 15.3). The image can be improved

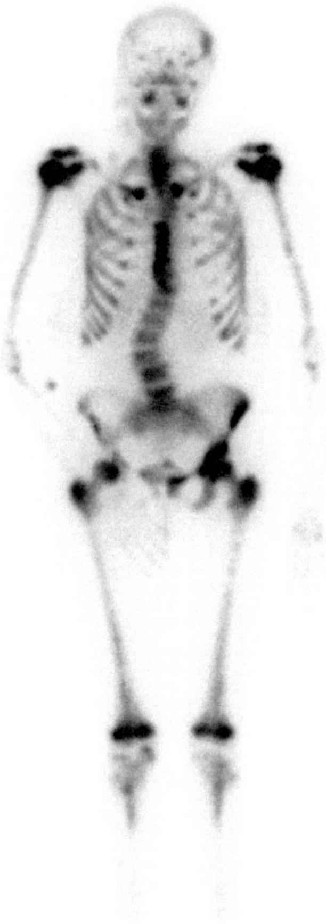

Fig. 15.4 Bone scan in myelofibrosis. Bone blood flow is a portal system with bony elements and marrow supplied in series rather than in parallel. Increased flow to marrow therefore brings increased amounts of tracer to bone giving rise to increased tracer accumulation in bone, even though the disease is in marrow

by acquiring it more than 3 h after tracer injection (phase 4). In contrast, in patients with metabolic bone disease, tracer clearance is rapid, and up to 90% of administered tracer may accumulate in the skeleton within 3 h of injection (Fig. 15.4). As small diffusible molecules, Tc-99m-diphosphonates enter '3rd' spaces, such as pleural effusions and ascites (Fig. 15.5).

Bone has a surprisingly high blood flow. It is a portal system insofar as incoming blood first serves the cortex and then the marrow. As explained in Chap. 2, the amount of tracer accumulating in a tissue is the product of perfusion and extraction efficiency. This simple rule and the bone's portal circulation explain how active bone marrow can lead to increased tracer accumulation in the cortex of the bone. Indeed, myelofibrosis may give a so-called superscan (Fig. 15.4), similar to that seen in disseminated bone metastases. Clearance into the interstitial space of tissue explains why bone scanning is used to diagnose inflammatory arthritis. Even if osteoblastic activity (which determines extraction efficiency) is not increased, bone uptake is increased when local perfusion is increased, as in synovitis (Fig. 15.6) and sinusitis (Fig. 15.7).

Metastatic bone disease is the most common indication for a bone scan, followed by orthopaedic problems, and less commonly to diagnose metabolic bone disease (especially Paget's disease) and occult fractures. The bone scan is non-specific, with abnormalities in general causing increased osteoblastic activity. The most common disease seen in the adult bone scan is degenerative joint disease. A general rule to distinguish joint disease from bone disease close to a joint is that uptake is increased on both sides of the joint in joint disease but only on one side in bone disease. In the paediatric bone scan, the dominant feature is normal high uptake in growth plates (Fig. 15.8). In contrast to the adult bone scan, the paediatric bone scan needs to be pristine to be called normal—any abnormality should raise the suspicion of significant disease.

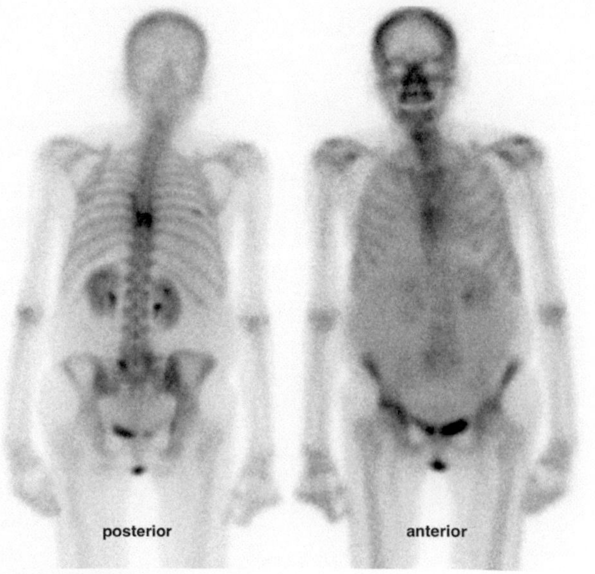

Fig. 15.5 Ascites in a patient with bone metastases. Note diffuse activity in the abdomen. Tc-99m-MDP is a small diffusible tracer and enters so-called 3rd spaces such as ascites and pleural effusion

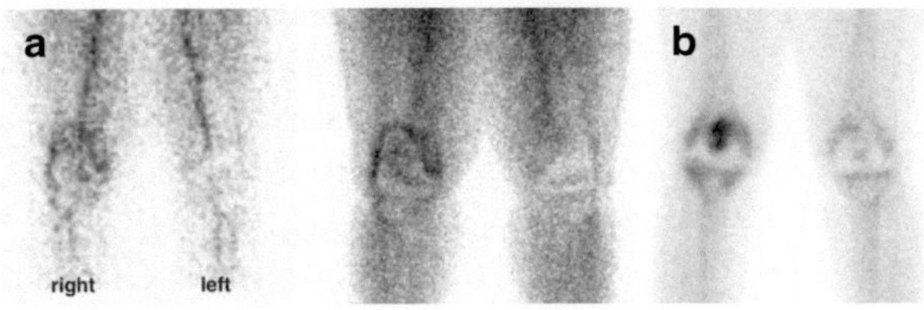

Fig. 15.6 A. Synovial hypervascularity shown in phase 1 (left panel) and phase 2 (right panel) in a patient with a painful right knee replacement. There is mild synovial hypervascularity in the left knee. B. Delayed image (phase 3) shows diffuse increased uptake in the right knee, compared to the left, resulting from the increased delivery of tracer to the region. There is also evidence of patellofemoral disease in the right knee

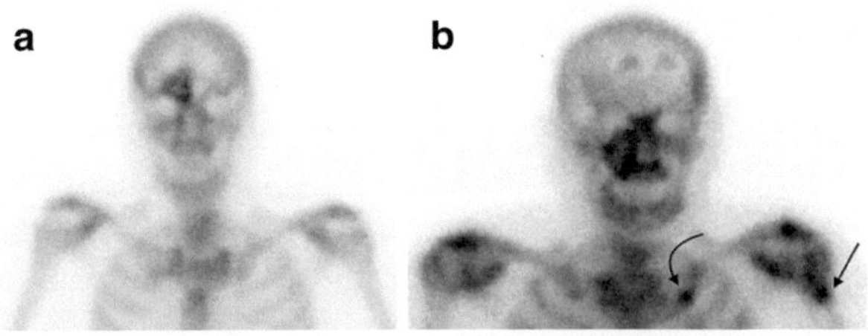

Fig. 15.7 Sinusitis in a bone scan: frontal (**a**); maxillary (**b**). Increased tracer accumulation is largely the result of increased blood flow in the mucosa lining the sinus. In **b**, note deposit in left humeral neck (straight arrow). Focus in left first rib (curved arrow) is more likely from enthesitis

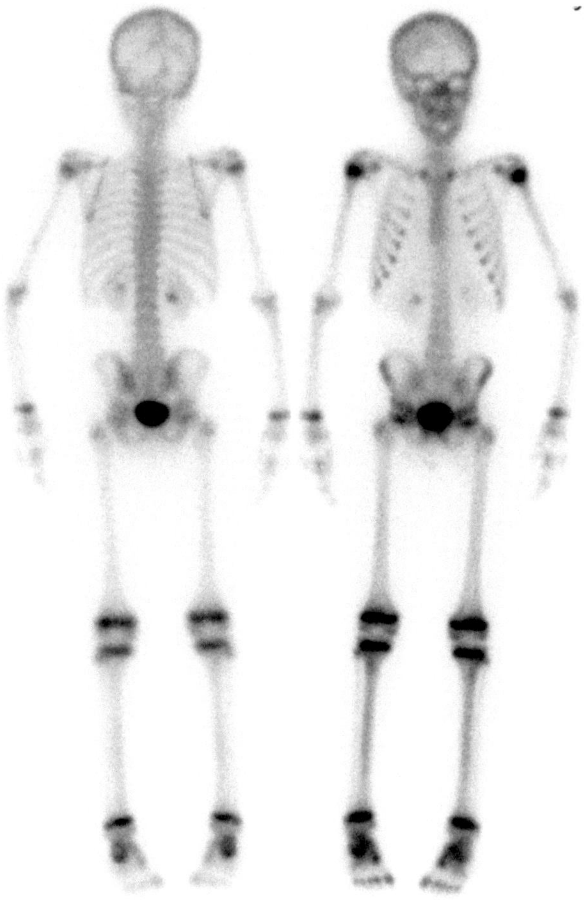

Fig. 15.8 Normal bone scan in a child showing prominent tracer accumulation in the growth plates

15.1 Reporting a Bone Scan

Adopting a reporting strategy is recommended that scrutinises every bone. Always correlate findings with diagnostic CT if available. If no prior CT, consider performing SPECT/CT. SPECT on its own is largely unhelpful.

Bone lesions of any cause generally induce an osteoblastic response and give foci of increased uptake in the bone scan. Increased tracer uptake is usually easy to recognise, but, in contrast, it is easy to miss absence of uptake in a bone—photopaenic lesions—as occurs in lytic lesions or following surgical excision of bone. Check both kidneys are functioning and make note of the distribution of soft tissue activity that may point to inflammation or lymphoedema. Soft tissue tumours, metastases, and infarcts (typically in brain and myocardium) accumulate Tc-99m-MDP (Fig. 15.9). Soft tissue uptake in the myocardium in elderly men, best imaged with Tc-99m-DPD, is not uncommon and suggests transthyretin amyloidosis (Fig. 15.10). In elderly patients, vertical linear uptake is usually seen in the femoral vessels from uptake in atheroma (Fig. 15.11). Radiotherapy abolishes bone tracer

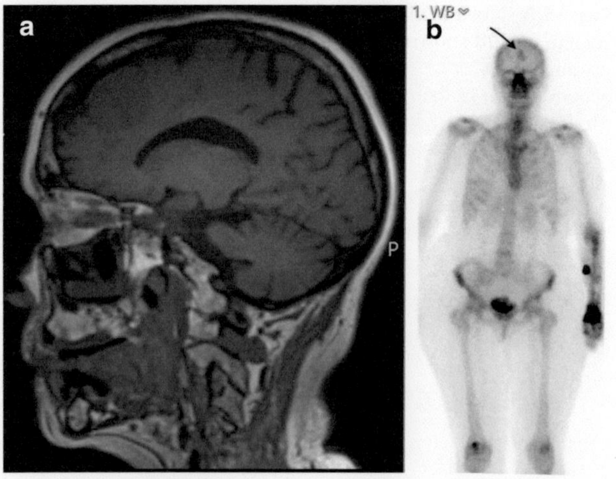

Fig. 15.9 Midline frontal meningioma (arrow) accumulating bone tracer. The intense tracer accumulation in the bones of the left arm, wrist and hand is the result of inadvertent partial intra-arterial tracer injection

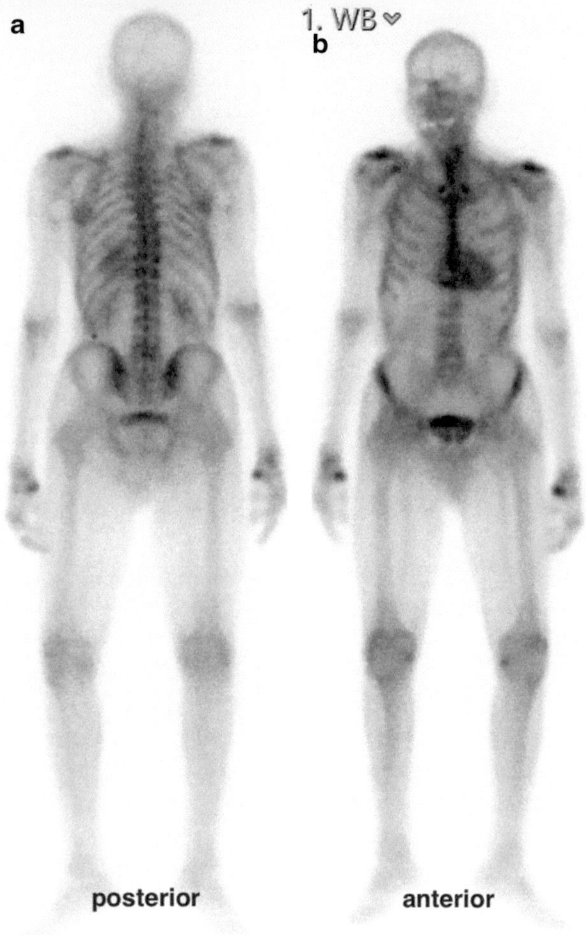

Fig. 15.10 Incidental finding of increased soft tissue accumulation of bone tracer in the myocardium of an elderly man with trans-thyretin (TTR) cardiac amyloidosis and prostate cancer. Note increased soft tissue uptake in the shoulders and especially hips, which is an accompanying feature of the disease. Cardiology referral was recommended

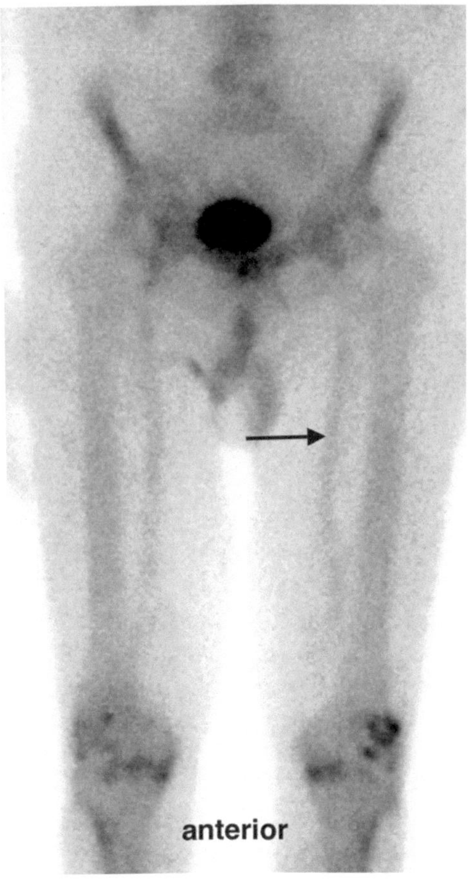

Fig. 15.11 Accumulation of bone tracer in the femoral vessels of an elderly man (arrow). This common finding in the elderly does not reflect blood pool activity in the femoral vessels but instead is the result of uptake in the atherosclerotic walls of the vessel. Note osteoarthritic changes in both knees

uptake, giving rise in treated breast cancer, for example, to a photopaenic anterior unilateral chest wall (Fig. 15.12). Causes of increased soft tissue uptake in kidneys (Fig. 15.13) include recent chemotherapy, hypercalcaemia (which may also give increased lung uptake), hepatic cirrhosis and iron overload. The fibroid uterus, prostate and calcified thyroid may also accumulate bone tracer (Figs. 15.14, 15.15, and 15.16).

Urinary contamination may be a problem (Fig. 15.17). Be careful not to misinterpret an apparent focus that arises from 'shine through', for example in the sternum from a prominent focus in the thoracic spine. When bones overlap, such as scapula and an underlying rib, an apparent focus may be generated from count summation. Count summation is demonstrated in Fig. 15.18, in which there appears to be a solitary left kidney on the delayed image. On careful inspection, however, there are too many counts from the lumbar spine, suggesting a structure anterior to it, which turned out to be an ectopic right kidney. Obese individuals may display apparent prominent skull uptake because of relatively less photon attenuation from overlying tissue compared with the central skeleton.

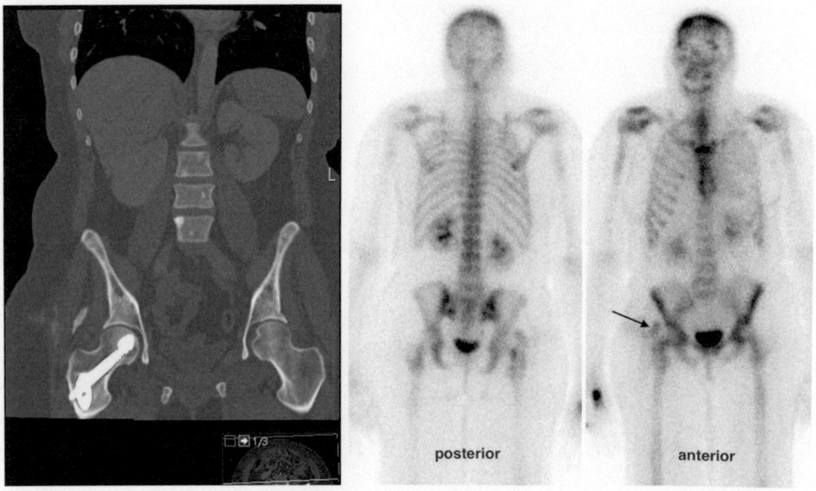

Fig. 15.12 Bone scan in a patient with breast cancer showing reduced tracer accumulation in the left anterior chest wall as a result of previous radiotherapy. Note that the sclerotic lesions on CT are not osteoblastic. Note also heterotopic ossification in region of right hip (arrow)

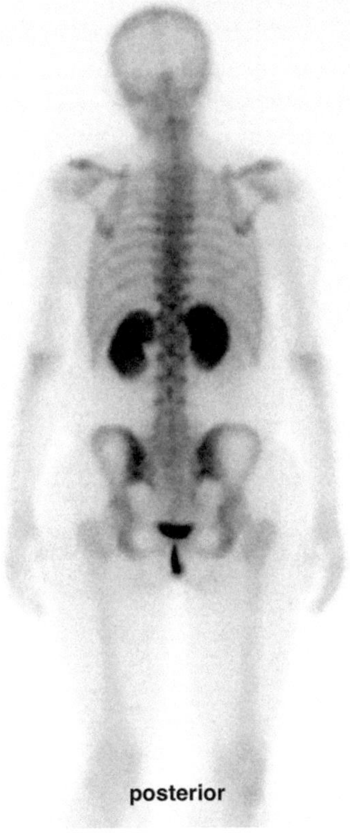

Fig. 15.13 Intense soft tissue accumulation of bone tracer in the kidneys resulting from recent chemotherapy in a woman with breast cancer. The probable mechanism is therapy-induced blockade of the MDR system of the tubular epithelium, allowing tubular reabsorption of filtered tracer

15.1.1 Bone Metastases

Metastatic bone deposits are usually sclerotic and produce an osteoblastic reaction (Fig. 15.19), or, less commonly, lytic (Fig. 15.20) or mixed sclerotic and lytic. If a deposit is included in a 3-phase bone scan, it will be seen to be hypervascular. Deposits may be solitary or involve multiple bones. The principal feature of bone metastases is their random distribution. The clue to competent reporting of a bone scan that suggests bone metastases is to think of benign conditions that may instead give the picture, such as degenerative disease, multiple fractures (Fig. 15.21), osteomalacia with pseudo-fractures, Paget's disease (Fig. 15.22), polyostotic fibrous dysplasia (Fig. 15.23) and SAPHO (Synovitis, Acne, Pustulosis, Hyperostosis, and Osteitis; Fig. 15.24). If the sternum looks odd, check for previous sternotomy, sternal fracture or direct invasion from breast cancer. A distribution of lesions that is non-random, for example several adjacent rib foci (usually fractures; Fig. 15.25) and involvement of all the elements of a single vertebra (Paget's disease; Fig. 15.26), argues against metastases. Lytic lesions may be seen on scintigraphy as photopaenic foci, although there is usually increased tracer accumulation sur-

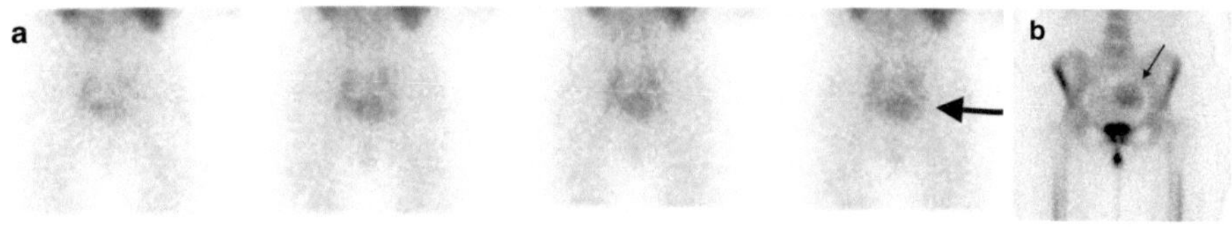

Fig. 15.14 (**a**) First few frames of phase 1 showing hypervascularity in a fibroid uterus (arrow), not to be confused with urinary activity in the bladder. Increased tracer accumulation in the uterus on delayed imaging (arrow) is shown in **b**

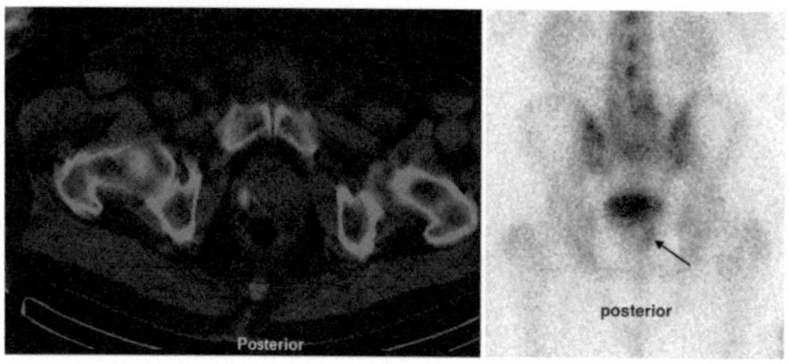

Fig. 15.15 Prostate may accumulate bone tracer, such as in this patient with prostate cancer (arrow). This may also be seen in chronic prostatic inflammation. Left panel: SPECT/CT; right panel: planar bone scan

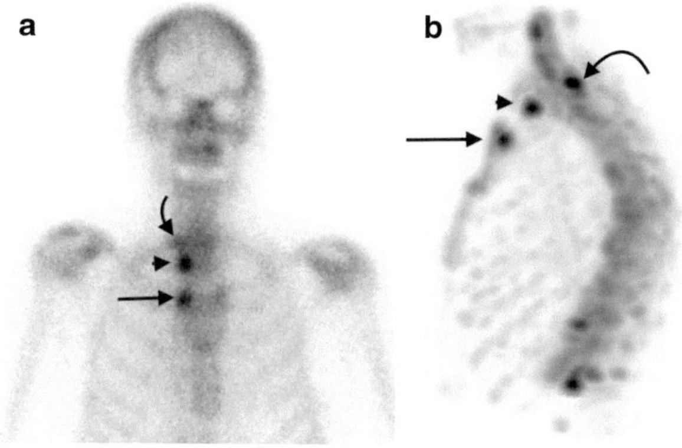

Fig. 15.16 Calcified thyroid gland (arrowhead). (**a**) Planar bone scan. (**b**) MIP from SPECT. Also shown are foci of increased uptake in right sternoclavicular joint (straight arrow) and right first costovertebral joint (curved arrow)

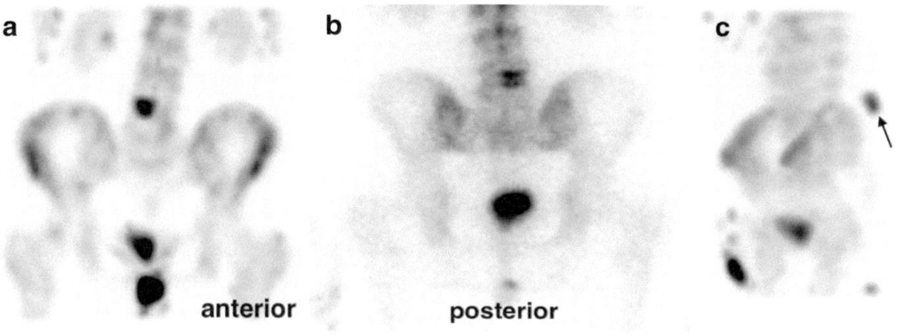

Fig. 15.17 Confusing urinary contamination. There is an apparent focus of increased tracer accumulation in the right side of vertebral body of L5 seen in anterior (**a**; MIP) and posterior (**b**; planar) views, but shown on SPECT to be contamination on the skin surface of the lumbar region (**c**; MIP). Contamination projected over the symphysis and posteroinferior to the pelvis is also clearly apparent from planar images

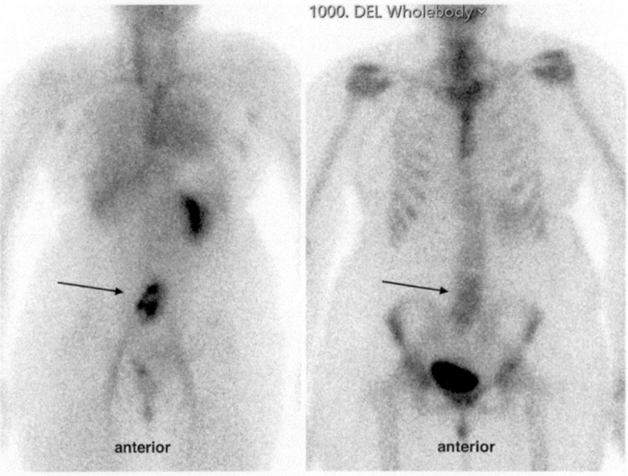

Fig. 15.18 The kidney at the pelvic brim (arrow) is clearly seen in the blood pool image (left panel) but is not clearly seen on the delayed image (right panel) because it overlaps the lower lumbar spine. Although it is projecting more counts over the lumbar spine than would usually be seen in the lumbar spine on the anterior view, one might be forgiven for reporting a non-functioning right kidney if a blood pool image was not available

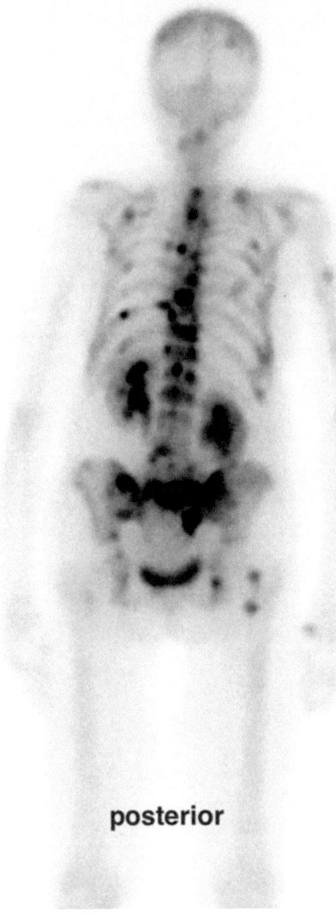

Fig. 15.19 Multiple osteoblastic bone metastases in a man with prostate cancer. Note their random distribution

rounding the 'cold' focus (Fig. 15.20). Multiple myeloma is an exception in that bone scans are mostly normal despite multiple lytic lesions. Cancers typically associated with lytic lesions are renal cell, thyroid and phaeochromocytoma. These cancers are also notable for their propensity to give long bone lesions without any in the central skeleton.

15.1.2 Orthopaedic Disease

Orthopaedic referrals usually require a 3-phase bone scan to assess bone vascularity from phases 1 and 2 (Fig. 15.2). The 3 principal causes of *discrete* prominent focal hypervascularity are avascular necrosis (Fig. 15.27), osteoid osteoma (Fig. 15.28) and recent fracture (Fig. 15.29). Bone metastases and Paget's disease also display focal increased blood flow (Fig. 15.30).

Do not use the term 'increased uptake' in phases 1 and 2 because in phase 1 the activity is in blood and in phase 2 it is in blood and the interstitial space. The whole point of phases 1 and 2 is that there is *no* bone uptake, although an abnormal focus that is very intense on delayed imaging may be visible in phase 2 simply because phase 3 accumulation has already started. For phase 3, SPECT/CT is routinely performed in

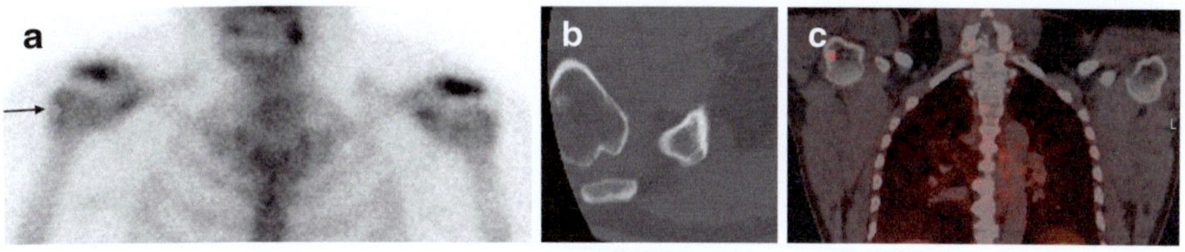

Fig. 15.20 Subtle lytic lesion in head of right humerus on planar bone scintigraphy (**a**; arrow), CT (**b**), and Ga-68-PSMA PET/CT (**c**)

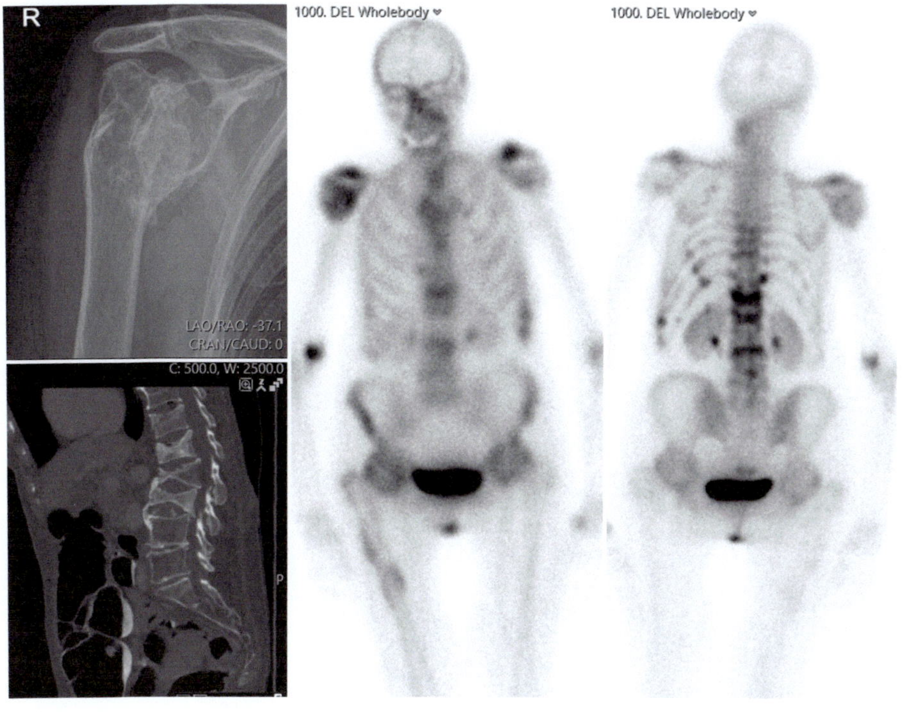

Fig. 15.21 Multiple fractures: head of right humerus, multiple ribs, and multiple compression fractures. There is synovitis in both hips and a right femoral nail. Multiple fractures can be confused with multiple bone metastases. The focus in the right elbow region is the injection site

Fig. 15.22 Paget's disease in several thoracic vertebrae. In the most inferior, uptake can be seen in the spinous process, in keeping with involvement of the entire vertebra, typical of Paget's disease

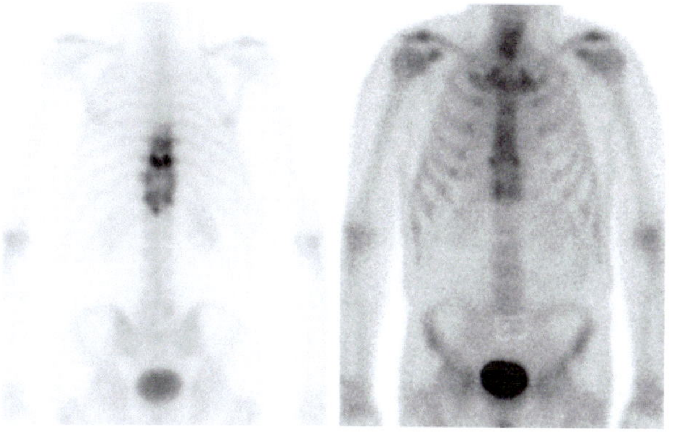

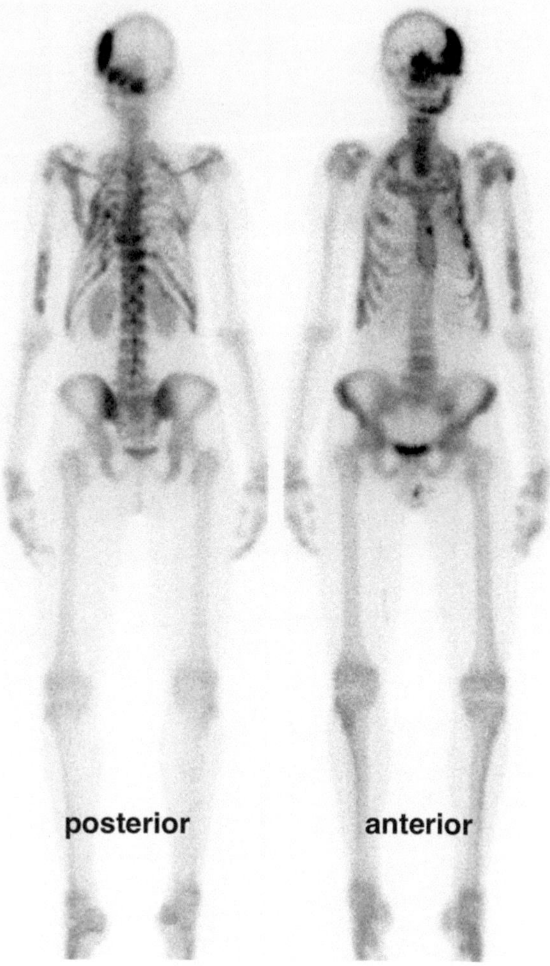

Fig. 15.23 Polyostotic fibrous dysplasia

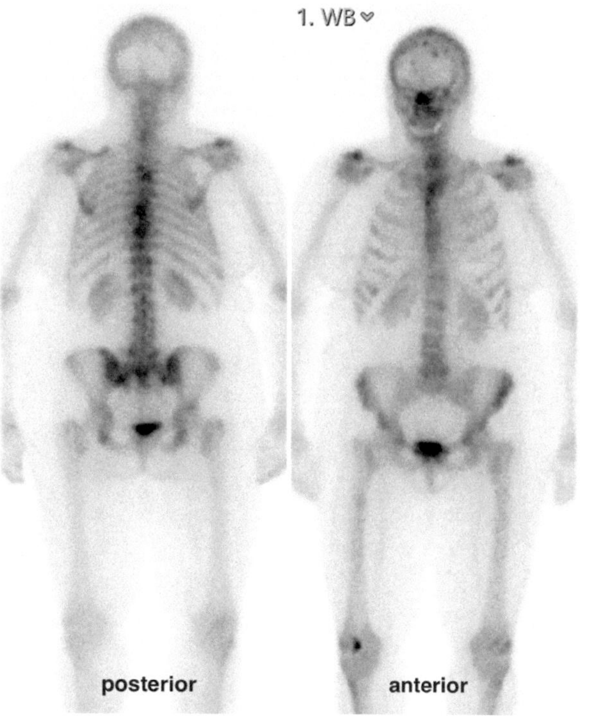

Fig. 15.24 Multiple bone lesions in SAPHO

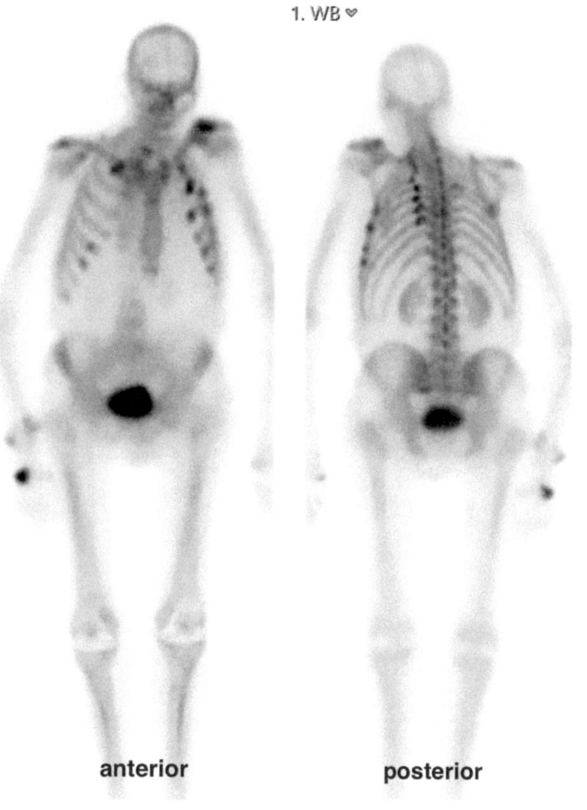

Fig. 15.25 Multiple bilateral rib fractures. Anterior end of right first rib is more likely from enthesopathy, a common site for it. Note unremarkable bilateral total knee replacements

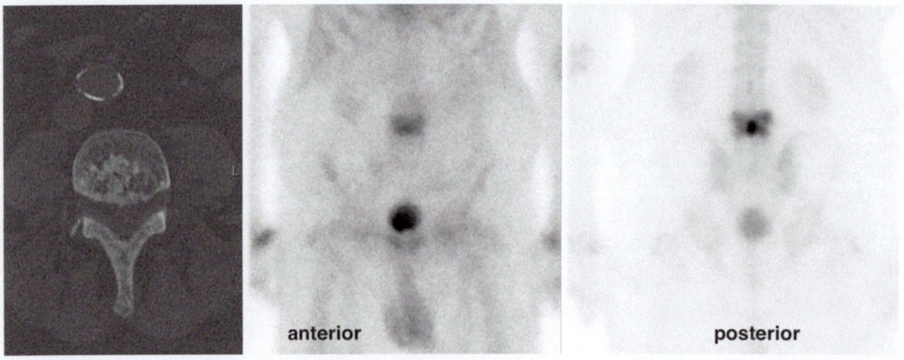

Fig. 15.26 Paget's disease throughout L4 vertebra. Note, for instance, prominent tracer accumulation in spinous process

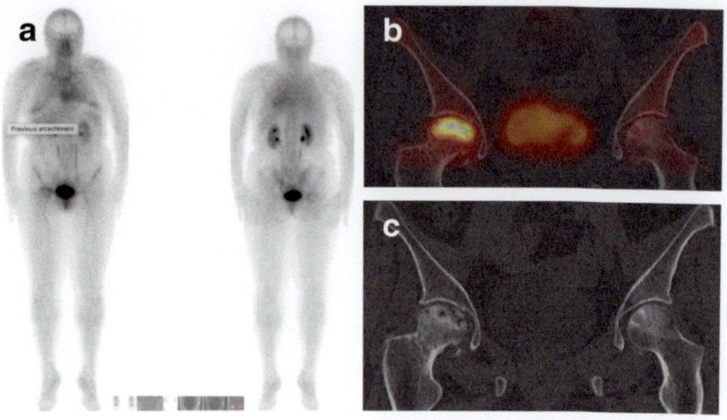

Fig. 15.27 Avascular necrosis of right femoral head seen to be hypervascular on the whole body blood pool image (**a**). SPECT/CT (**b**) and diagnostic CT (**c**) are also shown

Fig. 15.28 Osteoid osteoma in medial condyle of right tibia. (**a**) CT. (**b**) Focal discrete hypervascularity in the blood pool image (left panels) and increased uptake on delayed image

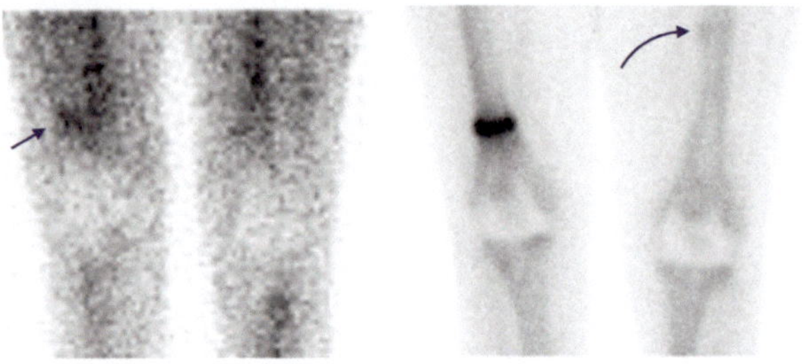

Fig. 15.29 Recent fracture of distal shaft of right femur. Frame from phase 1 shows focal hypervascularity at the fracture site (straight arrow; left panel). Image from phase 3 shows linear increased tracer accumulation typical of fracture (right panel). Note the healed fracture in midshaft of left femur (curved arrow)

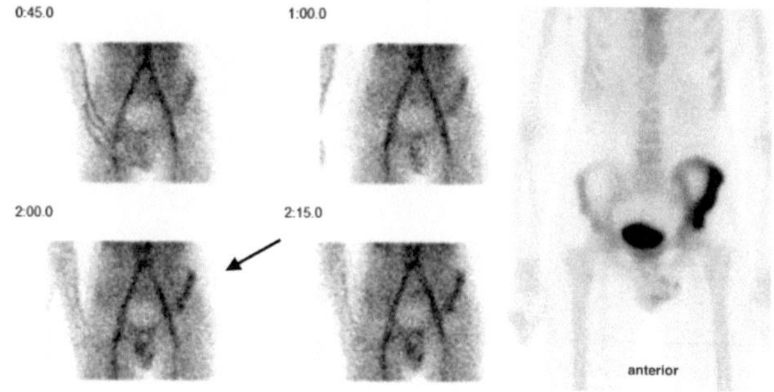

Fig. 15.30 Paget's disease is a metabolic abnormality, hence the hypervascularity in the left ilium on phase 1 imaging (left panel; arrow). Phase 3 image shows intense increased uptake in left ilium (right panel)

orthopaedic disorders to anatomically localise areas of abnormal tracer accumulation. Although the CT is low dose, it can be correlated with the bone scan findings.

Bone scans for bone infection, usually in relation to metalwork, are frequently requested but non-specific. Infected bone displays hypervascularity—usually diffuse rather than discrete—but it does not confirm infection. In suspected bone infection, therefore, the helpful outcome in phases 1 and 2 is no hypervascularity, which argues against infection. The best test for orthopaedic infection is In-111-leucocyte scintigraphy (Chap. 26), but unfortunately few centres nowadays offer cell-labelling services. Instead, patients are referred for FDG PET/CT, but this is also non-specific and cannot readily distinguish between infective and non-infective inflammation.

In knee replacements, synovitis is common and gives a typical triangular distribution of hypervascularity followed by generalised increased uptake on delayed imaging (Fig. 15.5). Loosening of joint replacements typically gives increased periprosthetic uptake. Association with increased vascularity suggests septic loosening (Figs. 15.31 and 15.32).

Orthopaedic surgeons often request bone scans to identify the pain generator in a painful spine. A focus of increased turnover is assumed to indicate a source of pain. Common examples include disc disease, pars defects and facet joint arthritis (Fig. 15.33).

15.1.3 Arthritis

The confirmation of inflammatory arthritis in patients with suggestive clinical features is a common indication for a bone scan. There is increased uptake on both sides of an inflamed joint because of increased blood flow, which delivers more tracer to the joint, thereby increasing tracer clearance into the bone (Fig. 15.6). Osteoarthritis is also inflammatory but can be distinguished from synovitis in joints that have characteristic synovial reflections on bone, such as the knee and hip. The synovium in the knee extends anterosuperiorly above the joint and gives the typical picture of a hot triangle in the blood flow phases of a bone scan (Fig. 15.6). Because it is in soft tissue, this triangle of activity is not seen in the delayed image which instead shows diffusely increased uptake throughout the

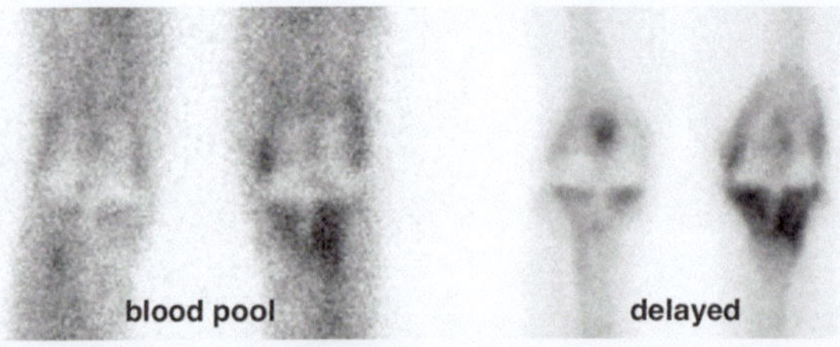

Fig. 15.31 There is increased periprosthetic tracer accumulation around the tibia in the delayed image of this left knee replacement (right panel) and markedly increased vascularity in the blood pool image (left panel), in keeping with septic loosening. Note synovial hypervascularity in both knees in keeping with bilateral synovitis

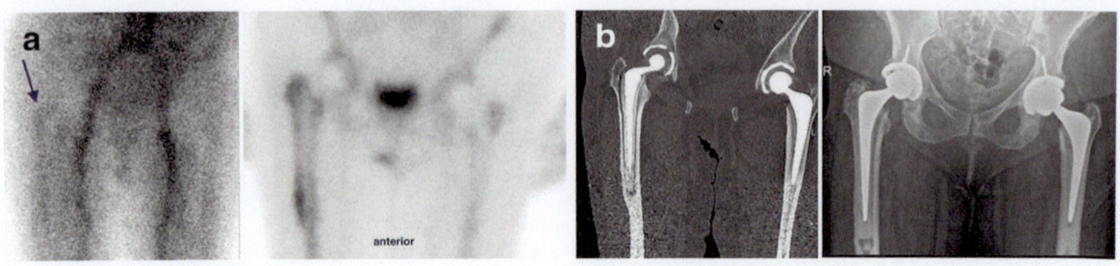

Fig. 15.32 Septic loosening of femoral component of right total hip replacement. Delayed planar image shows increased periprosthetic tracer accumulation (**a**; right panel) associated with hypervascularity on blood pool image (**a**; left panel; arrow) in keeping with infection. CT and plain X-ray show increased periprosthetic lucency (**b**)

Fig. 15.33 Bilateral L4/5 facet joint arthropathy (arrow)

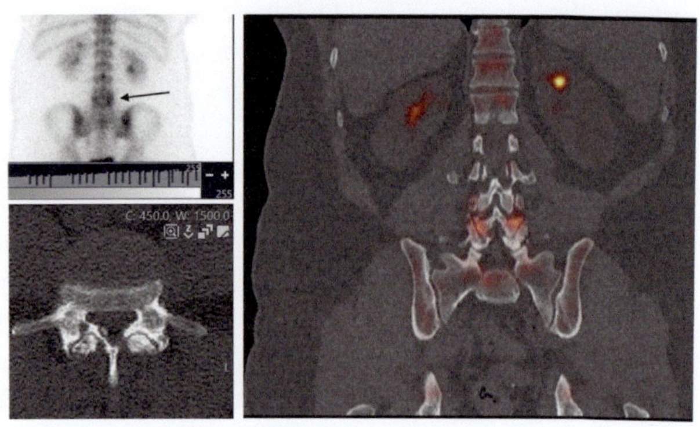

knee. On delayed imaging, because of the anatomy of the synovial attachment to bone, synovitis in the hip gives increased uptake encircling the femoral neck (Fig. 15.34). Increased uptake in osteoarthritis arises from bone disease rather than soft tissue inflammation, so hypervascularity and increased uptake at 3 h is confined to the articular surfaces. Distinguishing inflammatory from degenerative arthritis is more difficult in small joints, because increased blood flow may arise from either osteoarthritis or synovitis. On delayed imaging, however, osteoarthritis is more focal while synovitis is more diffuse.

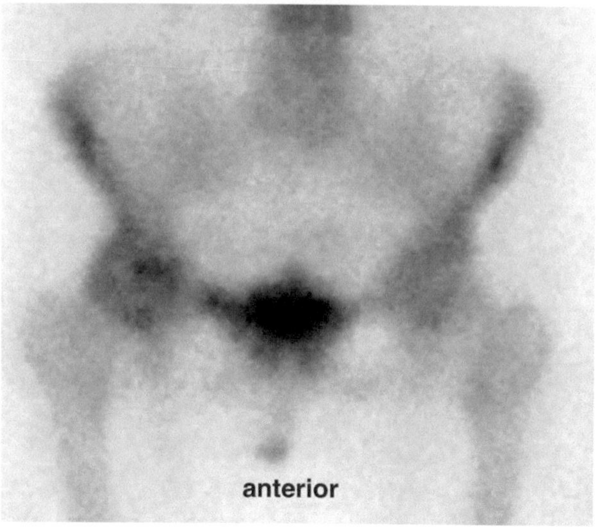

Fig. 15.34 Synovitis of the right hip. Note how the increased tracer accumulation on delayed imaging follows the synovial insertion rather than the articular surface, as in osteoarthritis. There is nevertheless also osteoarthritis in the hip

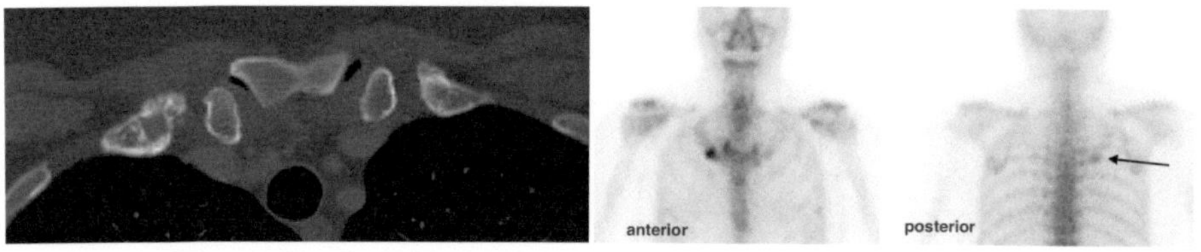

Fig. 15.35 Enthesopathy in the anterior end of the right first rib. Note 'shine-through' from the focus in the posterior projection (arrow)

Osteoblastic activity and tracer uptake are stimulated by muscular traction on bones, which is why the anterior ends of the first ribs (Fig. 15.35) and tuberosities of the humeral heads are often prominent. Such traction may be pathological, giving symptomatic enthesopathy. Calcaneal enthesopathy from plantar fasciitis or Achilles tendonitis is a common incidental finding in bone scans (Fig. 15.36).

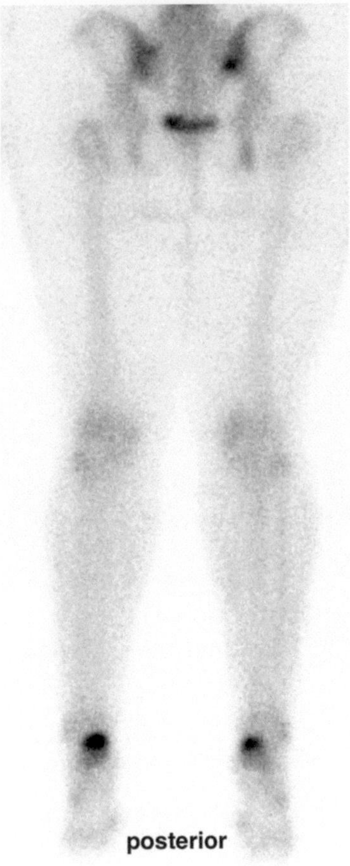

Fig. 15.36 Planar bone scan from the posterior projection showing bilateral Achilles tendonitis, right sacroiliitis and right ischial enthesopathy

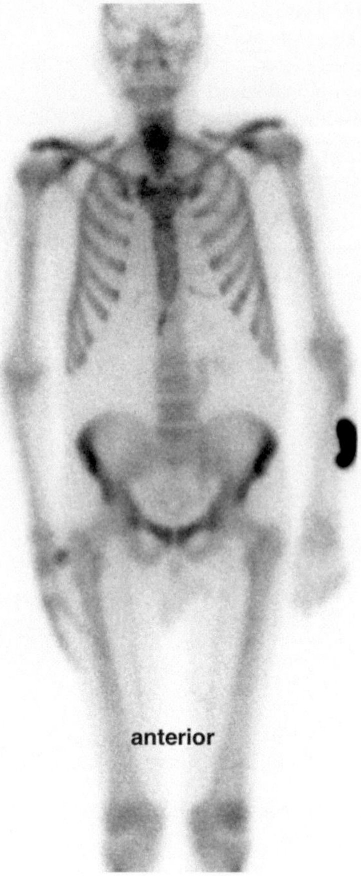

Fig. 15.37 Renal osteodystrophy. This man with prostate cancer shows minimal renal function yet target-to-soft tissue count density ratio is elevated, suggesting renal osteodystrophy. No bone metastases are demonstrated

15.1.4 Metabolic Bone Disease

Bone tracer accumulation is generally increased in metabolic bone disease, including osteomalacia (which may give multiple pseudofractures, mimicking disseminated metastases), renal osteodystrophy (Fig. 15.37), and hyperparathyroidism. Renal osteodystrophy can be suspected in a patient with renal impairment and a bone scan that does not display the expected poor bone definition that is characteristic of renal failure.

Paget's disease (Figs. 15.38, 15.39, and 15.40) and fibrous dysplasia (Figs. 15.23 and15.41) are regional forms of metabolic bone disease. In long bones, Paget's disease always extends from one end of the bone (Fig. 15.40), and in the spine, typically, but not always, involves the entire vertebra (Fig. 15.26). Hyperparathyroidism gives the 'tie' sternum and hot skull. All these are distinguishable from the so-called superscan of malignancy which typically shows heterogenous tracer uptake and relative sparing of skull and long bones (Fig. 15.42).

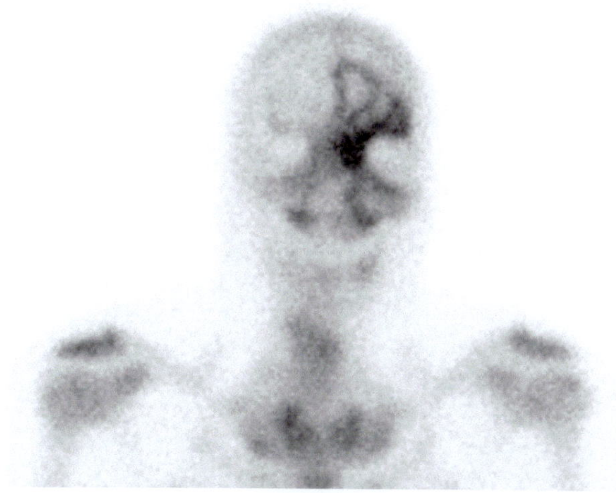

Fig. 15.38 Paget's disease in left frontal bone displaying the features of osteoporosis circumscripta

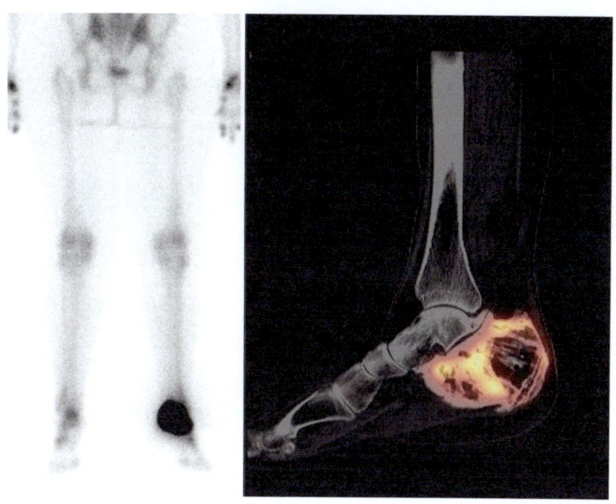

Fig. 15.39 Paget's disease involving the calcaneus. Left panel: planar bone scan; right panel: SPECT/CT. Note the involvement of the entire bone. Note also bilateral hip replacements

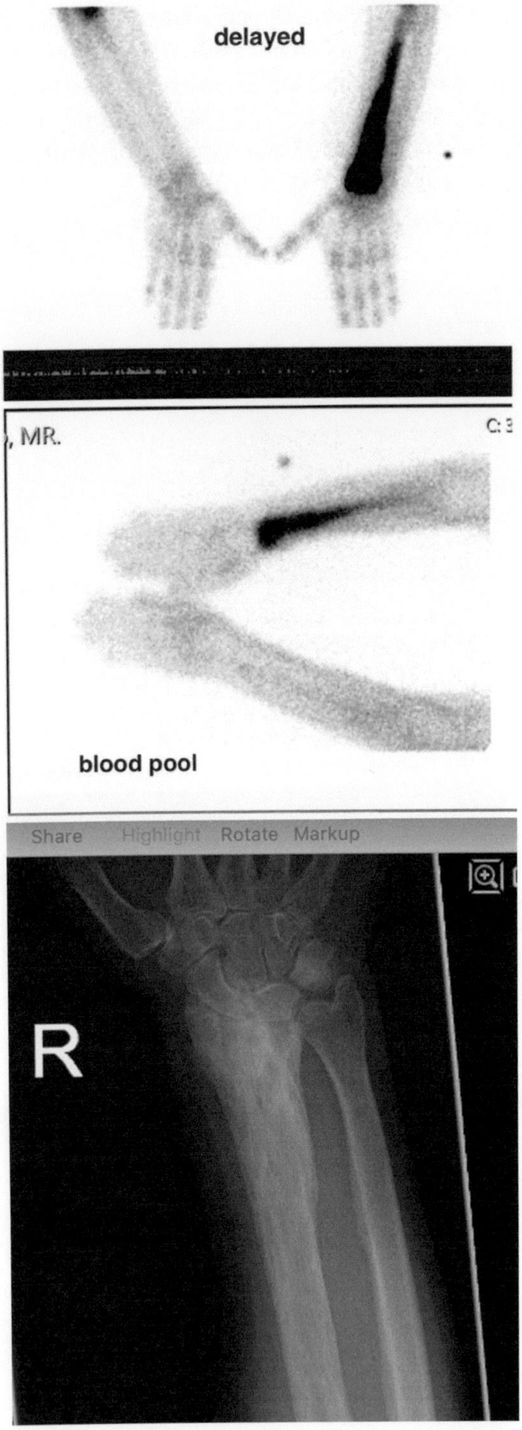

Fig. 15.40 Paget's disease is a metabolic abnormality, hence the hypervascularity on early blood pool image (middle panel). Paget's disease in long bones always extends to at least one end of the bone (upper panel)

Osteoporosis is diagnosed from DEXA scanning. It is not visible in bone scans but can be suspected when there are multiple fractures. Transient osteoporosis is a separate condition that typically involves the hip. It is distinguishable from hip joint disease because the increased uptake extends to involve the femoral head, femoral neck, and intertrochanteric region (Fig. 15.43). Osteoarthritis and synovitis do not extend to the intertrochanteric region. An obscure bone disease with a metabolic basis is hypertrophic pulmonary osteoarthropathy (Fig. 15.44), which affects the long bones of patients with intrathoracic disease, especially lung cancer.

15.1.5 Fractures

Recent fractures display prominent focal hypervascularity (Figs. 15.29, 15.45, and 15.46). On delayed imaging, they typically show increased uptake in a linear configuration. Long bone fractures may remain osteoblastic for many years because of ongoing remodelling, in contrast to rib fractures and spinal endplate fractures which resolve more rapidly. There may be multiple fractures which may be confused with disseminated metastases. Some fractures have characteristic features, such as fractures in the hemipelvis, of which there are almost always at least two (typically in inferior and superior pubic rami; Fig. 15.46), occasionally with increased uptake in the sacroiliac joints (sacroiliac diastasis). Honda (the vehicle logo) fractures comprise a horizontal linear sacral fracture along with bilateral vertical sacral ala fractures. Rib fractures occur in adjacent ribs, often several. If multiple rib fractures are randomly distributed but not accompanied by suspicious focal uptake elsewhere, suspect cough fractures (Fig. 15.47). Osteoporotic vertebral fractures are linear. Stress fractures give focal increased uptake associated

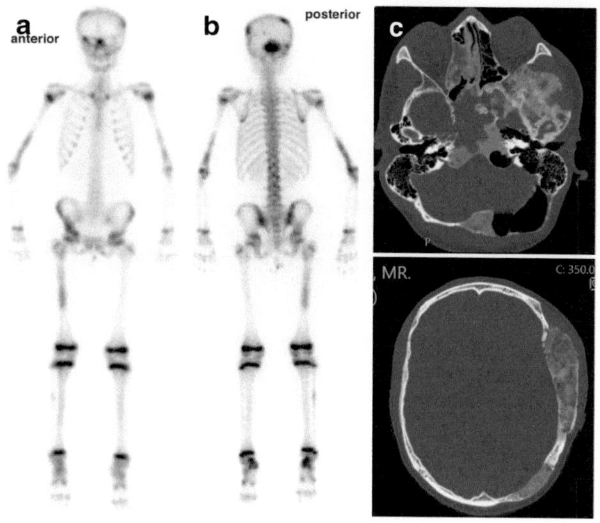

Fig. 15.41 Polyostotic fibrous dysplasia in a child. Note normal prominent uptake in growth plates

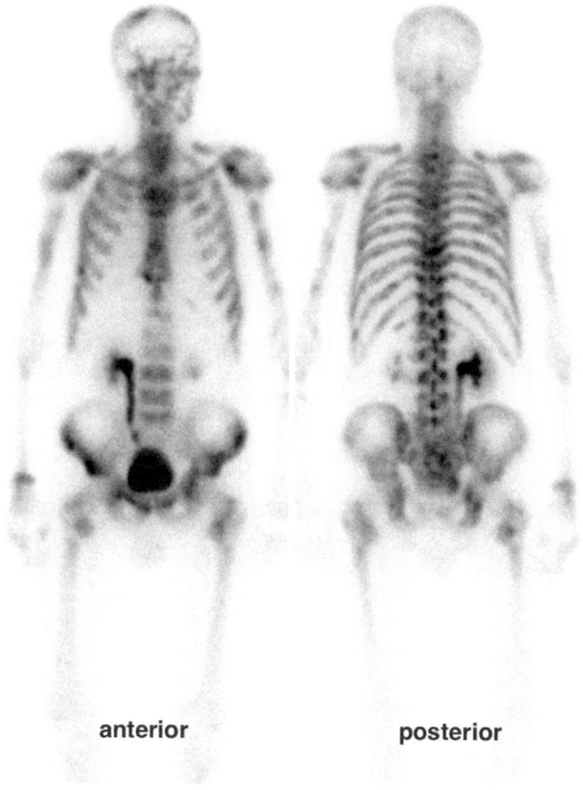

Fig. 15.42 Disseminated bone metastases. Note heterogeneity of tracer accumulation in the skeleton and relative sparing of long bones. The right renal tract is obstructed. There is a fracture in the right distal radius

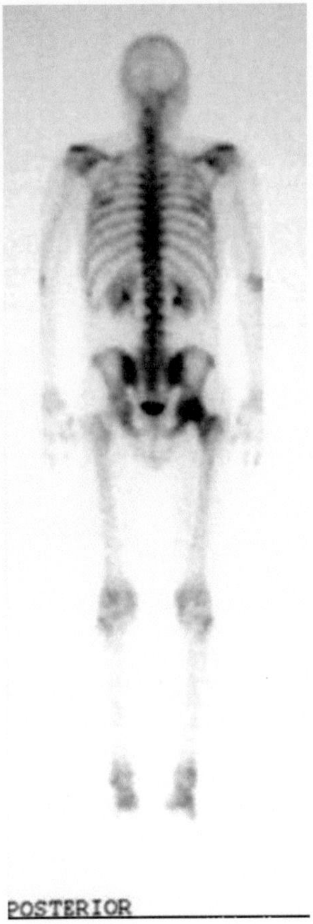

Fig. 15.43 Transient osteoporosis generally affects the hips of middle-aged men. The diagnostic clue, shown here, is involvement of the femoral head and neck, extending to the inter-trochanteric region. Regional osteoporosis gives a similar picture in the hip but is a separate condition

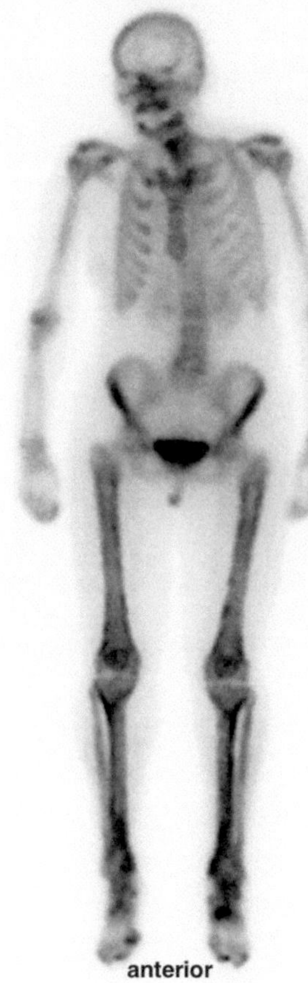

Fig. 15.44 Hypertrophic pulmonary osteoarthropathy. Note increased periosteal tracer accumulation in the long bones of the lower limbs. The condition is associated with lung disease, especially lung cancer

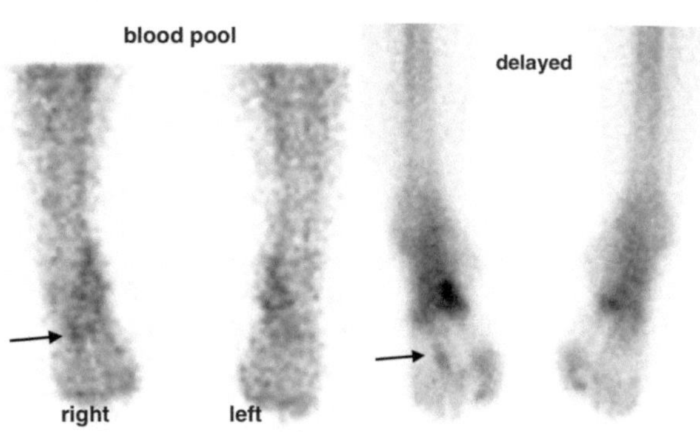

Fig. 15.45 Fracture of right 3rd metatarsal (right panel) associated with subtle focal hypervascularity in blood pool image (left panel). There is arthropathy in both tarsal regions, especially the right

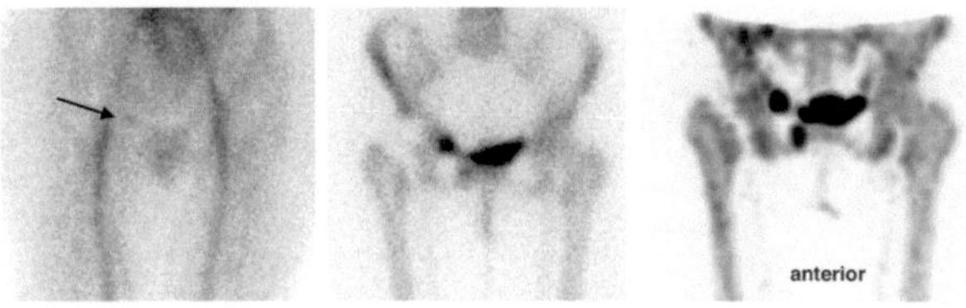

Fig. 15.46 Fractured pelvis showing focal increased tracer accumulation in right superior and inferior pubic rami in delayed planar image (**b**) and SPECT (**c**). Blood pool image (**a**) shows focal hypervascularity in the superior fracture (arrow)

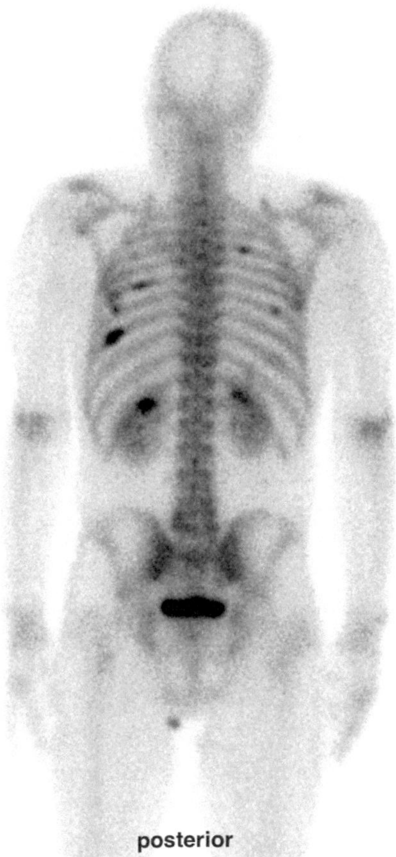

Fig. 15.47 Multiple foci of increased tracer accumulation in the ribs with no significant abnormal findings elsewhere suggest rib fractures resulting from a chronic cough. Focal activity projected over both 11th ribs is calyceal urinary activity. There is urinary contamination over upper left thigh

with focal hypervascularity on blood pool imaging (Fig. 15.48). Long bone stress fractures (focal) need to be distinguished from shin splints (linear). A rare fracture in the foot is a fracture of the Stieda bone (Fig. 15.49).

A common indication for a bone scan is a fracture following minimal trauma (often neck of femur). The referrer is not looking for confirmation of a fracture but instead abnormal uptake elsewhere for evidence that the fracture is pathological.

15.1.6 Avascular Necrosis (AVN)

AVN, paradoxically, is typically associated with prominent discrete increased blood flow that is the result of attempted bone healing. A common site is the femoral head (Fig. 15.27), especially in patients receiving steroids. Bleeding under the periosteum, as in sickle cell disease, is a strong osteoblastic stimulus that gives intense linear subperiosteal activity from blood tracking under the periosteum. Sickle cell disease is also associated with bone infarcts.

15.1.7 Benign Bone Tumours

The primary non-malignant bone tumour of most importance in nuclear medicine is osteoid osteoma, which is highly vascular and shows

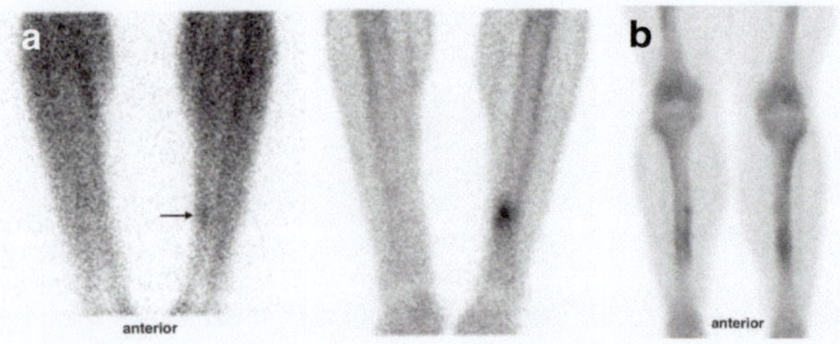

Fig. 15.48 Stress-related tibial injuries. (**a**) Planar delayed bone scan showing a stress fracture in left tibia (right panel) associated with focal hypervascularity in blood pool image (left panel; arrow). (**b**) Stress-related cortical injury with low-grade stress fracture in right tibia in a different patient with suspicion also of low-grade stress fracture in distal left tibia

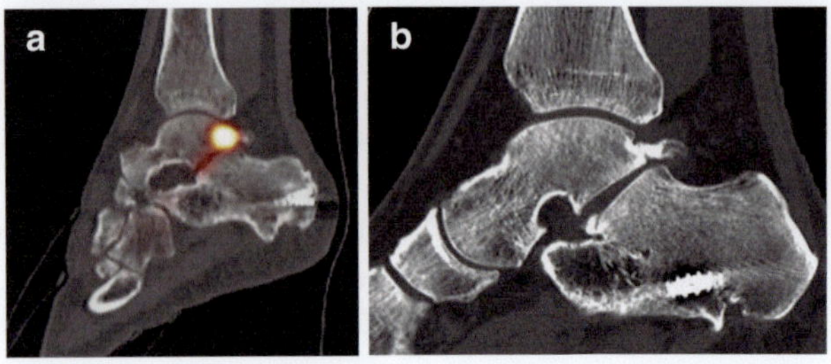

Fig. 15.49 SPECT/CT (**a**) and CT (**b**) showing fracture of a Stieda process. This process arises from the posterior aspect of the talus and is a normal variant. Note that the screw in the calcaneus is not associated with any increased osteoblastic activity

increased uptake on delayed imaging (Fig. 15.28). Otherwise, nuclear medicine has almost no role in the diagnosis of benign bone tumours, most of which show minimal increased uptake. Nevertheless, a working knowledge of primary bone tumours is helpful because one may appear serendipitously in a bone scan.

15.1.8 Paediatric Bone Scintigraphy

In contrast to adults, almost all of whom on bone scanning have some abnormal uptake—usually from degenerative disease—the normal bone scan in children should be pristine. Any abnormal uptake must be treated with suspicion. The normal paediatric bone scan is dominated by intense uptake in the growth plates throughout the skeleton (Fig. 15.8), each one of which shows declining uptake around the age at which the plates fuse. Childhood diseases commonly referred for bone scintigraphy include malignancies (osteosarcoma, Ewing's sarcoma, neuroblastoma), osteoid osteoma, osteomyelitis, avascular necrosis (especially Perthes' disease), slipped femoral epiphyses, fibrous dysplasia, juvenile rheumatoid arthritis, chronic recurrent non-bacterial osteomyelitis (Fig. 15.50), and, not to be forgotten, suspected fractures in non-accidental injury. Bone scans to image and quantify condylar hyperplasia are undertaken in adolescents with facial asymmetry (Fig. 15.51).

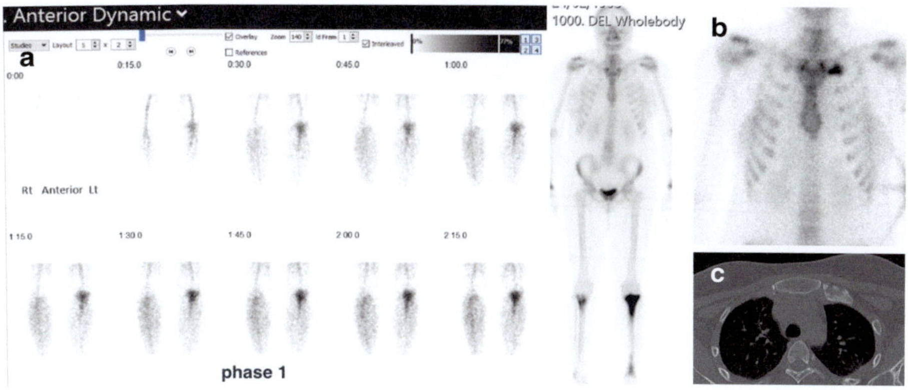

Fig. 15.50 (**a**) Chronic recurrent multifocal osteomyelitis involving both proximal tibias and distal left tibia in a young adult. Blood flow series (left panel) shows marked hypervascularity of the proximal left lesion. (**b** and **c**) Involvement of left first rib in another patient

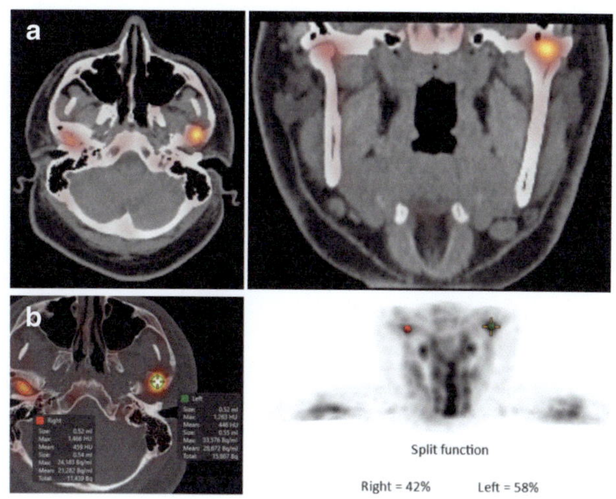

Fig. 15.51 (**a**) SPECT/CT in a young adult with condylar hyperplasia showing increased tracer accumulation in the left mandibular condyle compared with the right. (**b**) Differential uptake in the condyles

Further Reading

1. Buch K, Thuesen ACB, Brons C, Schwarz P. Chronic non-bacterial osteomyelitis: a review. Calcif Tissue Int. 2018;104:544–53.
2. Fogelman I. Skeletal uptake of diphosphonate: a review. Eur J Nucl Med. 1980;5:473–6.
3. Fogelman I, Pearson DW, Bessent RG, Tofe AJ, Francis MD. A comparison of skeletal uptakes of three diphosphonates by whole-body retention: concise communication. J Nucl Med. 1981;22:880–3.

16 Tc-99m-Sestamibi (MW 778 Da) and Tc-99m-Tetrafosmin (MW 895 Da)

These two agents are lipophilic, bind to plasma proteins and are taken up to a variable extent by all tissues because they target mitochondria in which glucose is used to synthesise ATP. They can be thought of as the single-photon equivalents of FDG and, not surprisingly therefore, have a range of indications broadly similar to FDG, namely imaging tumours and myocardium, but not the brain, as explained below. Although they have similar pharmacokinetics, Tc-99m-sestamibi is generally favoured for tumour imaging, while Tc-99m-tetrafosmin is favoured for myocardial imaging. Plasma clearances are rapid, with disappearance half-times from plasma of only a few minutes.

Both agents are recognised as xenobiotics by the multidrug resistance (MDR) system. This system is of physiological importance because its family members (also known as ABC transporters) function to prevent the entry of, or to eliminate, a wide range of environmental foreign substances called xenobiotics, examples of which include the constituents of air pollution and cigarette smoke. MDR proteins, which are widely distributed in nature and expressed in bacteria and neoplasms, comprise P-glycoprotein, multidrug resistance protein-1 (MRP-1), MRP-2, breast cancer-related protein and others. MDR expressed in tumours and bacteria confers resistance to chemotherapeutic agents (from where the family acquired its name). The transporters are prominently expressed in tissues that interface with the external environment, namely the bronchopulmonary epithelium, gastrointestinal tract, hepatocytes, and renal tubular epithelium, and are therefore expressed on the apical surfaces of cells facing the exterior (airways, gastrointestinal lumen, bile canaliculi and renal tubular lumen). MDR is also strongly expressed in the blood-brain barrier, preventing xenobiotics from entering the CSF and explaining why Tc-99m-sestamibi does not enter the brain. It does, however, accumulate in the choroid plexus and pituitary (Fig. 16.1).

The whole-body distribution of Tc-99m-sestamibi reflects firstly its relationship to glucose accumulation and secondly its affinity to the MDR system. In addition to pituitary and choroid plexus, it is conspicuous in salivary glands, thyroid, myocardium, liver, stomach and kidneys (Fig. 16.2). Like FDG, it accumulates in brown fat (Fig. 16.3). Because of MDR expression, it ‘washes out’ from stomach, liver and to a lesser extent the kidney. Although thyroid does not interface with the external environment, it nevertheless contains P-glycoprotein and eliminates Tc-99m-sestamibi. Salivary glands in contrast retain the tracer.

Tumours that have been imaged with Tc-99m-sestamibi include parathyroid adenoma (Fig. 16.4), breast cancer (Fig. 16.5), myeloma and renal oncocytoma. Tc-99m-sestamibi has also been used to image muscle ischaemia for the diagnosis of compartment syndrome. Be careful

A. M. Peters, M. Vadrucci, *Introduction to Nuclear Medicine for Trainees in Imaging and Imaging Sciences*, https://doi.org/10.1007/978-3-032-18364-4_16

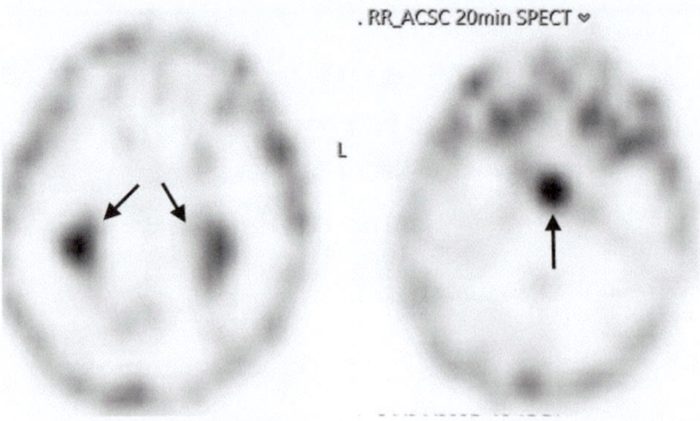

Fig. 16.1 The pituitary is outside the blood-brain barrier, so it accumulates Tc-99m-sestamibi (vertical arrow). The tracer also enters the ependymal cells that line the ventricles of the brain—the lateral ventricles in this example (diagonal arrows). Both tissues retain the tracer on delayed imaging, confirming the absence of MDR proteins in both the endothelia and ependymal cells. Lacrimal glands are also visible

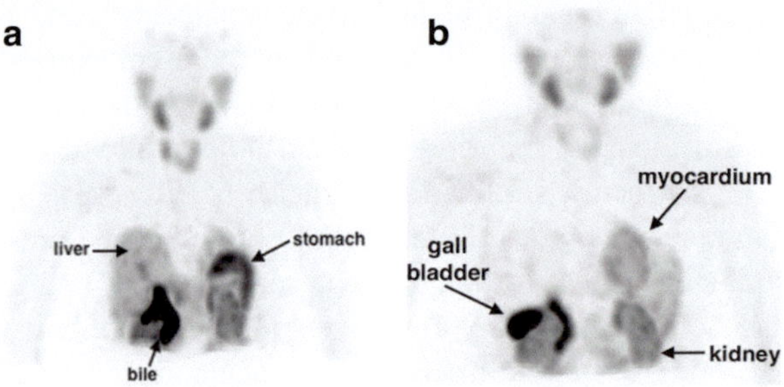

Fig. 16.2 Normal distribution of Tc-99m-sestamibi. (**a**) 20 min post-injection shows salivary glands, thyroid, myocardium, liver and kidneys. The activity partly obscuring the myocardium is likely stomach rather than biliary-secreted jejunal activity, which would not be expected to be seen as early as 20 min. (**b**) 90 min post-injection shows activity has left thyroid, stomach, liver and lesser extent kidneys, mediated by MDR proteins, but remains largely unchanged in salivary glands and myocardium. (Courtesy Alexander Gordon, King's College Hospital, London)

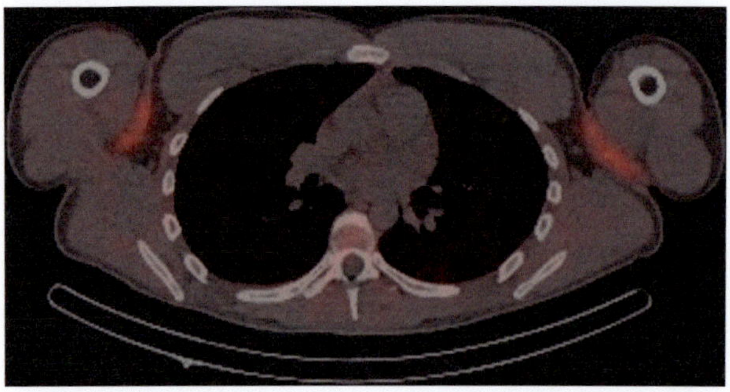

Fig. 16.3 As with F-18-FDG, Tc-99m-sestamibi may accumulate in brown fat, shown here in both axillae. Since they target intracellular metabolic machinery, these two tracers show similar whole-body distributions with the notable exception of the brain which does not accumulate Tc-99m-sestamibi because of the presence of MDR proteins in the blood-brain barrier

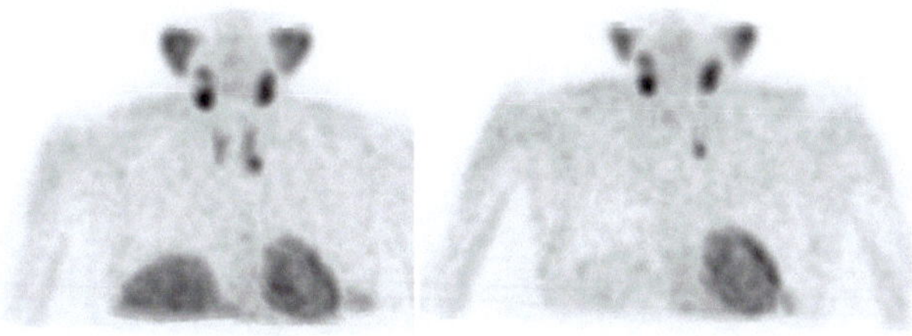

Fig. 16.4 Typical appearance of a parathyroid adenoma in the left lower position in a Tc-99m-sestamibi scan. Thyroid partially or completely eliminates activity between 20 min and 90 min post-tracer injection because it contains P-glycoprotein. At least 90% of parathyroid adenomas do not contain P-glycoprotein and lose only minimal activity between 20 and 90 min. An adenoma that contains P-glycoprotein risks a false negative outcome. Note the disappearance of hepatic activity between 20 and 90 min

Fig. 16.5 Tc-99m-sestamibi accumulation in breasts of a woman of reproductive age without breast cancer. The tracer has been used to image breast cancer but as shown here is non-specific

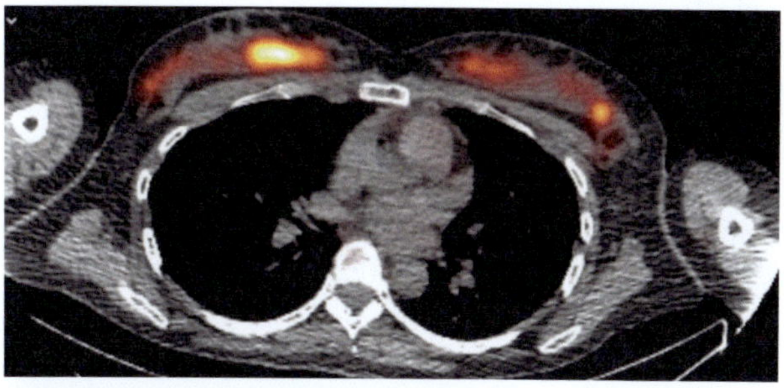

Fig. 16.6 Accumulation of Tc-99-sestamibi in an axillary lymph node (arrow) as a result of a 'tissued' injection. SPECT/CT (left panel); MIP (right panel)

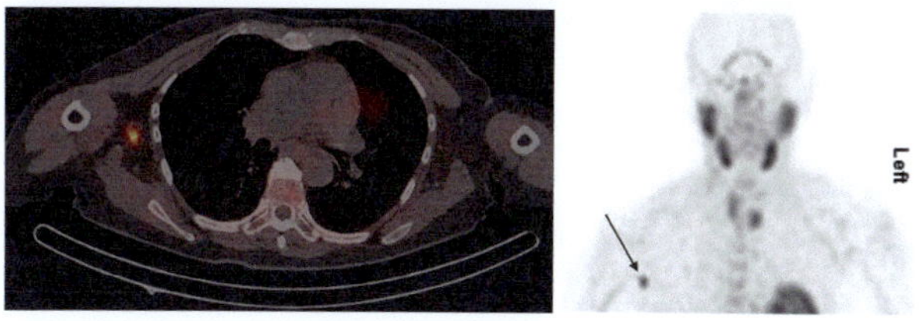

not to misinterpret lymph node activity in the axilla as tumour if the tracer, when injected, has been 'tissued' (Fig. 16.6). As well as Tc-99m-sestamibi, several radiopharmaceuticals, mostly PET-labelled, have been developed to image MDR expression in cancers and predict their response to therapy.

16.1 Locating a Parathyroid Adenoma

Tc-99m-sestamibi scintigraphy is not used to diagnose hyperparathyroidism but instead to identify a parathyroid gland harbouring an adenoma. Imaging is performed at 20 min and

90 min post-injection. The thyroid accumulates Tc-99m-sestamibi on early imaging but eliminates it by the time of delayed imaging (Fig. 16.4). Most parathyroid adenomas in contrast do not express MDR and therefore remain visible on delayed imaging. About 10% of parathyroid adenomas, however, express P-glycoprotein and, like the thyroid, may disappear on delayed imaging, giving rise to a potential false negative.

A thyroid adenoma may resemble a parathyroid adenoma and be indistinguishable from it. SPECT/CT is therefore important because parathyroid adenomas are usually posterior to the pole of a thyroid lobe. Intrathyroidal parathyroid adenoma is also a potential problem in this scenario, although very rarely. Ultrasonography is helpful and should be recommended. Thyroid Tc-99mO_4 imaging may help make a distinction between thyroid and parathyroid adenoma (Figs. 16.7 and 16.8).

Ectopic parathyroid adenoma, usually mediastinal, should be excluded in an otherwise negative scan for parathyroid adenoma in the neck (Fig. 16.9). Ectopic adenoma may rarely be in the upper neck and confused with normal Tc-99m-sestamibi accumulation in a submandibular gland. The salivary glands should therefore also be inspected. Parathyroids may be implanted in soft tissue and later harbour an adenoma (Fig. 16.10).

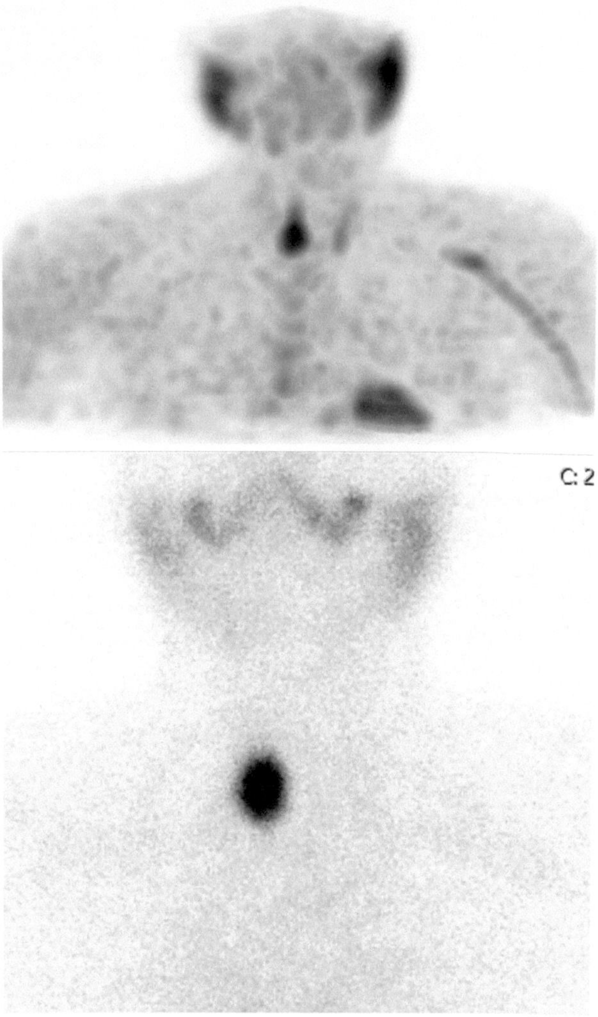

Fig. 16.7 Thyroid adenoma masquerading as a parathyroid adenoma. Upper panel: Tc-99m-sestamibi scan; lower panel: Tc-99mO_4 scan showing autonomous hot nodule with suppression of tracer accumulation in left lobe and upper pole of right lobe. Note partially tissued injection on the left, with axillary lymph node uptake in the Tc-99m-sestamibi scan

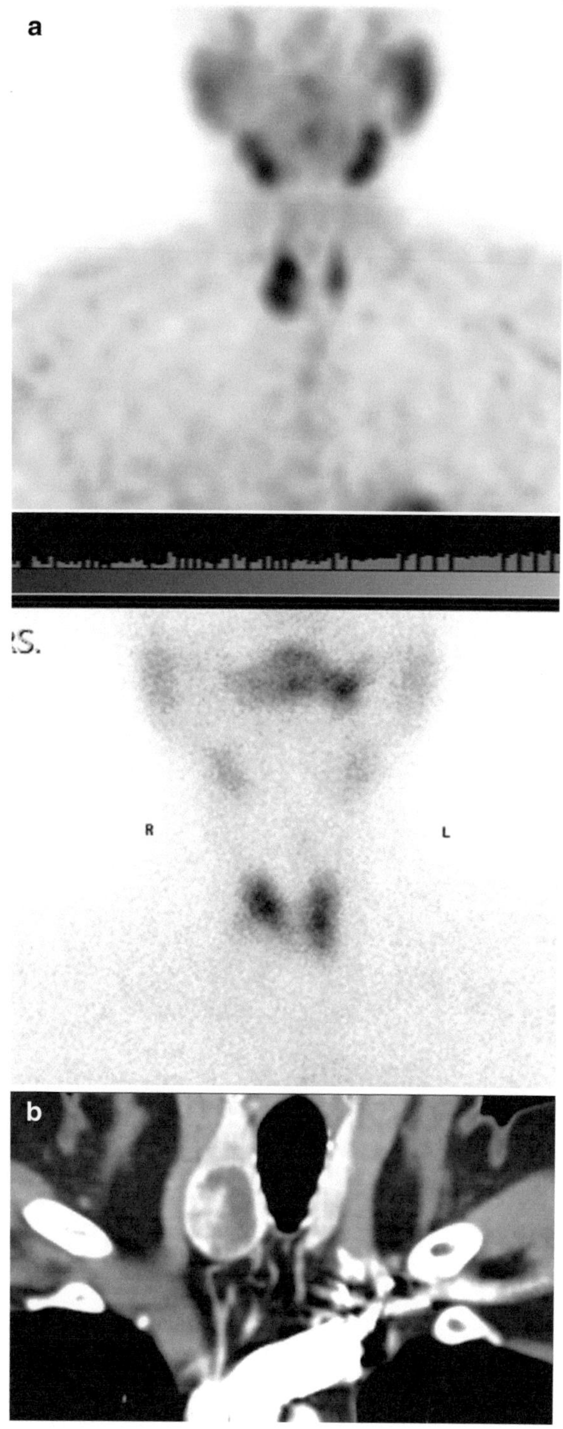

Fig. 16.8 Tc-99m-sestamibi scan (**a**, upper panel) raises strong suspicion of parathyroid adenoma in right lower position. Tc-99mO_4 scan (**a**, lower panel) shows absent tracer accumulation in lower pole of right lobe of thyroid raising suspicion of thyroid nodule instead. Latter is confirmed with CT (**b**) which shows a cystic thyroid nodule

Fig. 16.9 Ectopic parathyroid adenoma (**a**) immediately posterior to the sternomanubrial junction on SPECT/CT (**b**)

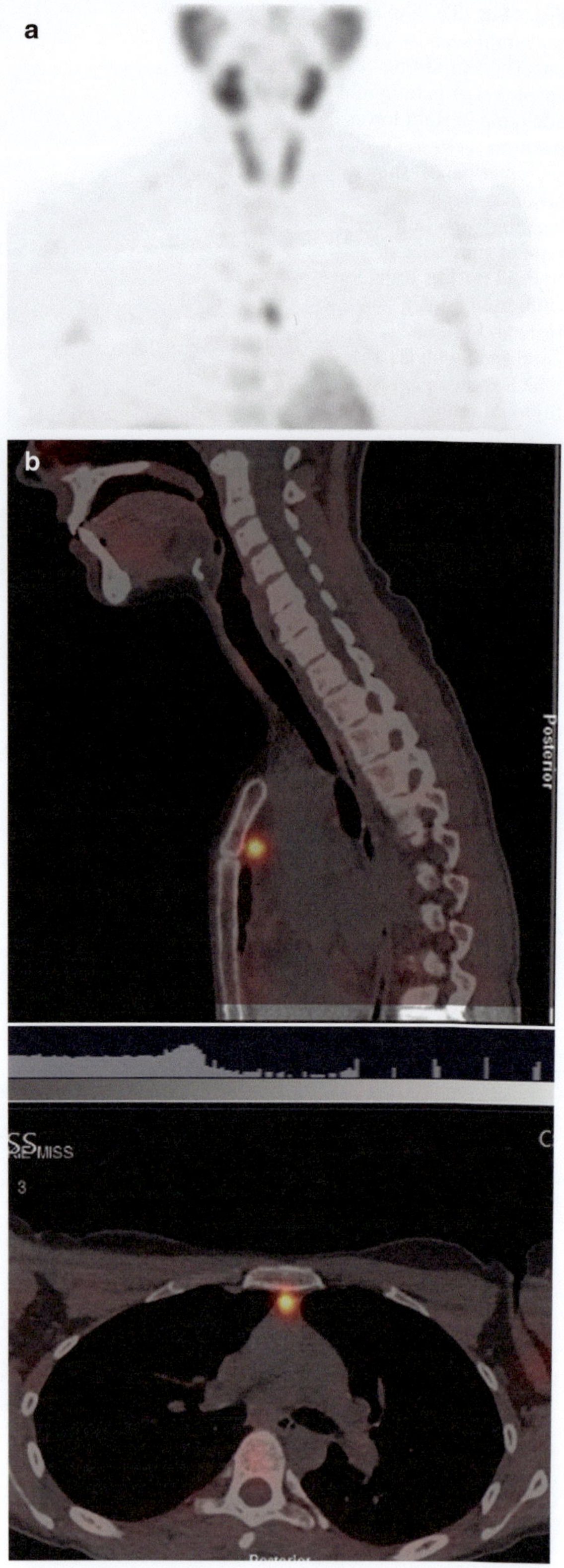

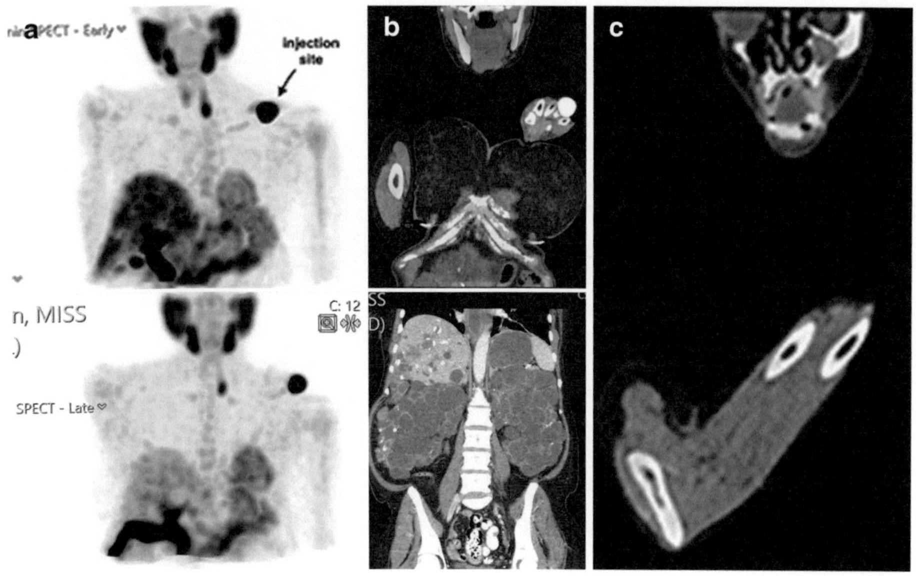

Fig. 16.10 Tc-99m-sestamibi scan showing parathyroid adenoma in left lower position (**a**) in a patient with renal failure from polycystic kidney disease (**b**). The patient previously had a parathyroid implant in the forearm which was therefore included in the field of view. This positioning resulted in a prominent focus—the injection site (arrow)—being projected over the left shoulder (**a**–**c**)

16.2 Myocardial Perfusion Scintigraphy (MPS)

MPS with Tc-99m-tetrofosmin or Tc-99m-sestamibi is undertaken in two stages: firstly, following myocardial stressing and secondly at rest on the same or later day. Resting myocardial blood flow (MBF) is about 100 ml/min/100 ml, increasing to about 300 following stress, and distributed to the left ventricular myocardium by 3 major arteries: left anterior descending supplying the anterior and anteroseptal wall, right coronary serving the inferior and inferoseptal wall, and circumflex supplying the lateral wall. Myocardial stressing was previously achieved by bicycle ergometer exercise, but this has been replaced by pharmacological agents including adenosine, regadenoson, dipyridamole and dobutamine (Fig. 16.11).

There are four adenosine receptors: A1, A2A, A2B and A3. Adenosine is a vasodilator in the myocardium but a vasoconstrictor in other tissues, such as kidney and spleen. The myocardial adenosine receptor responsible for vasodilatation is A2A. Regadenoson is a selective A2A agonist and gives an increment in MBF similar to adenosine. Regadenoson was introduced for MPS because it can be given as a single iv injection. Adenosine, on the other hand, has a very short half-life in blood and is given as an i.v. infusion over 6 min. Dipyridamole works by prolonging the half-time in blood of endogenously produced adenosine. Dobutamine increases MBF by increasing myocardial energy requirements; i.e. it is inotropic. Nowadays, most nuclear medicine departments use adenosine or regadenoson for stressing.

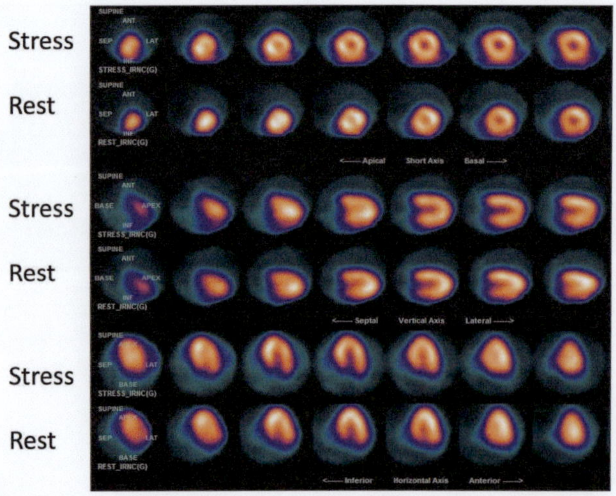

Fig. 16.11 Normal Tc-99m-tetrafosmin myocardial perfusion scintigraphy. In essence, the short axis is transaxial, vertical axis is sagittal and horizontal axis is coronal. Viewing from left to right, transaxial slices go from apex to base, sagittal from septum to lateral wall and coronal from inferior to anterior walls. Note that left ventricular volume is slightly higher following stress. Note also that the right ventricular wall is not visible, although it may be visible when the right ventricle hypertrophies, as in pulmonary hypertension. (Courtesy of Parthiban Arumugam, Manchester Royal Infirmary)

When a major coronary artery is narrowed, commonly from atheroma, the arterioles in the territory it supplies undergo vasodilatation to maintain regional perfusion. Because they are already dilated at rest the territory is unable to increase its perfusion following administration of a vasodilator. The region therefore appears normal at rest but shows up as a defect following stress because of increased flow to other territories. It is therefore called a reversible defect and is the hallmark of myocardial vascular disease (Figs. 16.12 and 16.13). 'Inducible ischaemia' is a popular term in reports, but the ischaemia is already present before the vasodilator is administered. A previous myocardial infarct, in contrast, shows as a defect at both rest and stress—a fixed defect (Fig. 16.14).

SPECT can delineate the count rate void created by the left ventricular cavity. Using dynamic gated imaging, this enables measurement of left ventricular ejection fraction and represents the inverse of a MUGA study, which gives ejection fraction by measuring the counts contained in the left ventricular cavity in diastole and systole following injection of Tc-99mO_4-radiolabelled red cells (Chap. 20).

16.2.1 Reporting a Myocardial Perfusion Study

Firstly, check that stressing has been adequate. Following adenosine or regadenoson there should be an increase in heart rate and blood pressure. Then evaluate tracer accumulation throughout the myocardium, looking for reversible or fixed defects. The skill in reporting MPS lies largely in the identification of artefacts of which there are several. The female breast attenuates the signal and causes breast attenuation artefacts in the anterior wall. Inferior wall attenuation artefacts are seen in large individuals, usually men. Left bundle branch block may cause problems especially by producing artefactual reversible defects in the septum.

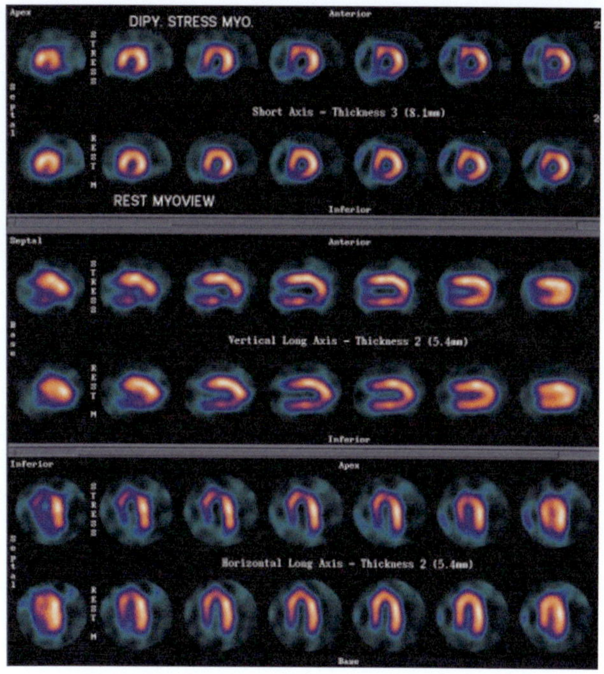

Fig. 16.12 Myocardial perfusion scintigraphy with Tc-99m-tetrafosmin. SPECT acquired following stress is shown in top rows of each panel and SPECT at rest in the bottom rows. There is a reversible defect in the infero-septal region indicating disease in the right coronary artery. (Courtesy of Parthiban Arumugam, Manchester Royal Infirmary)

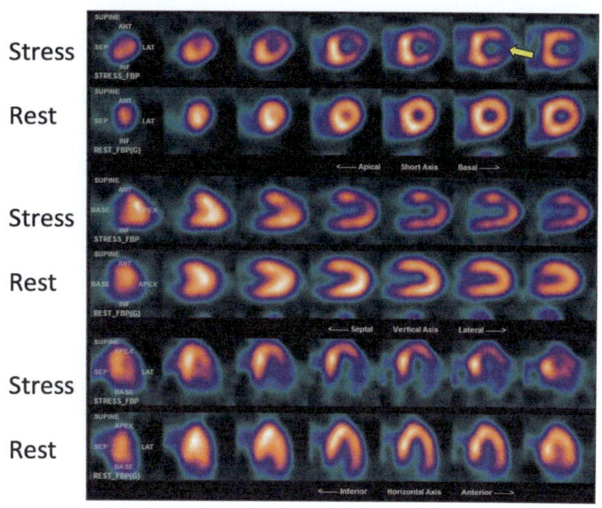

Fig. 16.13 Tetrafosmin myocardial SPECT. There is a reversible defect in the lateral wall indicating disease in the circumflex artery. (Courtesy of Parthiban Arumugam, Manchester Royal Infirmary)

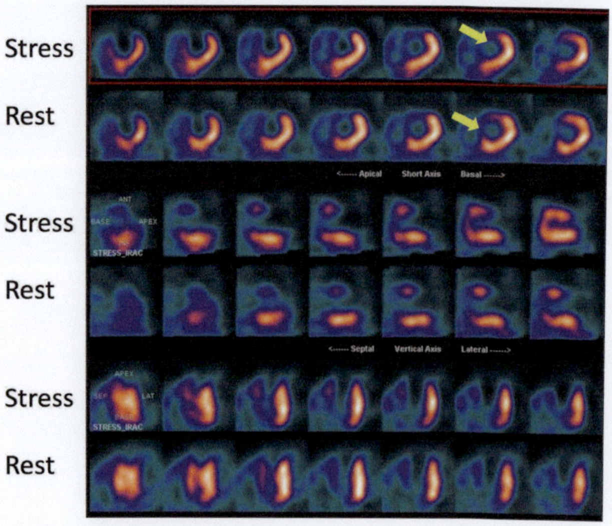

Fig. 16.14 Tetrafosmin myocardial SPECT. There is a fixed defect in the antero-septal region, in keeping with infarct and indicating disease in the right left anterior descending artery. (Courtesy of Parthiban Arumugam, Manchester Royal Infirmary)

16.3 Other Applications

Tc-99m-sestamibi is useful for diagnosing amiodarone-induced thyrotoxicosis (AIT). Thyroid scintigraphy with Tc-99mO_4 is almost always unhelpful because excess iodine from the drug prevents tracer accumulation. In type 1 AIT, the thyroid accumulates Tc-99m-sestamibi because there is retained cellular integrity, but in type 2 AIT, which is a form of thyroiditis, there is very little accumulation.

Further Reading

1. Dizdarevic S, Peters AM. Imaging of multidrug resistance in cancer. Cancer Imaging. 2011;11(1):1–8. https://doi.org/10.1102/1470-7330.2011.0001.
2. Kabasakal L, Halaĉ M, Nisli C, Oguz O, Onsel C, Civi G, Uslu I. The effect of P-glycoprotein function inhibition with cyclosporine A on the biodistribution of Tc-99m sestamibi. Clin Nucl Med. 2000;25:20–3. https://doi.org/10.1097/00003072-200001000-00005.
3. Wang J, Zhang R. Evaluation of ^{99m}Tc-MIBI in thyroid gland imaging for the diagnosis of amiodarone-induced thyrotoxicosis. Br J Radiol. 2017;90:20160836.
4. Whitman J, Allen IE, Bergsland EK, Suh I, Hope TA. Assessment and comparison of ^{18}F-fluorocholine PET and ^{99m}Tc-sestamibi scans in identifying parathyroid adenomas: a metaanalysis. J Nucl Med. 2021;62:1285–91.
5. Wong M, Evans S, Rivory LP, et al. Hepatic Technetium Tc 99m–labeled sestamibi elimination rate and *ABCB1* (*MDR1*) genotype as indicators of ABCB1 (P–glycoprotein) activity in patients with cancer. Clin Pharmacol Therap. 2005;77:33–42.

Tc-99m-Hexamethylpropylamine Oxime (HMPAO) (MW 385 Da)

17

HMPAO is a lipophilic chelator of Tc-99mO_4. Following i.v. injection, Tc-99m-HMPAO is cleared from blood rapidly and becomes widely distributed in the body, freely entering cells on account of its lipophilicity. It is therefore an example of a chemical microsphere and was developed to image the distribution of cerebral blood flow (Fig. 17.1). Later, its properties as a lipophilic chelator were exploited to label autologous leucocytes for white cell scanning (Chap. 26). Tc-99m-HMPAO is used to diagnose cerebral atrophy in the dementias and to identify epileptogenic foci in epilepsy but has been largely replaced for brain imaging by FDG PET/CT.

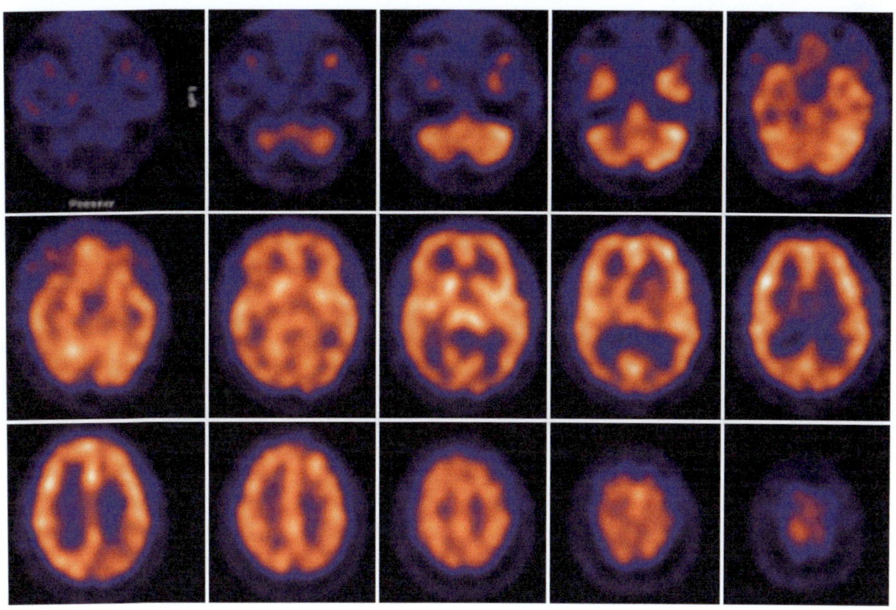

Fig. 17.1 Normal Tc-99m-HMPAO brain SPECT. The tracer behaves as a chemical microsphere so that its distribution portrays distribution of blood flow

A. M. Peters, M. Vadrucci, *Introduction to Nuclear Medicine for Trainees in Imaging and Imaging Sciences*, https://doi.org/10.1007/978-3-032-18364-4_17

Further Reading

1. Neary D, Snowden JS, Shields RA, et al. Single photon emission tomography using 99mTc-HM-PAO in the investigation of dementia. J Neurol Neurosurg Psychiatry. 1987;50:1101–9.

Tc-99m-Labelled Aerosols 18

Almost any radiopharmaceutical can be nebulised into an aerosol for inhalation. This is routinely performed, for example, with Tc-99m-DTPA for imaging the distribution of ventilation in ventilation-perfusion (VQ) lung scanning. Tc-99m-DTPA aerosol imaging is inexpensive and usually performs adequately, although it requires patient co-operation. In airway disease, it tends to form aggregates that deposit in the central airways as a result of turbulent airflow, reducing the amount of activity delivered to distal small airways.

Following inhalation, aerosolised radiopharmaceuticals cross the blood-gas barrier at widely differing rates. Tc-99m-DTPA diffuses through the inter-epithelial junction pores in the bronchoalveolar epithelium of the distal airways and disappears from normal lung exponentially with a clearance half time of about 80 min. In cigarette smokers, the clearance half-time decreases to as little as 20 min and activity appears in the kidneys and urine (Fig. 11.4). If the patient is not a smoker, this may provide a clue as to the presence of interstitial lung disease. It remains unexplained how cigarette smoke markedly increases the transfer rate in otherwise healthy individuals. It may be the result of decreased alveolar fluid, which would increase concentration of inhaled tracer, driving it into pulmonary capillary blood. Because it is lipophilic, Tc-99m-HMPAO rapidly crosses the blood-gas barrier following inhalation. In contrast, Tc-99m-sestamibi crosses very slowly with a half-time of 120 min because it is excluded by the bronchopulmonary MDR transporters, specifically MRP-1 (Fig. 18.1). In contrast to Tc-99m-DTPA, the transfer rate of Tc-99m-sestamibi in smokers is decreased because of upregulation of MRP-1. Despite this advantage over Tc-99m-DTPA, Tc-99m-sestamibi has not been utilised for VQ scanning.

The other two agents routinely used for ventilation imaging in VQ scanning are Kr-81m and *Technegas*. *Technegas* can be thought of as Tc-99m-labelled smoke as it is generated by raising the Tc-99mO_4 solution in the *Technegas* generator to a very high temperature. It performs better than Tc-99m-DTPA but still has problems in COPD patients because of central airway deposition. The optimal agent for ventilation imaging is Kr-81m (Chap. 23).

A. M. Peters, M. Vadrucci, *Introduction to Nuclear Medicine for Trainees in Imaging and Imaging Sciences*, https://doi.org/10.1007/978-3-032-18364-4_18

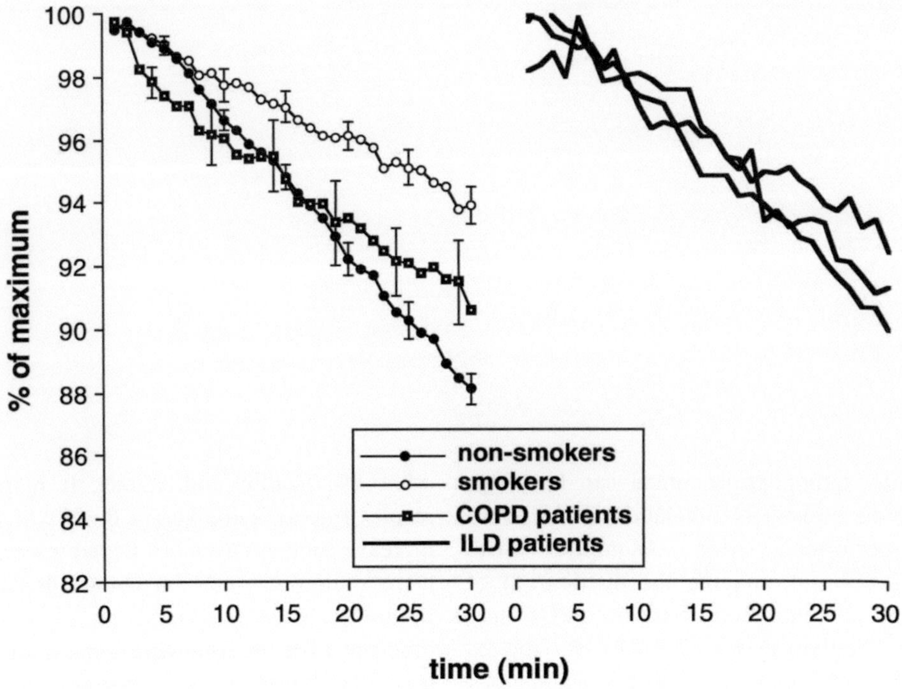

Fig. 18.1 Clearance from the lung of inhaled aerosol containing Tc-99m-sestamibi. In contrast to inhaled Tc-99m-DTPA, clearance is delayed in healthy cigarette smokers compared with healthy non-smokers. Also, in contrast to inhaled Tc-99m-DTPA, clearance is not accelerated in patients with interstitial lung disease (ILD). There is a slightly faster clearance in chronic obstructive airways disease (COPD; ex-smokers). (From Ruparelia P, et al. Pulmonary elimination rate of inhaled ^{99m}Tc-sestamibi radioaerosol is delayed in healthy cigarette smokers. *Br J Clin Pharmacol* 2008;65:611–614)

Further Reading

1. Beadsmoore C, Cheow HK, Szczepura K, Ruparelia P, Peters AM. Healthy passive cigarette smokers have increased pulmonary alveolar permeability. Nucl Med Commun. 2007;28:75–7.
2. Bourke SJ, Banham SW, McKillop JH, Boyd G. Clearance of 99mTc-DTPA in pigeon fancier's hypersensitivity pneumonitis. Am Rev Respir Dis. 1990;142:1168–71.

19 Tc-99m-Labelled Liquid and Semisolid Meals

The rate at which radiolabelled liquid and semisolid meals leave the stomach following oral ingestion is a routine measure of gastric function, usually performed to exclude gastroparesis, and less often to assess symptoms that may be the result of abnormally accelerated gastric emptying associated with the clinical syndrome of 'dumping'. Tc-99mO_4 is complexed with a semisolid meal, such as mash, which is consumed by the patient. Dynamic imaging or sequential image acquisition at 5 min intervals over 60 min is then undertaken. If the stomach empties more than 50% of the consumed activity by 60 min, most departments will terminate the study and call it normal, but if less than 50%, further static post-ambulation images are acquired (Fig. 19.1). In dumping syndrome, often seen in diabetics, the stomach empties rapidly, emptying half of its radioactive contents in less than 25 min (Fig. 19.2). A liquid meal leaves the stomach more rapidly than a semisolid meal and is preferred for the detection of gastro-oesophageal reflux, especially in paediatrics.

When reporting a gastric emptying study, the dynamic series of images should be viewed to check firstly for retention of swallowed activity in the distal oesophagus (Figs. 19.3 and 19.4) and secondly for gastro-oesophageal reflux (Fig. 19.5). Comment also on subsequent rate of intestinal transit. Rarely duodenal obstruction will be encountered in superior mesenteric artery syndrome, in which the third part of the duodenum is compressed between the aorta and superior mesenteric artery. Alternatively, rapid intestinal transit may explain why the patient has chronic diarrhoea (Chap. 25). In paediatrics, liquid meal gastric emptying is used to image gastro-oesophageal reflux. This requires a more rapid dynamic frame rate. Delayed static imaging over the lungs up to 24 h post-ingestion may show evidence of aspiration.

A. M. Peters, M. Vadrucci, *Introduction to Nuclear Medicine for Trainees in Imaging and Imaging Sciences*, https://doi.org/10.1007/978-3-032-18364-4_19

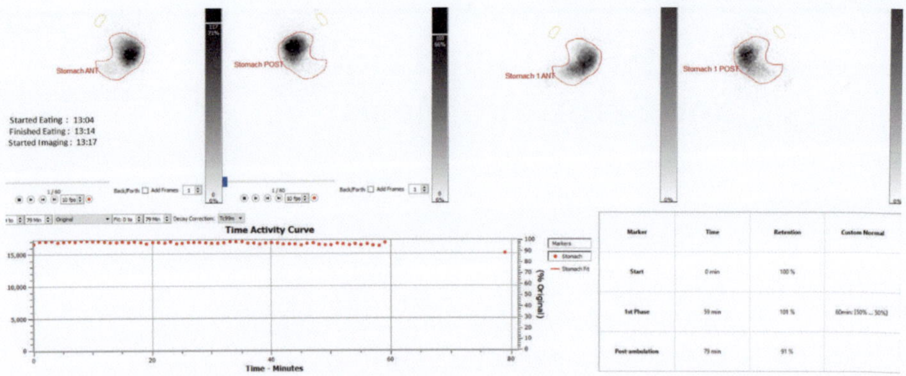

Fig. 19.1 Markedly delayed gastric emptying following consumption of a Tc-99m-labelled semisolid meal. There is negligible emptying over the initial 60 min dynamic image acquisition. Post-ambulation retention at 79 min post-meal was 91%. The delay is predominantly within the fundus

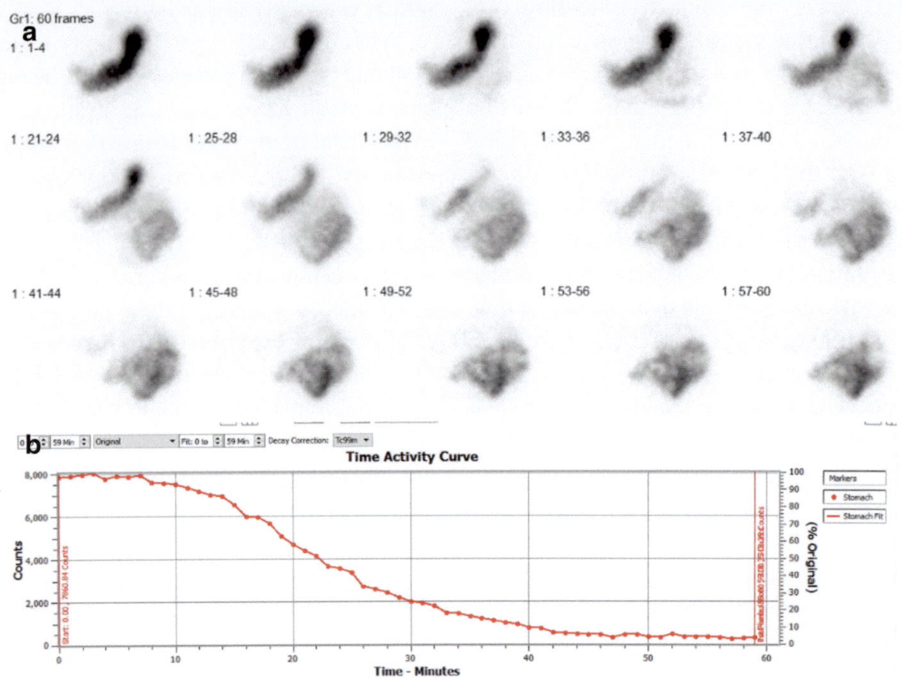

Fig. 19.2 Abnormally rapid gastric emptying (**a**) leading to symptoms described as 'dumping syndrome', often seen in diabetic patients. Half-emptying time was 22 min and 60 min retention was <5% (**b**)

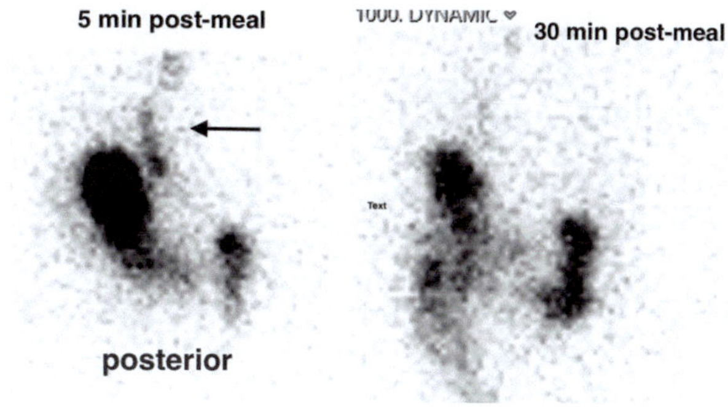

Fig. 19.3 Residual activity in distal oesophagus moving into the stomach during the 60 min dynamic image acquisition may lead to an erroneous 60 min retention value

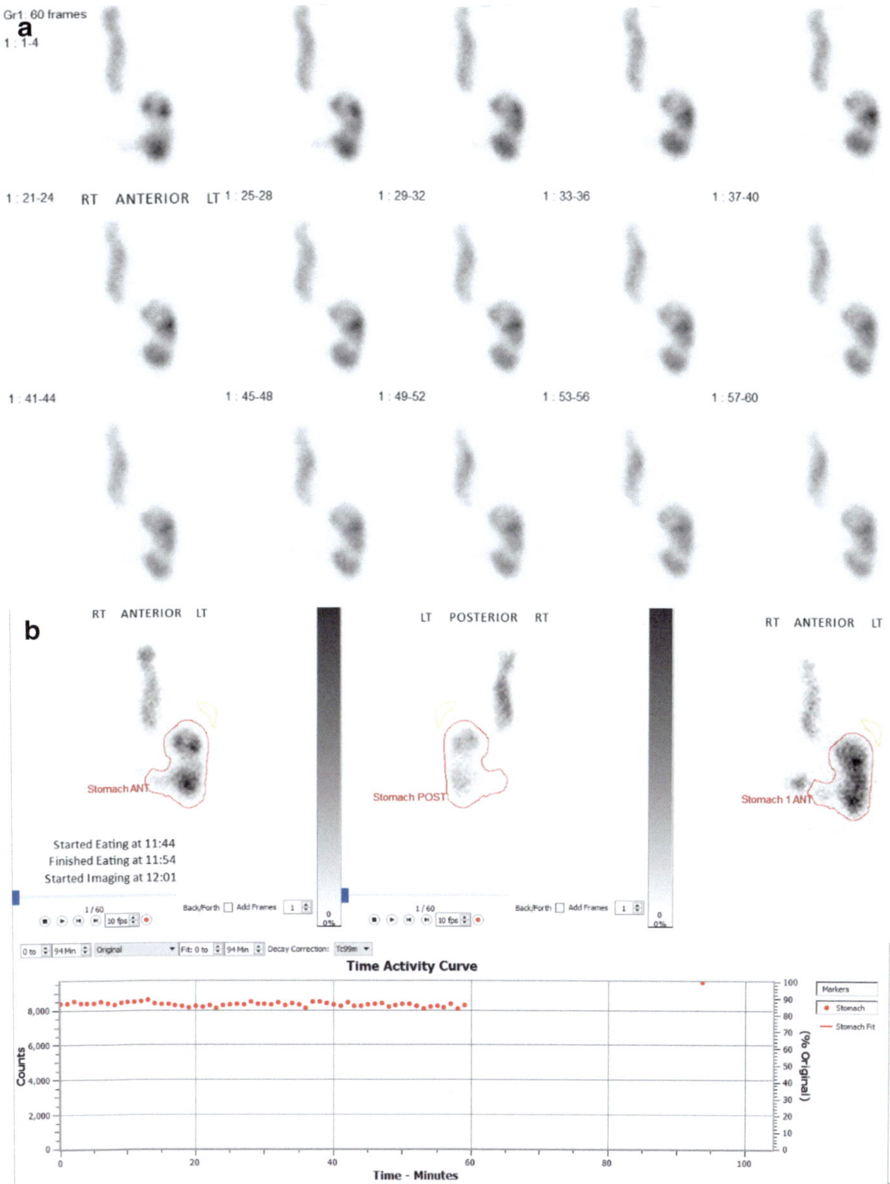

Fig. 19.4 Gastro-oesophageal obstruction in a patient with achalasia and post-POEM procedure (**a**). Subsequent gastric emptying is markedly delayed (**b**)

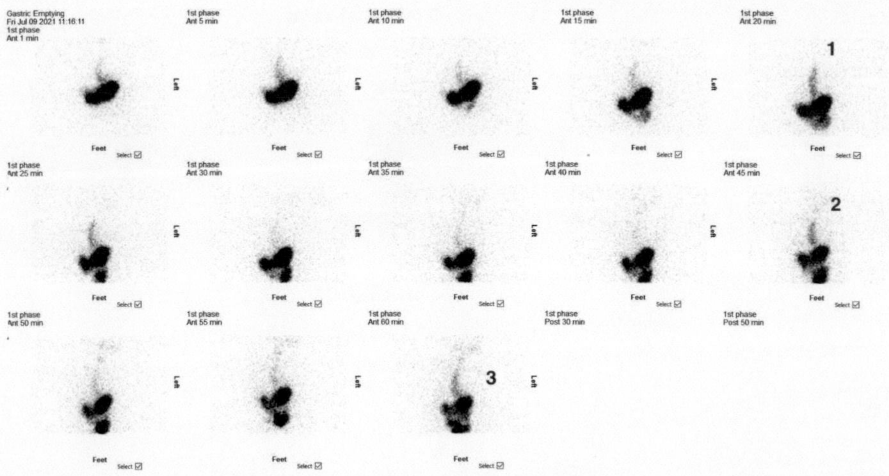

Fig. 19.5 Gastro-oesophageal reflux occurring during a gastric emptying study. Discounting the first frame of the dynamic image sequence, there were 3 episodes of reflux, labelled 1, 2 and 3

Further Reading

1. Bharucha AE, Camilleri M, Forstrom LA, Zinsmeister. Relationship between clinical features and gastric emptying disturbances in diabetes mellitus. Clin Endocrinol. 2009;70:415–20.
2. Patrick A, Epstein O. Review article: gastroparesis. Aliment Pharmacol Ther. 2008;27:724–40.

20 Tc-99m-Labelled Red Blood Cells

Red blood cells can be labelled with several radionuclides, including Cr-51, In-111 and Tc-99m, in vitro, or with radio-iron, in vivo. Cr-51 has a half-life of sufficient duration (27 days) to enable measurement of red cell lifespan, but this is now largely of historical interest. Tc-99m-labelled red cells are used to localise sites of bleeding, especially in the intestinal tract, measure left ventricular ejection fraction, and, occasionally, image haemangiomata.

There are two approaches to labelling red cells with Tc-99mO_4. Both first require exposure of the cells to stannous chloride, which 'tins' them. Tc-99mO_4 readily exchanges between aqueous media and red cells. After penetrating a 'tinned' red cell, however, Tc-99mO_4 is converted in the presence of the stannous ion to a chemical form in which it cannot escape from the cell. The first and preferred labelling approach is to draw a peripheral venous blood sample and perform the labelling procedure entirely in vitro. This enables the labelled cells to be 'washed' to remove unbound tracer before being returned to the patient. The second and technically simpler approach is to inject the stannous salt i.v. and 'tin' the entire circulating red cell population. Tc-99mO_4 administered i.v. then labels all the red cells in vivo, although with a level of labelling efficiency that leaves free Tc-99mO_4 in the circulation. A variant of this approach is to inject stannous ion i.v. then draw blood into a syringe containing Tc-99mO_4, gently mix and inject the blood back into the patient. This technique also leaves free Tc-99mO_4 which accumulates in the stomach (Chap. 10) and enters the proximal small bowel, potentially complicating the detection of upper gastrointestinal bleeding.

20.1 Imaging Occult Intestinal Bleeding (OIB)

This is one of the most challenging tests in nuclear medicine—for the patient, nuclear medicine technologist/radiographer and department. There are several imaging approaches to OIB that combine general radiological techniques, such as angiography, with red cell scintigraphy. As for scintigraphy, conventional practice is to start with a 60 min dynamic acquisition followed by periodic static imaging at 1- or 2-hourly intervals, and again at 24 h. If no bleeding is seen in the dynamic study, static imaging may show that bleeding has taken place but, unfortunately, not necessarily from where in the gastrointestinal tract because intestinal transit of blood may be rapid. To capture an episode of bleeding, several periods of dynamic acquisition make more sense but are demanding for the patient as well as the nuclear medicine department. A bleed can be identified, and approximately located, as a focus that appears during a dynamic sequence and is then seen to move distally within the intestinal lumen, either later in the dynamic sequence or in

A. M. Peters, M. Vadrucci, *Introduction to Nuclear Medicine for Trainees in Imaging and Imaging Sciences*, https://doi.org/10.1007/978-3-032-18364-4_20

a subsequent static image. Imaging at 24 h post-injection is generally unhelpful because the site of bleeding remains unknown and gut activity may simply be free Tc-99mO_4.

Because OIB is usually intermittent, red cell scans are almost always negative. One option is to induce bleeding with heparin, although understandably this is not widely practised. Scintigraphic localisation is relatively crude, so another option is to immediately send the patient for angiography if bleeding is identified on the red cell scan.

20.2 Left Ventricular Wall Motion and Left Ventricular Ejection Fraction

Tc-99m-labelled red cells are used to image the beating heart and measure left ventricular (LV) ejection fraction, especially in patients receiving potentially cardiotoxic drugs such as Herceptin for breast cancer. The technique is called multiple gated image acquisition (MUGA). The patient's ECG is linked to the gamma camera computer and dynamic image acquisition is performed over an individual cardiac cycle with a frame time of one sixteenth of the duration of the cycle, giving 16 frames per cycle. All the first of the 16 frames are then added together so that if there are 350 beats in 5 min, there will be 350 first frames to be summed to give a single composite first frame image. Then all subsequent 350 s frames are summed and so on to give one composite dynamic sequence of 16 frames portraying the cardiac cycle. The R-R interval may be divided into 32 frames to give more detailed data. Wall motion can then be viewed, and LV ejection fraction calculated from the time-activity curve of the composite cycle (Fig. 20.1). To achieve the best separation of right and left ventricles, imaging is acquired from the left anterior oblique projection. The lower limit of normal LV ejection fraction is not well defined but is around 50%. High LV ejection fractions, >75%, are seen in hypertrophic cardiomyopathy. However, in this disease, end-diastolic LV volume is reduced so that stroke volume is reduced rather than increased.

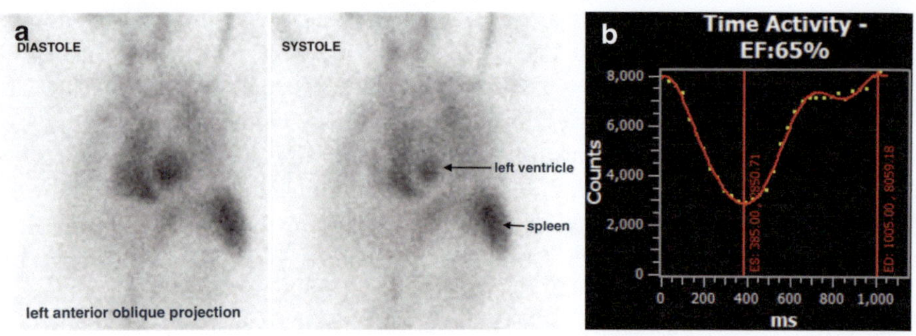

Fig. 20.1 Multiple gated acquisition (MUGA) with Tc-99m-radiolabelled blood cells to image left ventricular wall motion (**a**) and measure left ventricular ejection fraction (**b**)

20.3 Tc-99m-Labelled Denatured Red Blood Cells

Denatured red blood cells are used to image splenunculi (Fig. 20.2). The spleen concentrates erythrocytes that have been denatured by heating, chemical damage, or exposure to an anti-erythrocyte monoclonal antibody. For routine clinical application, heat denaturing is the usual approach. It involves heating a small sample of autologous red cells at 49.5 °C for 20 min before in vitro labelling with Tc-99m. Heating makes the red cells stiff and leads to their retention in the spleen following i.v. injection.

Undamaged red cells normally transit the spleen with a mean transit time of about one minute. This is longer than in any other tissue because of the spleen's role in removing effete red cells from the circulation. All blood cells entering the spleen are required to negotiate the sinus endothelium, which contains intercellular gaps of a size that allows red cells with normal deformability to pass but retains aged red cells that have become stiff or contain inclusion bodies. Aged red cells are destroyed, and their haem iron is recycled. Red cells with inclusion bodies, on the other hand, are caught up in the intercellular gaps and the inclusion body 'snipped' off while the cells are trapped in the sinus, after which they are free to re-circulate. Because they are stiff, heat damaged red blood cells (HDRBC) are held up in the spleen. On average, a HDRBC has a 65% probability of leaving the spleen after a residence time of 10–15 min, or a 35% probability of being retained for destruction. The clearance rate of HDRBC from the circulation is therefore biexponential, the first exponential reflecting the splenic accumulation rate of HDRBC, and therefore splenic blood flow, and the second reflecting splenic reticuloendothelial function.

SPECT/CT for imaging splenunculi should be performed at a time post-injection that depends on whether an intact spleen is present. With a spleen present, imaging can be undertaken 40 min post-injection, but if the patient is asplenic, the residence time of the HDRBC in the circulation is prolonged and imaging delayed to 60 min. Overheating of the cells promotes localisation in liver. Under-heating prolongs residence time in the circulation, potentially giving rise to a false positive outcome if the tumour competing with the splenunculus in the differential diagnosis has a high blood volume (Fig. 20.3).

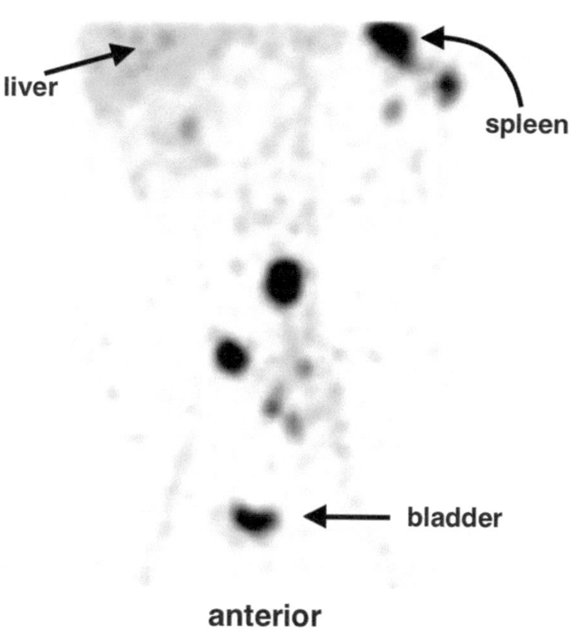

Fig. 20.2 Multiple splenunculi in the abdomen imaged with Tc-99m-labelled heat-damaged red blood cells

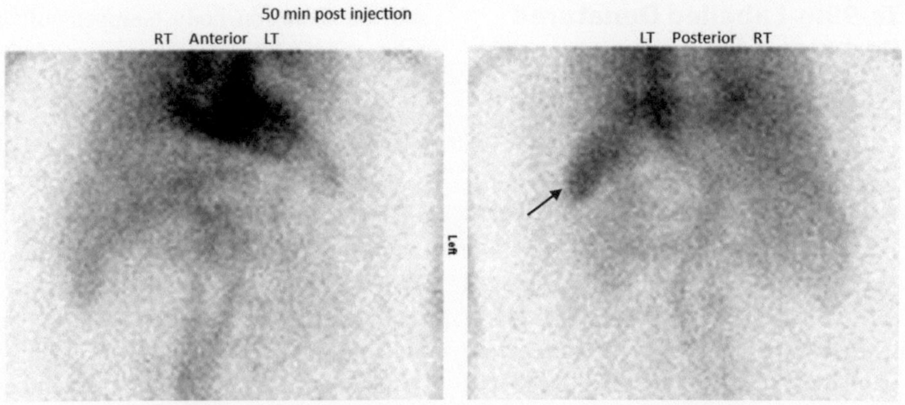

Fig. 20.3 For a Tc-99m-labelled heat-damaged red blood cell scan, it is important for the radiopharmacy lab to exactly follow the damaging protocol, which is 49.5 °C for 20 min. In this case, the cells are insufficiently damaged. Even at 50 min post-injection there is excessive activity still in the circulation and the spleen (arrowed) is poorly visualised

Further Reading

1. Grady E. Gastrointestinal bleeding scintigraphy in the early 21st century. J Nucl Med. 2016;57:252–9.
2. Peters AM, Ryan PF, Klonizakis I, et al. Kinetics of heat damaged autologous red blood cells. Mechanism of clearance from blood. Scand J Haematol. 1982;28:5–14.

21 Tc-99m-Labelled Proteins

21.1 Tc-99m-Labelled Human Serum Albumin (HSA; MW 68 kDa) and Polyclonal Human Immunoglobulin (MW 150 kDa)

Tc-99m-HSA was originally developed as a blood pool agent and used for MUGA studies as described above under Tc-99m-labelled erythrocytes. It can also be used for lymphoscintigraphy (Chap. 22). Tc-99m-polyclonal IgG (HIG) can also be used for lymphoscintigraphy. Its lymph node extraction efficiency is about 50% compared to about 70% for Tc-99m-nanocolloid. It may be used for imaging inflammation, in which positive images result from the increased capillary permeability of inflammation rather than specific binding of IgG at the site of inflammation.

21.2 Tc-99m-Macroaggregated Albumin (MAA)

Tc-99m-MAA consists of a suspension of microparticles of denatured HSA varying in diameter from 10 to 100 μm. The particles are too large to pass through the pulmonary circulation and when injected intravenously micro-embolise in the pulmonary arterioles (diameter 10–100 μm). (Note that there are far fewer numbers of pulmonary arterioles compared with pulmonary capillaries.) Numbers of particles injected ranges between 200,000 and 500,000, which is enough to statistically ensure that the distribution of the particles is identical to the distribution of pulmonary blood flow.

Tc-99m-MAA has two uses: firstly, to image pulmonary embolism and secondly to quantify anatomical right-to-left shunting (Fig. 21.1). The first is covered in Chap. 23 under ventilation/perfusion imaging. Disorders for which the second use is indicated include hepatopulmonary syndrome (HPS), pulmonary arteriovenous malformations and right-to-left shunting in congenital heart disease in which pulmonary blood pressure exceeds systemic pressure (Eisenmenger syndrome). In HPS, the shunts are preferentially located in the lower zones of the lungs which, because of the effect of gravity on the distribution of pulmonary blood flow, results in greater breathlessness in the upright position (platypnoea). Patients with suspected HPS should therefore be injected with Tc-99m-MAA upright rather than supine.

After shunting from right to left, Tc-99m-MAA is distributed according to the proportion of cardiac output received by individual organs. This in itself has previously been studied in a research setting using Tc-99-MAA injected into a left-sided heart chamber. The following percentages received by organs are approximately 10% for each kidney, 15% for the brain, 5% for the resting myocardium, 5% for the spleen, and 17.5% for the splanchnic bed. The liver only

A. M. Peters, M. Vadrucci, *Introduction to Nuclear Medicine for Trainees in Imaging and Imaging Sciences*, https://doi.org/10.1007/978-3-032-18364-4_21

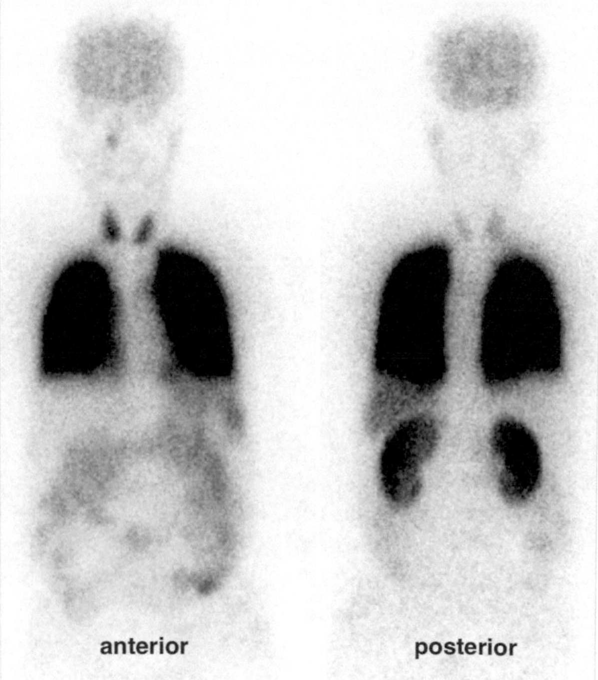

Fig. 21.1 Tc-99m-MAA whole-body scan in a patient with advanced liver disease and hepatopulmonary syndrome showing an anatomical right-to-left shunt of 35%. Note relative paucity of hepatic activity, which arrives exclusively via the hepatic artery because of entrapment of particles in tissues draining into the portal vein

receives about 7.5% which arrives via the hepatic artery, the portal input having been cleared of tracer in the splanchnic bed and spleen.

Right-to-left shunting of Tc-99m-MAA is quantified by comparing counts in the lungs with whole body counts from which lung counts have been subtracted. The lower limit of normal is 10%. Quite what this 10% represents is uncertain because MAA particles of 5–10 μm will embolise in pulmonary capillaries rather than pulmonary arterioles, so it is likely due to very small fragments or free Tc-99mO_4. Alternatively, the assumption can be made that the right kidney receives 10% of cardiac output and the counts within it compared with administered counts. The right kidney is chosen over the left because no activity arrives in the liver via the portal vein, thereby minimising interfering background liver activity.

21.3 Monoclonal Antibodies

Radiolabelling monoclonal antibodies (MABs) or their Fab fragments, opened a wide spectrum of potential applications in scintigraphy—personalised imaging to suit the pathology. Only one, however, *Leukoscan*, has enjoyed clinical use. *Leukoscan* is the Tc-99m-labelled Fab fragment of a monoclonal antibody that binds NCA-90, an antigen on the cell surface of neutrophils involved in neutrophil adhesion to activated endothelium. It is claimed the MAB targets foci of infection and inflammation by first binding to circulating neutrophils. However, like other labelled proteins that have been used to image inflammation, such as polyclonal immunoglobulin and human serum albumin, it probably enters inflammatory foci by passively diffusing through compromised endothelium into an expanded local interstitial space. Thus, target-to-background ratio is no higher than with Tc-99m-labelled albumin. Moreover, circulating activity has been shown not to be blood cell associated.

Further Reading

1. Abrams G, Nanda N, Dubovsky E, Krowka MJ, Fallon M. Use of macroaggregated albumin lung perfusion scan to diagnose hepatopulmonary syndrome: a new approach. Gastroenterology. 1998;114:305–10.
2. Skehan SJ, White JF, Evans JW, et al. Mechanism of accumulation of ^{99m}Tc-sulesomab in inflammation. J Nucl Med. 2003;44:11–8.

22 Tc-99m-Labelled Nanocolloids

Like Tc-99m-MAA (macroaggregated albumin; Chap. 21), Tc-99m-nanocolloids are made from human serum albumin. Particle size, however, is much smaller than MAA (≤80 nm versus 10–100 μm), so after i.v. injection nanocolloids traverse the lungs, enter the circulation and are cleared into the macrophages of the reticuloendothelial system (liver, spleen and bone marrow). The distribution between liver, spleen and bone marrow depends to some extent on particle size, although with any size the great majority accumulates in the liver. Sulphur colloid has a larger size and is more selective for the liver but is no longer available in the UK. The smaller sized Tc-99m-nanocolloids (*NanoColl, NanoTop, NanoScan*) have a slight selectivity for bone marrow. Because hepatic extraction efficiency is about 90%, Tc-99m-nanocolloids have a rapid plasma clearance of approximately 800 ml/min (ignoring marrow clearance; spleen drains into liver). For a plasma volume of 3000 ml, this translates to a mean Tc-99m-nanocolloid residence time in the circulation of only about 3000/800 or ~4 min.

Tc-99m-nanocolloids are used in five clinical scenarios.

22.1 Imaging the Liver

It is sometimes difficult with cross-sectional imaging to distinguish between hepatic tumours and the benign condition of focal nodular hyperplasia (FNH). Unlike focal liver lesions, such as hepatocellular carcinoma, FNH accumulates colloid and can therefore be positively identified.

22.2 Imaging the Spleen

A diagnostic problem is the distinction between intraabdominal tumours and splenunculi. Although this distinction is best resolved with labelled heat-damaged erythrocytes (Chap. 20), splenunculi can be imaged with Tc-99m-nanocolloid when such erythrocytes are not available. The main disadvantage of Tc-99m-nanocolloid in this setting is that the splenunculus is likely to be invisible if it is close to the liver. Moreover, sensitivity is less compared with Tc-99m-HDRBC because most of the tracer accumulates in the liver (Fig. 22.1).

A. M. Peters, M. Vadrucci, *Introduction to Nuclear Medicine for Trainees in Imaging and Imaging Sciences*, https://doi.org/10.1007/978-3-032-18364-4_22

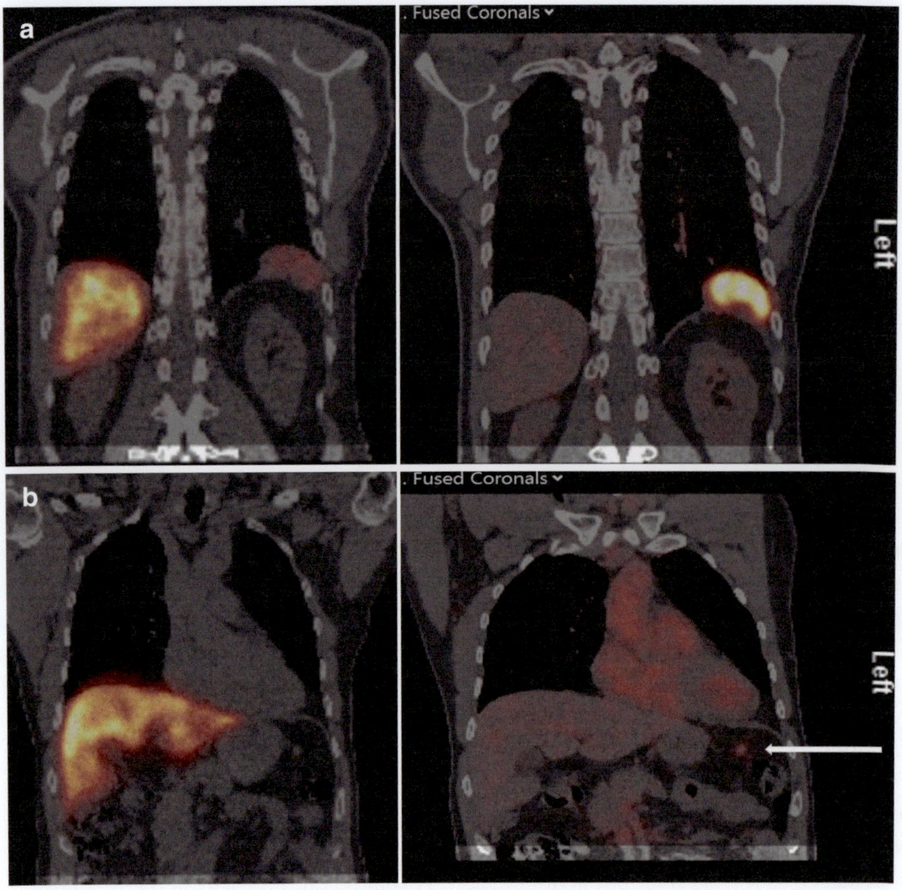

Fig. 22.1 Tc-99m-labelled heat-damaged red blood cell (HDRBC) SPECT/CT in comparison with Tc-99m-nanocolloid SPECT/CT in the same patient searching for splenunculi. Two separate coronal slices are shown (**a** and **b**). The HDRBC scan (in right panels) shows that the spleen is above the diaphragm and that the focus in the left upper quadrant is a small splenunculus. In the colloid scan (left panels), in contrast, the spleen is less prominent and tracer uptake in the splenunculus is barely apparent

22.3 Imaging the Bone Marrow

Intramedullary bone malignancy is a rare indication for bone marrow imaging, but Tc-99m-nanocolloid has been used, for example, to image lymphoma, which gives defects of uptake. A more common application is to identify bone marrow in conjunction with radiolabelled leucocytes—which accumulate in marrow physiologically—as part of a white cell scan (Chap. 26).

22.4 Imaging the Lymphatic System

Tc-99m-nanocolloid injected directly into a tissue, avoiding blood vessels, enters lymphatic vessels and is carried to the draining lymph nodes where it is taken up by lymph node macrophages. Tc-99m-nanocolloid in the interstitial space enters lymphatic vessels rather than blood capillaries because lymphatic vessel endothelium is fenestrated, thereby permitting passage of the particles, which are too large to diffuse through blood capillary endothelium. This forms the basis of two imaging techniques: firstly, lymphoscintigraphy to determine the cause of a chronically swollen limb and, secondly, sentinel node imaging (SNI) in cancer.

22.5 Imaging Chylous Leaks

An occasional clinical request made of Tc-99m-nanocolloid is to image chylous leaks from the thoracic duct. However, because it is efficiently extracted from lymph as it passes through a chain of lymph nodes, little or no Tc-99m-nanocolloid enters the thoracic duct following injection into a lower extremity. So, it makes little sense for imaging thoracic duct leaks. Tc-99m-human serum albumin may have an advantage in this setting as its lymph node extraction efficiency is lower.

22.5.1 Lymphoscintigraphy

Lymphoscintigraphy is performed for limb swelling suspected to be the result of lymphoedema. Referrals are more often for lower than upper limb swelling. Limbs may be swollen from excess fat, which is known as lipoedema, or excess fluid, which is known as oedema. When oedema is caused by lymphatic dysfunction, it is known as lymphoedema. The causes of oedema can be appreciated from the Starling equation which describes net water movement, J, across blood capillaries, as follows.

$$J = K_f.A.\left[\left(P_i - P_e\right) - \sigma.\left(\pi_i - \pi_e\right)\right]$$

where K_f is the capillary filtration coefficient, A is capillary surface area, subscripts i and e refer to intravascular and extravascular, P is hydrostatic pressure and Π is oncotic pressure. The variable, σ, is the reflection coefficient, which depends on capillary permeability to protein. Hepatic sinusoids, for example, are permeable to macromolecules, so σ approaches zero and oncotic pressure is ineffective. For tissues with tight endothelial junctions that exclude macromolecules, in contrast, σ approaches unity.

The hydrostatic pressure difference between intravascular and interstitial spaces (which drives capillary water into the interstitial space) exceeds the oncotic pressure difference generated by the respective blood and interstitial protein concentrations (which drives water back from the interstitial space to the capillary) *throughout the length of the capillary* so that *net* water movement is always towards the interstitial space. Macromolecules are too large to move across the endothelium by molecular diffusion. (Molecules diffuse at a rate inversely proportional to the cube root of their molecular weight.) Via convective transport, however, the moving water 'drags' macromolecules into the interstitial space where they are needed for various functions, including immune function. Because there is no net water movement from interstitial space to blood, macromolecules are unable to return to the blood capillary from the interstitial space and instead enter lymphatic vessels which are much more permeable than blood capillaries, at least in limbs. Net fluid transfer from capillaries to interstitial space—the capillary filtration rate—is therefore equal to lymph flow.

Lymphoscintigraphy is not appropriate for the investigation of oedema in patients with heart failure (which increases P_i), hypoalbuminaemia (which decreases Π_i) or capillary leak syndromes (which increase K_f and reduce σ). Venous disease, which increases P_i, is also regarded as an exclusion criterion, although lymphoscintigraphy may occasionally be requested to confirm it in the lower limbs.

The term *latent* lymphoedema—coined to identify patients at risk of lymphoedema—arose from the observation that only 25% of breast cancer patients undergoing axillary clearance surgery develop upper limb lymphoedema (breast cancer-related lymphoedema), consistent with the notion of constitutional lymphatic weakness. Surgical procedures in the lower limb may also precipitate lymphoedema in those at risk. Abnormal lymphoscintigraphy in a non-swollen limb suggests that the limb is at risk of swelling. Normal lymphoscintigraphy in a swollen limb remains unexplained. The widely used terms primary lymphoedema (de novo) and secondary lymphoedema (secondary to disease or an intervention) rather miss the concept of constitutional lymphatic weakness.

Lymphatic and venous drainage in a limb occurs in two compartments: epifascial and subfascial (muscle). Capillary filtration rate per ml of tissue is two to three times higher in resting muscle than in the epifascia. The two trunks merge immediately before reaching the axillary or ilioinguinal lymph nodes. Because of the fascial envelope, the subfascial compartment is unable to swell when its lymphatic drainage is compromised, so, via connecting vessels, excess lymph enters the epifascial compartment, which swells instead.

There are three possible injection sites: subcutaneous, intradermal and intramuscular (calf in lower limb or forearm in upper limb). Tracer is deposited in the epifascial compartment from s.c. injection and into the subfascial compartment following i.m. injection. Intradermal injection is superficial. It raises a blister and under pressure forces tracer into the skin, resulting in rapid delivery to the lymphatics with which the skin is generously furnished. For lymphoscintigraphy, s.c. injection is preferred because it challenges the lymphatic system to mobilise the tracer and deliver it the loco-regional lymph nodes. For imaging lymph nodes, as in SNI (see below), in contrast, i.d. injection is preferred because it rapidly delivers a higher proportion of the injected dose to the drainage basin. Intramuscular injection is used to image subfascial drainage in cases where this is suspected to be abnormal.

22.5.1.1 How to Report Lymphoscintigraphy

Lower Limbs

Tracer is routinely injected subcutaneously into a webspace in both feet followed by half-body imaging (from toes to upper chest) immediately and again at 2–2.5 h (Fig. 22.2). Later imaging is generally not necessary. Some departments also

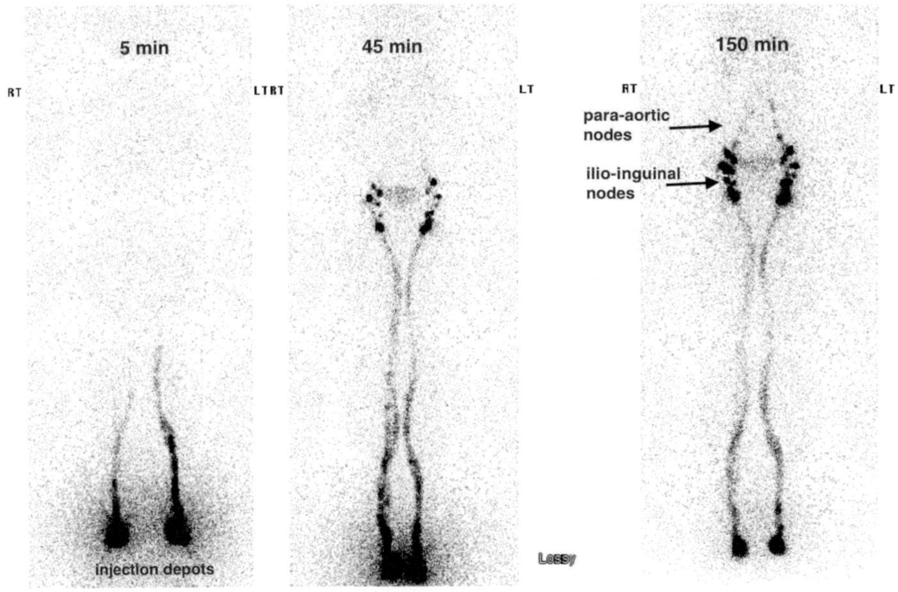

Fig. 22.2 Normal lower limb lymphoscintigraphy (5, 45 and 150 min post-injection; **a**–**c**). Subcutaneous injection into the webspace of an extremity delivers tracer to the epifascial compartment of the limb. This compartment drains via the epifascial lymphatic trunk, which, in the lower limbs, 'shadows' the saphenous vein, in contrast to the deep or subfascial compartment, which takes a deeper course and 'shadows' the femoral vein. Urinary activity is the result of free Tc-99mO_4 or colloid breakdown products

image at 45–60 min, but this adds little further useful information. The immediate image confirms that no tracer has been inadvertently injected into a blood vessel, otherwise there is immediate appearance of liver activity (Fig. 22.3). When this happens, the study is likely to need repeating.

Lymphoedema occurs in a limb when lymph production rate exceeds lymphatic drainage capacity. Lymphoedema is rarely the result of lymphatic obstruction, but instead is much more commonly the result of a constitutional 'weakness' of lymphatic function, and is therefore frequently bilateral. Avoid using the word 'obstruction' in your report unless the patient has a disease known to cause obstruction, such as in filariasis.

The epifascial lymphatic trunk 'shadows' the saphenous vein, while the trunk draining the subfascial compartment 'shadows' the femoral vein. Interpretation of the 150 min image follows the 3-D rule: delay, diversion and damage, all of which are abnormal. Reduced tracer delivery to the ilioinguinal nodes—*delay*—can be appreciated from imaging (Fig. 22.4) but should be confirmed with quantification as described below. Tracer may enter skin, traditionally called 'dermal backflow' (Fig. 22.5), or drain via the deep subfascial route whereupon popliteal lymph nodes will be visualised (Fig. 22.6), both scenarios being described as *diversion*. These two abnormal routes are often seen together (Fig. 22.7). There are usually no lymph nodes in the epifascial compartment, although rarely one may be visualised and should not be confused with a popliteal node. *Damage* to lymphatic vessels may follow previous trauma or cellulitis and appear as grossly dilated lymphatic vessels or as a lymph 'lake', formed when tracer leaks out of the damaged vessel and produces a diffuse, ill-defined accumulation of tracer (Fig. 22.8).

Fig. 22.3 Visualisation of hepatic activity in the immediate post-injection half body scan indicates inadvertent partial injection of the tracer into a blood vessel. This usually requires rescheduling of the study

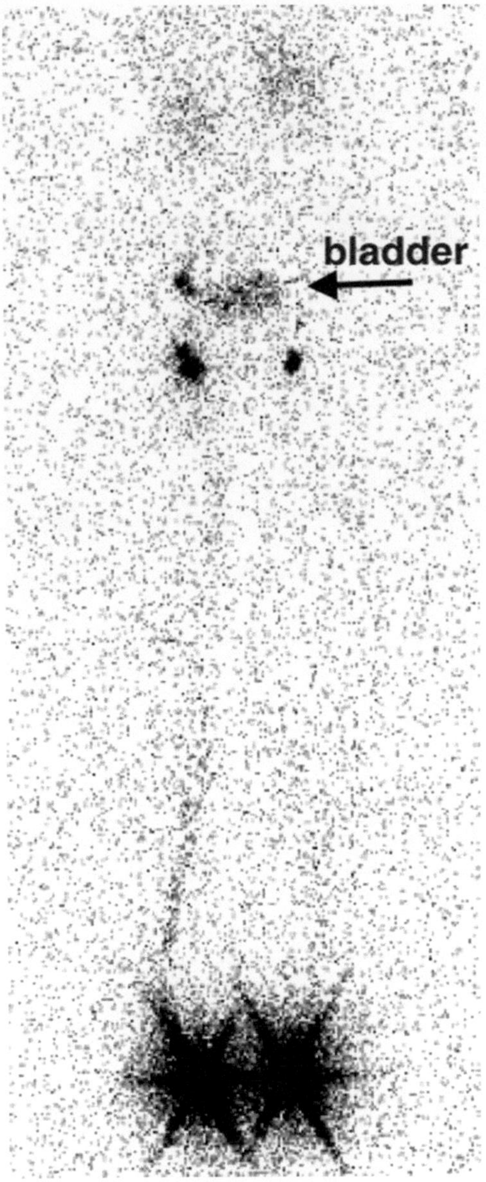

Fig. 22.4 Lymph delay. Minimal activity has reached ilioinguinal nodes by 120 min post-injection

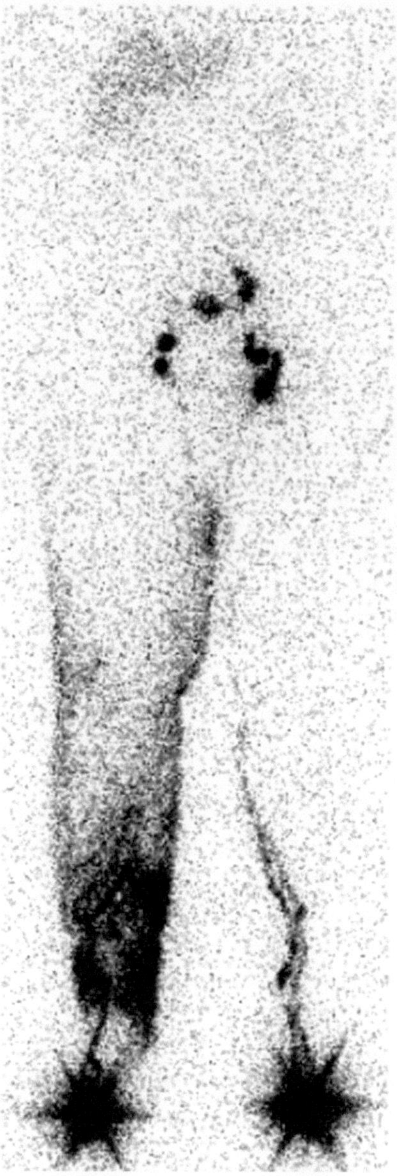

Fig. 22.5 Gross diversion of tracer through the skin of the right lower limb indicating severe lymphatic dysfunction

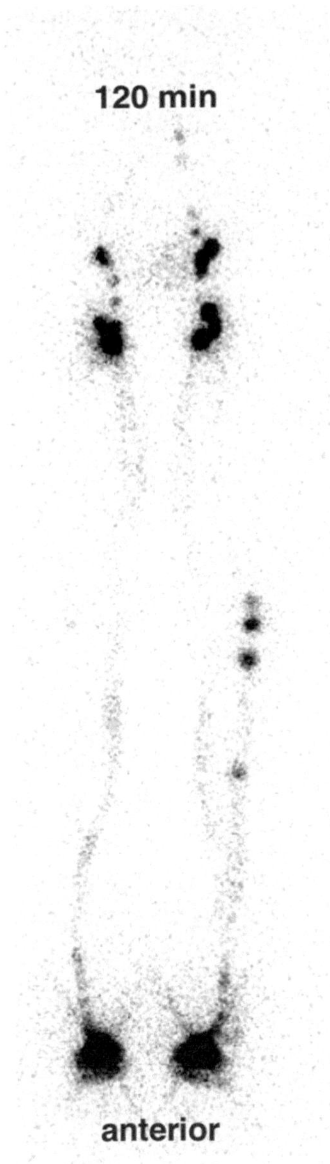

Fig. 22.6 Diversion of tracer into the deep system, shown by visualisation of four popliteal nodes, which is abnormal

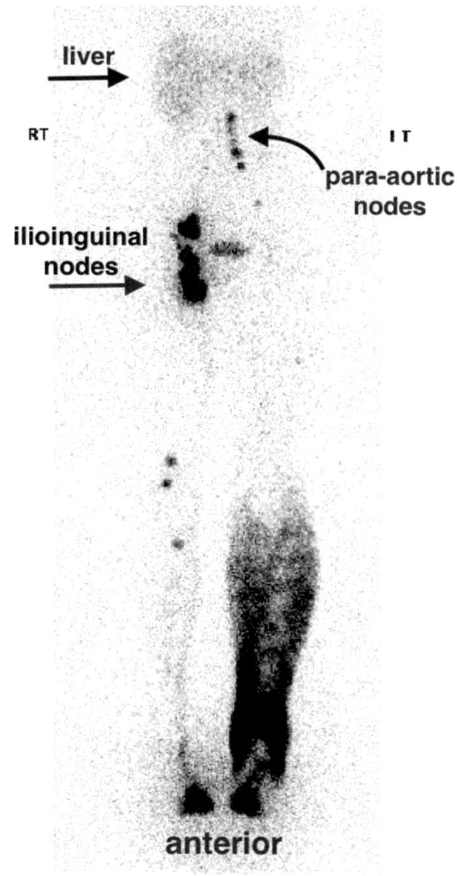

Fig. 22.7 Grossly abnormal lymphoscintigraphy with diversion of tracer into skin of left lower limb and deep system of right lower limb. Note how tracer on the left appears to have bypassed ilioinguinal nodes and accumulated instead in left para-aortic nodes. This raises the possibility of previous lymph node rsection

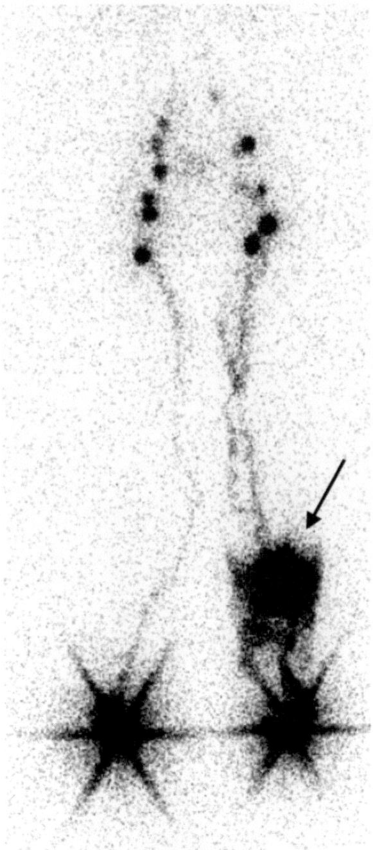

Fig. 22.8 Prominent lymph lake (arrow) resulting from previous injury to lymphatic vessels, typically from cellulitis or soft tissue trauma, allowing lymph to leak from lymphatic vessels. No other abnormal findings

Because of raised pressure at the venous end of blood capillaries, lymph production rate is increased in venous disease, resulting in visualisation of inguinal nodes in the immediate post-injection image, lymphatic vessel collaterals and abundant activity in ilioinguinal nodes (Fig. 22.9). If this picture is accompanied by signs of lymphatic dysfunction, such as diversion, it indicates that the lymphatic system is failing to cope with the increased lymph flow, a condition called phlebolymphoedema. Since a diagnosis can be made from lymphoscintigraphy, venous disease is becoming an indication for lymphoscintigraphy rather than an exclusion criterion. Lymphoscintigraphy is warranted in patients with a clinical diagnosis of lipoedema because excess fat may interfere with lymphatic drainage.

Hepatic activity seen on delayed imaging, but not on immediate imaging, has no clear explanation. It is generally attributed to intact colloid entering the thoracic duct, but, because of efficient lymph node extraction, which in an individual lymph node is about 70%, this seems unlikely. Moreover, hepatic activity varies with the manufacturer of the tracer. The preparation called *Nanoscan* gives no liver activity in almost all cases ruling out intact colloid entering the thoracic duct. Activity is sometimes seen in neck lymph nodes (Fig. 22.10), suggesting thoracic

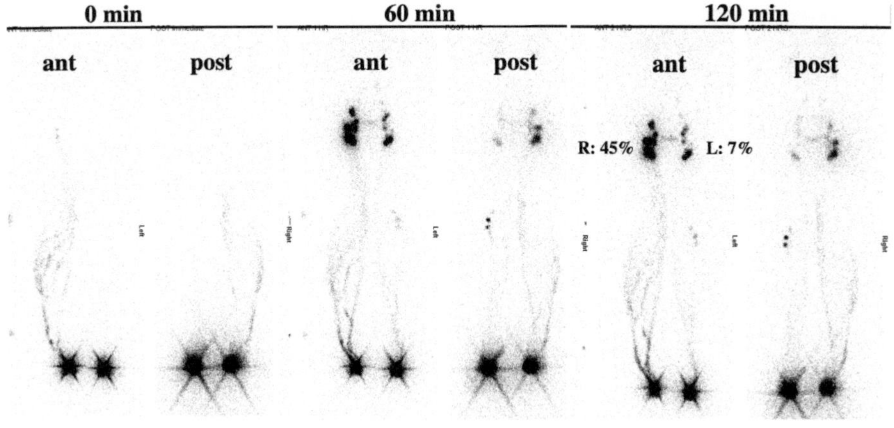

Fig. 22.9 Venous disease, seen here in the right lower limb, typically has three features: visualisation of inguinal nodes in the immediate post-injection image, lymphatic vessel collateralisation and increased ilioinguinal nodal accumulation at 120–150 min (>30% of administered activity)—all markers of increased capillary filtration and therefore lymph flow. There is lymphatic dysfunction on the left with visualisation of three popliteal nodes

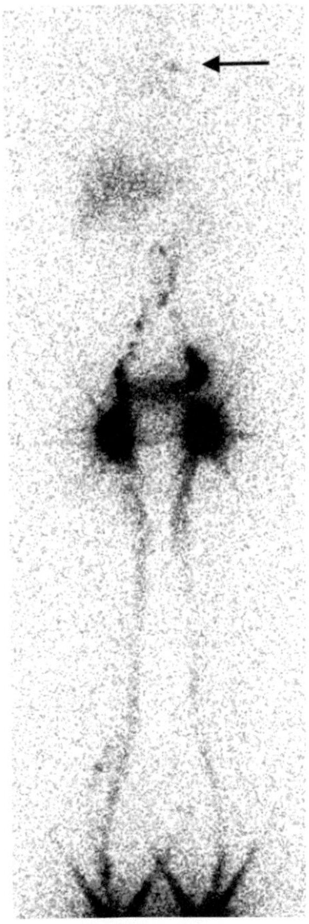

Fig. 22.10 Faint visualisation of a lymph node in the neck (arrow) indicates thoracic duct transit either of intact nanocolloid or more likely fragments thereof. This explains at least one route for activity to reach the liver, the other potential routes being anatomical lymphovenous communications and direct transfer of colloid fragments from lymph to blood within lymph nodes

duct transit of colloid breakdown products (Fig. 22.11), which may also arise in, and enter blood within, lymph nodes. Delayed prominent liver activity is more often seen when lymphoscintigraphy is abnormal, raising the possibility that lymphovenous communications open as a compensatory response (Fig. 22.12).

Upper Limbs

Abnormal features in upper limb lymphoscintigraphy are limited to delay and skin diversion because transit of tracer through the nodes at the elbow (trochlear nodes) is normal (Figs. 22.13 and 22.14). The commonest cause of lymphoedema in the upper limb is axillary lymph node clearance for treatment of breast cancer (Fig. 22.15). Breast cancer-related lymphoedema is seen in only 25% of patients undergoing axillary clearance, emphasising the constitutional nature of lymphoedema. This is also emphasised by the occasional appearance of four-limb lymphoedema (Fig. 22.16).

22.5.1.2 Quantification in Limb Lymphoscintigraphy

There are two approaches to quantification in lymphoscintigraphy—firstly, the rate of clearance of activity from the injection site and, secondly, the quantification of activity arriving in ilioinguinal or axillary nodes as a percentage of the injected activity. There is no established normal range for clearance rate. The normal range

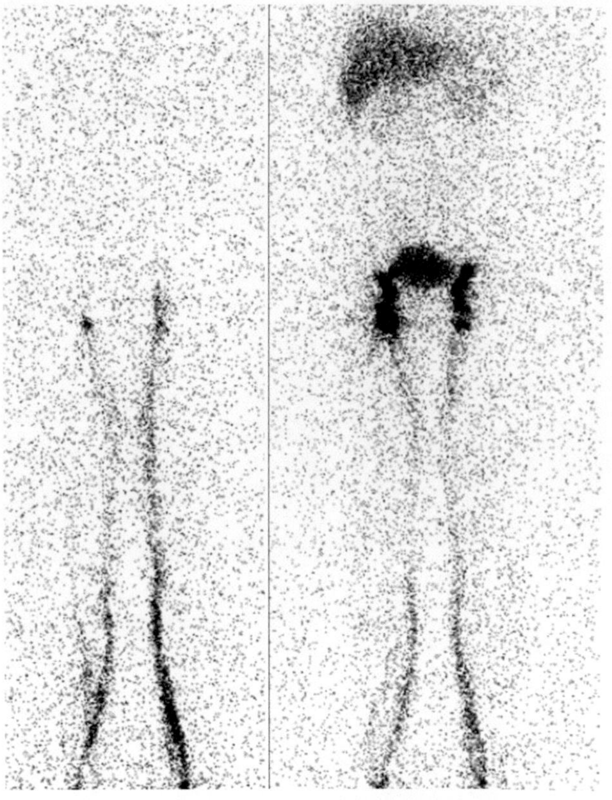

Fig. 22.11 Probable hepatic accumulation of Tc-99m-nanocolloid breakdown products. There is no hepatic activity in the immediate image. In the delayed image, however, there is prominent hepatic activity but no para-aortic activity. No clear evidence of lymphatic dysfunction to suggest lymphovenous communications, as there is in Fig. 22.12. It is therefore suggested that breakdown products were formed in lymph nodes and transferred directly to blood capillaries in the nodes

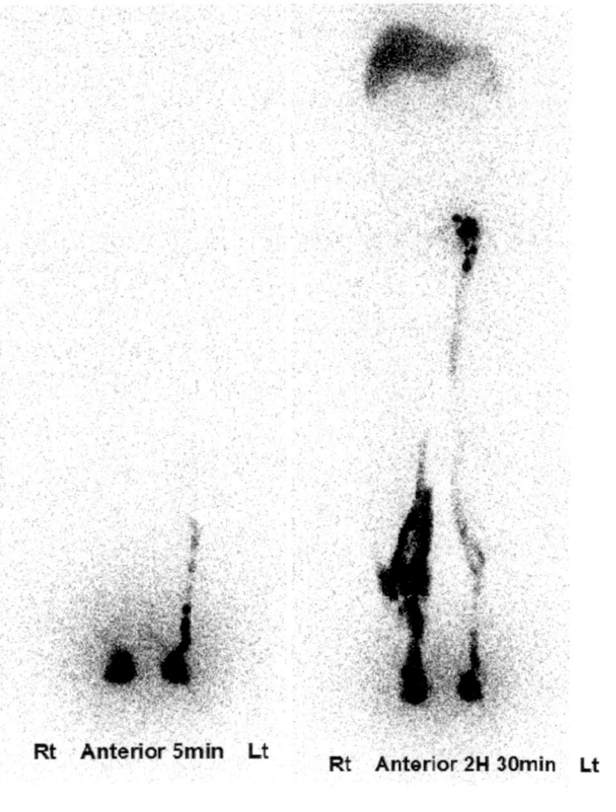

Fig. 22.12 Hepatic activity is usually faint or absent. When it is prominent on delayed imaging but absent at 5 min, it raises the suspicion of lymphovenous communications. The sites of such communications are usually not apparent, but they are encountered more often in abnormal lymph scans, such as this one, which shows gross lymphatic vessel dilatation on the right and absent tracer accumulation in ilioinguinal nodes

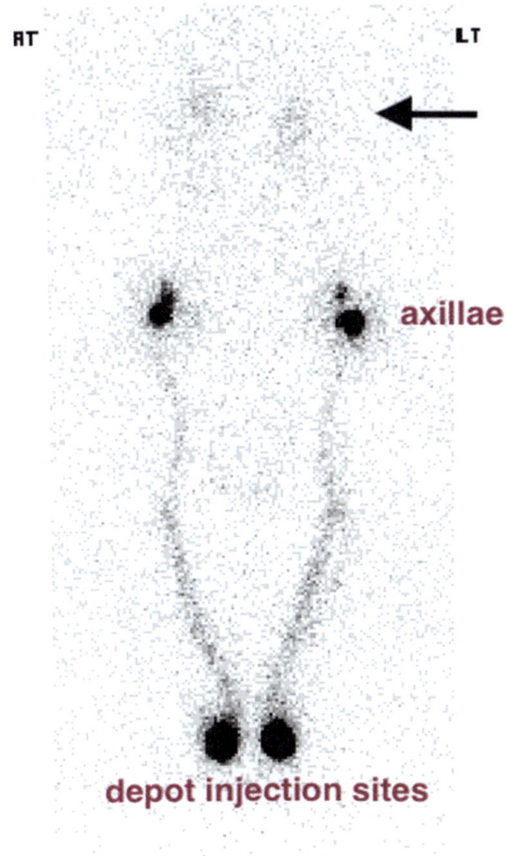

Fig. 22.13 Normal upper limb lymphoscintigraphy. Note reverse patient orientation (kidneys arrowed)

for ilioinguinal activity is 8–30%. Values below 8% suggest lymphatic dysfunction while those above 30% suggest venous disease. There is no normal range for axillary quantification. Ideally, in the lower limbs, these two quantitative approaches can be combined, thereby expressing nodal activity as a percentage of the activity *leaving* the injection depot, and therefore accounting for activity in transit in the lymphatic vessels of the limb (Fig. 22.17).

22.5.2 SNI

SNI is used in several cancers, most frequently breast cancer. Tc-99m-nanocolloid is injected into the peri-areolar skin of the breast. Intradermal injection is chosen over deeper intraparenchymal injection because it delivers tracer rapidly to the axillary lymph nodes. It is argued, however, that intraparenchymal injection more closely follows the route of malignant cells. The injection is made several hours before axillary dissection. Using a hand-held probe during surgery, the surgeon identifies the 'hottest' lymph node, deemed the sentinel node, and resects it. If the sentinel node is free of disease, it is concluded that the axilla is free of disease and axillary clearance surgery avoided. Some departments image the

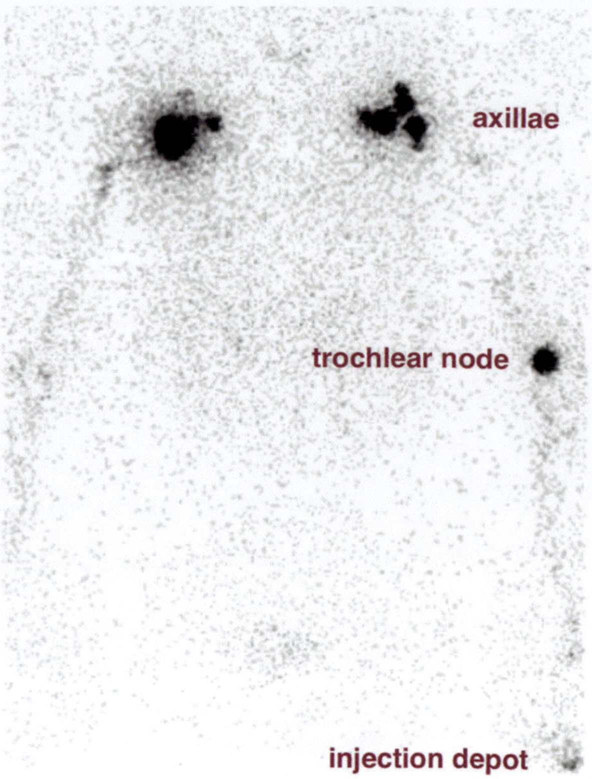

Fig. 22.14 Trochlear nodes at the elbow are a normal finding in upper limb lymphoscintigraphy

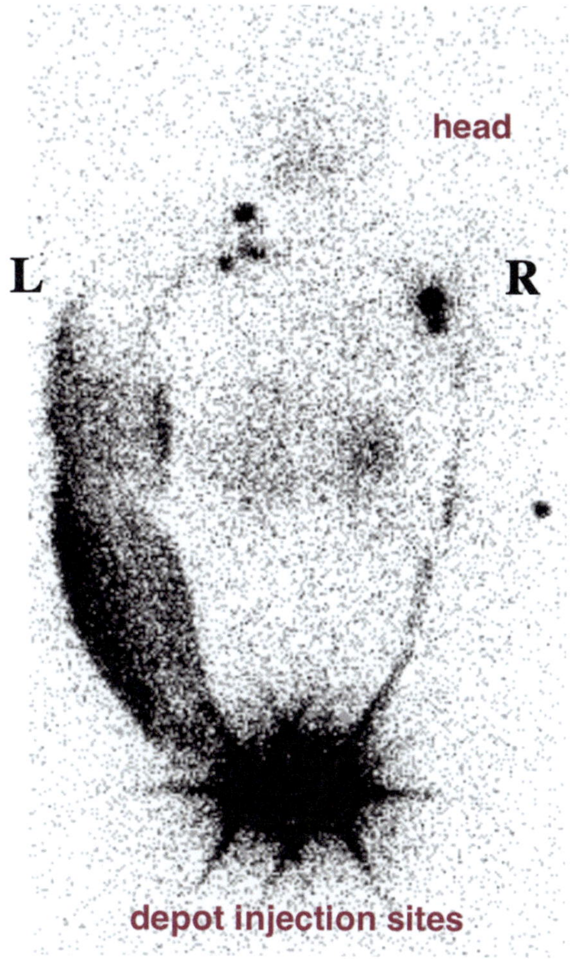

Fig. 22.15 Skin diversion in the left forearm of a patient with breast cancer-related lymphoedema. Note absence of lymph node activity in the left axilla. Cervical nodes are seen instead. The dot on the right is a radioactive marker which conventionally indicates the right side of the patient

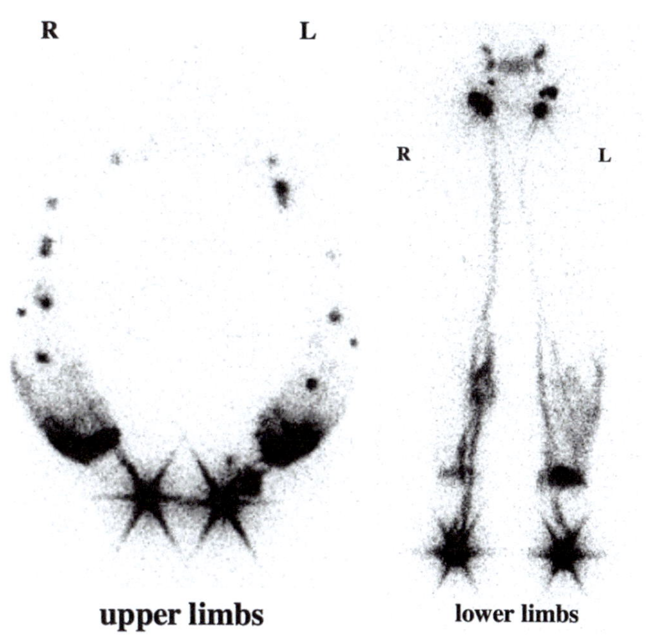

Fig. 22.16 Four-limb lymphoedema, the occurrence of which emphasises the constitutional nature of lymphoedema

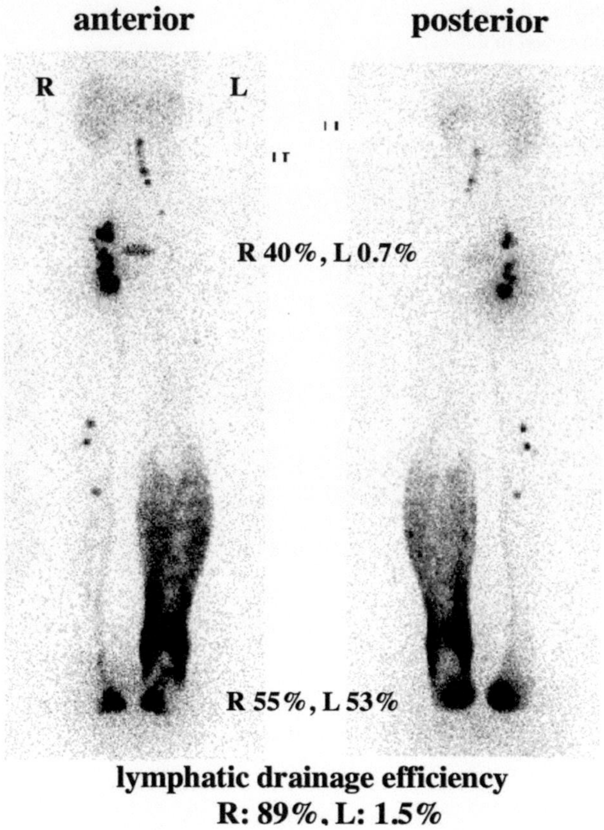

Fig. 22.17 Same patient as in Fig. 21.7. Depot retention is compared with ilioinguinal nodal quantification. Depot retention on the right is 55%, meaning 45% has left the depot. On the left, depot retention is 53%. Ilioinguinal nodal activity on the right is 40% of administered activity, meaning that 89% of activity leaving the depot has reached the ilioinguinal nodes (i.e. 40/45). In contrast, the corresponding value on the left is only 1.5%. This is called the lymphatic drainage efficiency and gives a quantitative measure of how efficiently the lymphatic system transports tracer leaving the depot. Thus, on the left, almost all of the activity leaving the depot is held up in the skin of the leg

axilla to identify the sentinel node prior to surgery, and nodes further down the chain (lower echelon nodes). Imaging may also determine whether the drainage basin includes the internal mammary nodes.

Further Reading

1. Peters AM, Mortimer PS. "Latent" and "constitutional" lymphedema, useful terms to complement the terms "primary" and "secondary" lymphedema. J Vasc Surg Venous Lymphat Disord. 2021 Sep;9(5):1089–92.
2. Stanton AWB, Modi S, Mellor RH, Levick JR, Mortimer PS. Recent advances in breast cancer-related lymphedema of the arm: lymphatic pump failure and predisposing factors. Lymphat Res Biol. 2009;7:29–45.

Part V

Miscellaneous Radiopharmaceuticals

In addition to Tc-99m, there are many other radionuclides used in nuclear medicine practice, the most important of which are Kr-81m, Se-75, In-111 and the radionuclides of iodine, especially I-123. Others that are no longer used are nevertheless covered in this part because of their historical interest.

Noble Gases

23

23.1 Krypton-81m (Half-Life 13 sec; 190 keV)

Kr-81m is an inert (noble) gas with an ultra-short half-life of 13 sec. It is the generator-produced, metastable daughter of Rb-81, which decays by electron capture to stable Kr-81 via Kr-81m. Rb-81 has a half-life of 4 h, so a Rb-81m generator has a lifespan of 1 day. The generator is connected to an air cylinder. Air in the exit portal contains Kr-81m, which is continuously inhaled by the patient. Continuous inhalation of a long-lived inert radioactive gas, such as Xe-133, gives an image of regional lung volume. Kr-81m, however, because of its very short half-life, gives an image of regional distribution of ventilation, as can be shown from the Fick principle.

$$dM / dt = V.C_{\mathrm{i}} - \left[\left(V / V'\right) + \lambda\right].M \qquad (23.1)$$

where C_i is the Kr-81m concentration in inspired air, M is the amount of Kr-81 in a lung ROI, V' is volume of the lung in the ROI (ml), V is ventilation (ml/min) and λ is the decay constant of Kr-81m (0.05 sec^{-1}; i.e., 5% decay per second). Note that V/V' is ventilatory turnover with unit of min^{-1}.

The gas is inspired to steady state, which, because of the short half-life, is reached rapidly, whereupon $dM/dt = 0$. Equation 23.1 can therefore be rearranged accordingly

$$M = \frac{V.C_{\mathrm{i}}}{V / V' + \lambda} \qquad (23.2)$$

For Xe-133, λ is negligible, so Eq. 23.2 reduces to

$$M = V'.C_{\mathrm{i}} \qquad (23.3)$$

and M reflects regional lung volume. For Kr-81m, however, V/V' is negligible compared with λ, so Eq. 23.2 reduces to

$$M = V.C_{\mathrm{i}} / \lambda \qquad (23.4)$$

and M reflects regional ventilation.

Kr-81m is the ideal agent for ventilation imaging in VQ lung scanning. Thus, it is easy for patients to inhale and gives high-quality images because its short half-life allows high doses to be administered. It has a photon energy higher than that of Tc-99m, so the Q signal does not interfere with V images. During planar imaging, the air delivery can be switched on and off, and V and Q imaged without moving the patient, going from projection to projection. Or SPECT can be performed, first on either perfusion or ventilation, then immediately on to the other, or simultaneously by dual photon acquisition. Finally, the patient breathes the gas in the supine position, the same in which the Tc-99m-MAA is administered, thereby matching the effects of gravity on Q.

A. M. Peters, M. Vadrucci, *Introduction to Nuclear Medicine for Trainees in Imaging and Imaging Sciences*, https://doi.org/10.1007/978-3-032-18364-4_23

In small children, ventilatory turnover (V/V') is more rapid than in adults and not so low compared with λ. The Kr-81m signal is therefore slightly weighted towards depicting regional lung volume. It is nevertheless still ideal for VQ imaging in children.

23.2 Xenon-133 (Half-Life 5.2 Days; Decays by Beta Minus Emission to Cs-133; Gamma Energy 81 keV)

Xe-133 is the other noble gas to find a role in nuclear medicine—historically a very important role. It was originally given over a limited number of breaths for *V* imaging in VQ lung scanning.

Administered in solution, its other role is measurement of tissue perfusion. The inert gases are lipid and water soluble, and rapidly diffusible. Following bolus injection into an artery, Xe-133 rapidly enters the entire space of the organ (including intracellular space) so that venous (C_v) and tissue (C_t) concentrations equalise almost instantly. It is then washed out of the organ at a rate that depends on organ perfusion, as shown below, with the minus sign indicating that dM/dt, the rate at which activity leaves the organ, declines over time. After washout from the tissue, the tracer is trapped in the lung and exhaled. There is therefore no recirculation.

$$\begin{aligned} dM/dt &= -Q \cdot C_V \\ &= -Q \cdot C_t \\ &= \frac{-Q \cdot M}{V''} \end{aligned} \tag{23.5}$$

where V'' is tissue volume.

dM/dt is a function of M, so Eq. 23.5 is exponential and tissue perfusion is measured as the rate constant, Q/V'', with which the tissue radioactivity declines.

Following the same principles for ventilation imaging described above, Kr-81m can also be given in solution as a continuous arterial infusion to provide real-time imaging of changes in the regional distribution of tissue blood flow, such as in the myocardium for which it has been widely used in research studies.

In addition to inert gases, the other group of agents used for VQ scanning are aerosols of nebulised tracer, such as Tc-99m-DTPA, or an agent called *Technegas* (Chap. 18).

23.2.1 Reporting a VQ Lung Scan

The pulmonary circulation is a low-pressure system, and so distribution of pulmonary blood flow is influenced by gravity. For VQ scintigraphy, Tc-99m-MAA should therefore be injected with the patient supine, otherwise relatively few particles will reach the apices (Fig. 23.1). First, correctly identify the ventilation and perfusion scans. The *V* scan from an aerosol usually has activity in the mouth, and some may be seen in airways, stomach and kidneys. The *Q* scan may show aggregates of Tc-99m-MAA as focal hot spots (Fig 23.2).

The diagnostic feature of pulmonary embolism (PE) in a VQ scan is a perfusion defect of segmental shape and size that is not matched on the ventilation scan—the unmatched perfusion defect (Figs. 23.3 and 23.4). Matched VQ defects are seen in airway disease, including asthma, the pathophysiological explanation for which is that pulmonary blood flow supplying a hypoxic region of lung

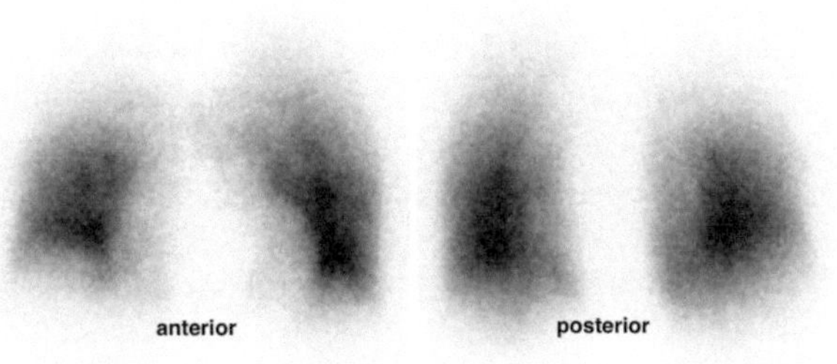

Fig. 23.1 Poor visualisation of upper zones as a result of injection of Tc-99-MAA with the patient sitting rather than supine

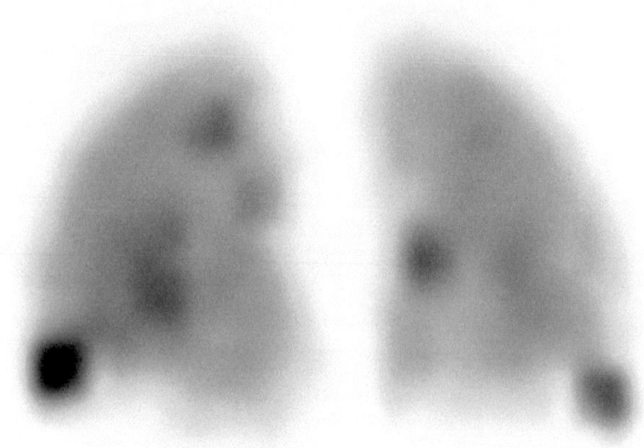

Fig. 23.2 Multiple 'hot spots' in a perfusion lung scan resulting from aggregates of Tc-99m-MAA

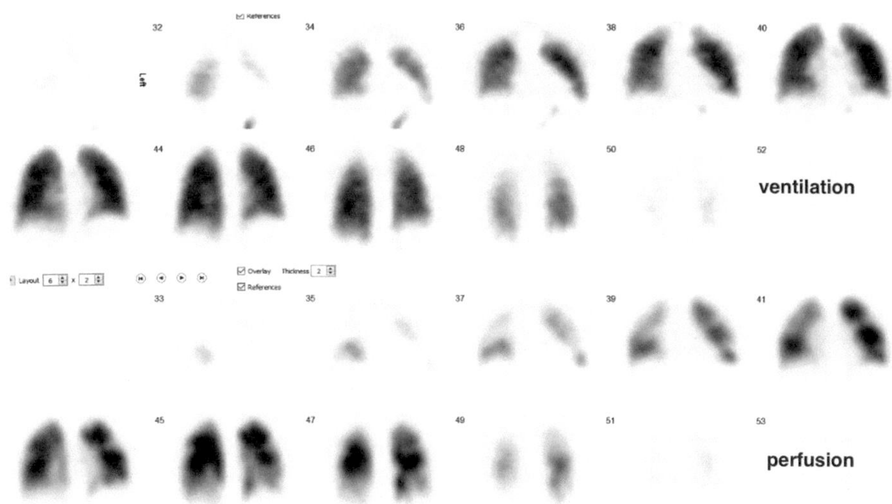

Fig. 23.3 Coronal slices of SPECT VQ lung scan showing bilateral mismatched perfusion defects typical of pulmonary embolism

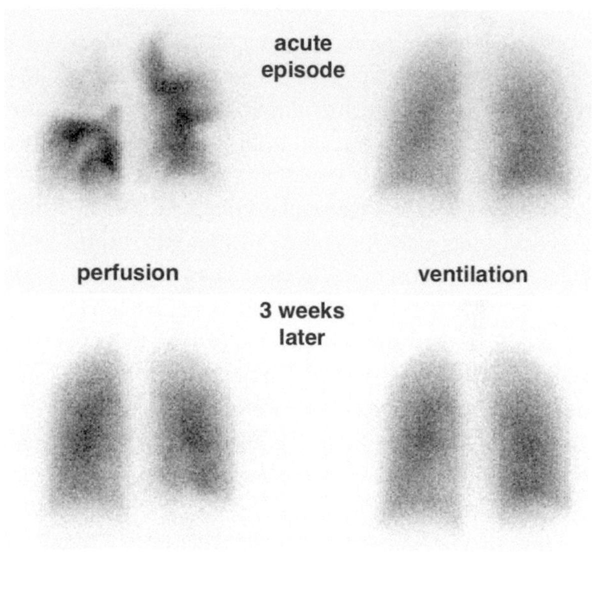

Fig. 23.4 Planar lung VQ lung scan showing resolution of acute pulmonary embolism. During the acute episode of breathlessness and chest pain, the VQ scan shows mismatched perfusion defects. Scan 3 weeks later shows complete resolution of the perfusion defects

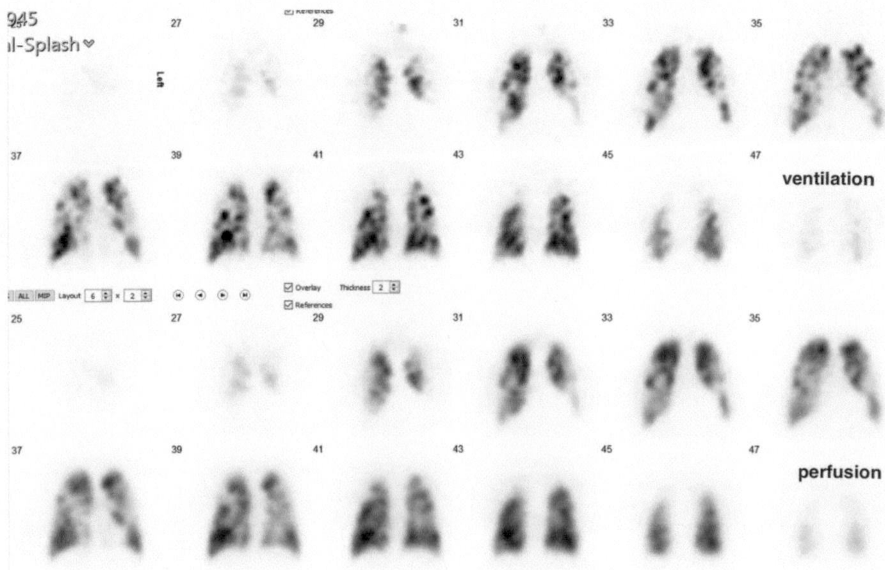

Fig. 23.5 Multiple matched ventilation and perfusion defects typically seen in chronic obstructive pulmonary disease. There are no mismatched perfusion defects to suggest pulmonary embolism

shuts down to avoid physiological right-to-left shunting that would otherwise produce hypoxaemia (Fig. 23.5). This is called hypoxic vasoconstriction. Pleural effusion (Fig. 23.6) causes lung compression and abolishes regional *V* but allows some perfusion to continue, giving rise to 'reversed' mismatching. The resulting physiological right-to-left shunting should be mentioned in the report as it may account for the breathlessness that gave rise to the clinical suspicion of pulmonary embolism in the first place. Lung consolidation also causes reversed mismatching because alveolae are full of exudate, but the pulmonary capillaries remain open. A less well-recognised cause of reversed mismatching is left ventricular enlargement. This causes lung compression and right-to-left shunting in the supine position, explaining the orthostatic breathlessness of left ventricular failure.

Focal lung pathology, such as tumours, bronchiectasis and abscesses, gives matched defects (Fig. 23.7). Lung cancer, however, may give lobar or whole lung mismatched perfusion defects because of compression of a major branch of the pulmonary artery (Fig. 23.8). Pulmonary infarcts, although considered to be the cause of pleuritic chest pain—a common presenting feature of patients suspected of having acute PE are rarely seen in VQ scanning, probably because the nutrient blood supply of the lung is predominantly through the bronchial circulation. The cause of pleuritic chest pain is therefore unclear. Patients presenting with pleuritic chest pain as their only symptom rarely have PE! With high-quality ventilation imaging—usually requiring Kr-81m—a pulmonary infarct gives a focal perfusion defect larger than the corresponding ventilation defect, i.e., a mismatched penumbra (Fig. 23.9).

Using Tc-99m-labelled aerosol or *Technegas*, *V* imaging must be performed before *Q* because the administered dose for perfusion needs to be higher to 'flood' the residual ventilation signal. In pregnant women, perfusion-only lung scanning is often performed to reduce radiation exposure to the foetus from urinary activity in the bladder. A normal *Q* scan reliably excludes PE but, if it is abnormal, *V* imaging is performed the following day. Because hypoxic vasoconstriction is reversible, however, the distribution of ventilation may change. If ventilation returns to normal overnight, a positive scan will be wrongly diagnosed. So, a delayed *V* scan is not ideal, hence the value of Kr-81m.

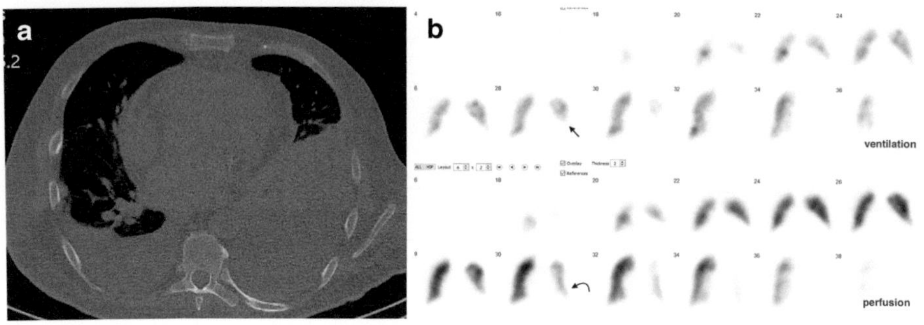

Fig. 23.6 Left pleural effusion (CT; **a**) causing reversed mismatching (coronal SPECT; **b**). Lower lobe perfusion (curved arrow) continues in face of reduced ventilation (straight arrow), thereby creating a right-to-left 'physiological shunt' and accounting for the patient's breathlessness

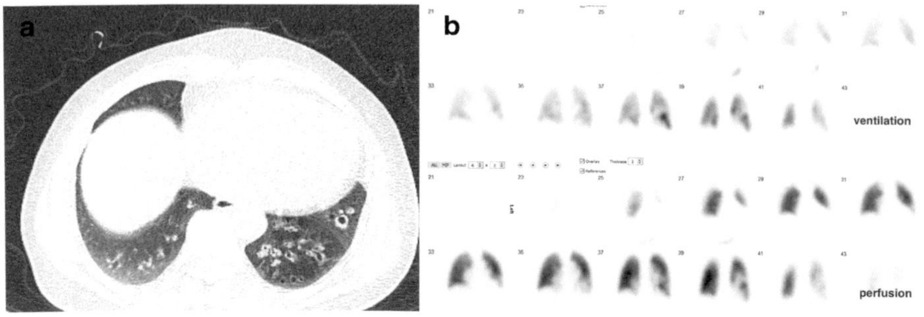

Fig. 23.7 Bronchiectasis, more prominent in left lower lobe, shown on low-dose CT (**a**) giving rise to matched reduced ventilation and perfusion on coronal VQ SPECT (**b**)

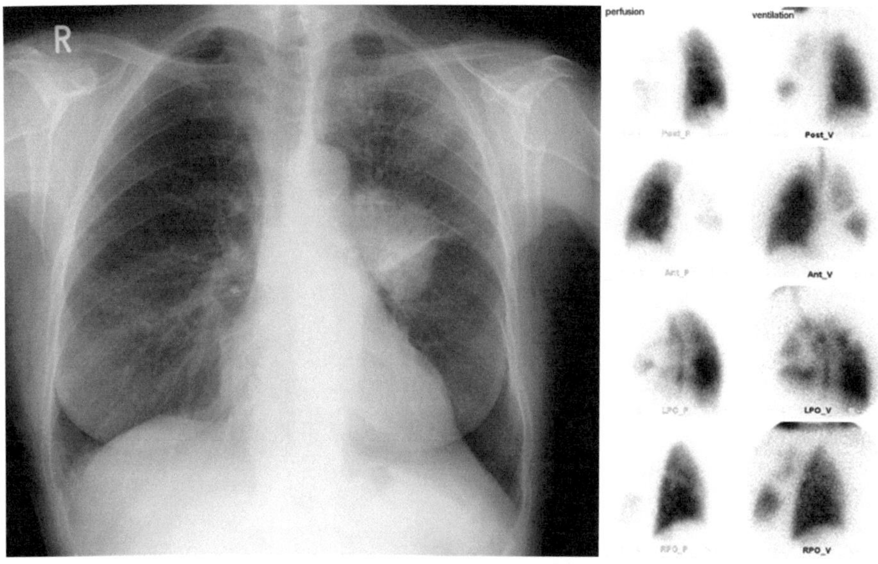

Fig. 23.8 Bronchial carcinoma (left panel) causing almost complete loss of perfusion to the left lung (right panel). Ventilation is also reduced but not by as much

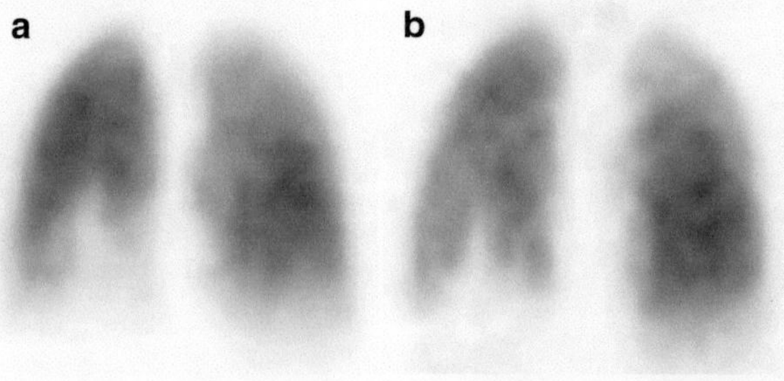

Fig. 23.9 Pulmonary infarction is a rare complication of pulmonary embolism probably because the structural elements of the lungs are supplied by the bronchial artery rather than pulmonary artery. Given its rarity, it does not adequately explain pleuritic chest pain, which, in contrast, is a common reason for referral for a VQ scan. In this patient, there is a matched defect but the perfusion defect (**a**) is clearly larger than the ventilation defect (**b**) in keeping with infarction

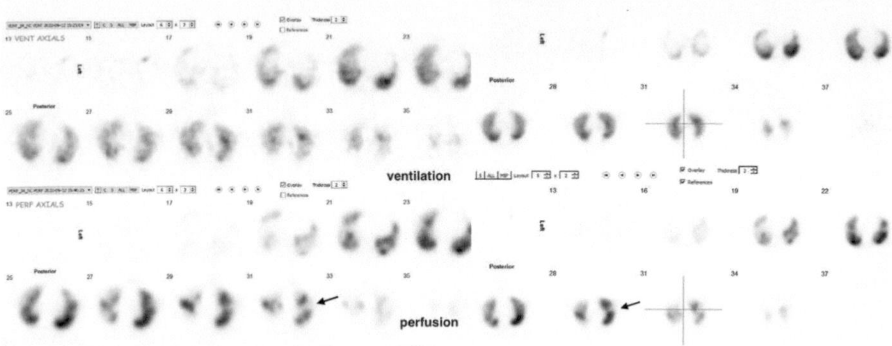

Fig. 23.10 When acute pulmonary embolism fails to resolve, it is called chronic pulmonary embolism. These two axial SPECT VQ lung scans showing bilateral mismatched perfusion defects were recorded 3 years apart and illustrate chronic pulmonary embolism, which may lead to pulmonary hypertension (CTEPH). VQ scintigraphy is unable to distinguish between acute and chronic pulmonary embolism

An embolic perfusion defect that fails to resolve is called chronic PE. When chronic pulmonary emboli are multiple, pulmonary hypertension may develop. Chronic and acute PE are indistinguishable on VQ scanning (Fig. 23.10). Recommending follow-up VQ scintigraphy within 2–3 weeks of a diagnosis of pulmonary embolism is therefore reasonable to check for resolution (Fig. 23.4). Lack of resolution suggests pre-existing chronic rather than acute embolism as the cause of the mismatched perfusion defect.

Causes of mismatched perfusion abnormalities other than PE include (a) interstitial lung disease in which fibrosis, usually bilateral and predominantly involving the lower lobes, obliterates alveolar septal capillaries (Fig. 23.11), (b) emphysema for the same reason, (c) sequestered lung which receives no pulmonary blood supply and (d) bronchial carcinoma. Upper lobe diversion of pulmonary blood flow in heart disease may also give the impression of mismatched reduced perfusion in the lower lobes (Fig. 23.12).

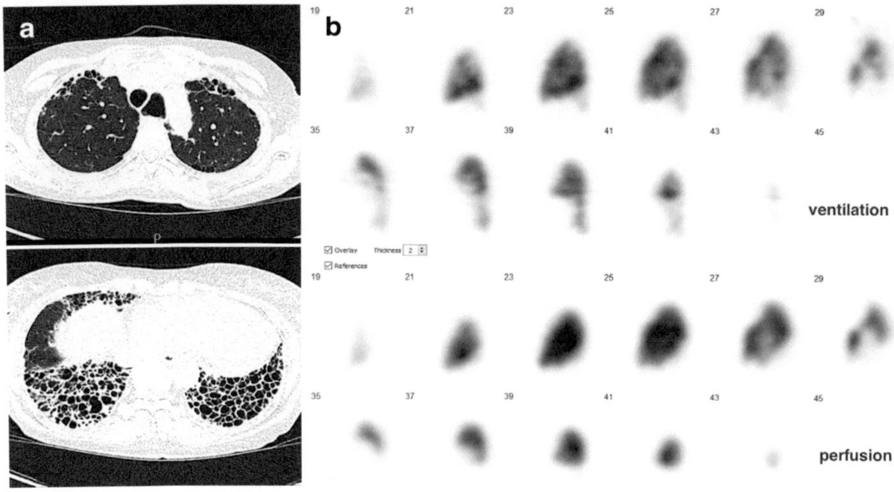

Fig. 23.11 Interstitial lung disease involves lower lobes and reduces perfusion more than ventilation because of obliteration of pulmonary alveolar capillaries. (**a**) CT (upper panel: upper zones; lower panel: lower zones). (**b**) Sagittal VQ SPECT, showing reduced perfusion in lower lobes with maintenance of some ventilation

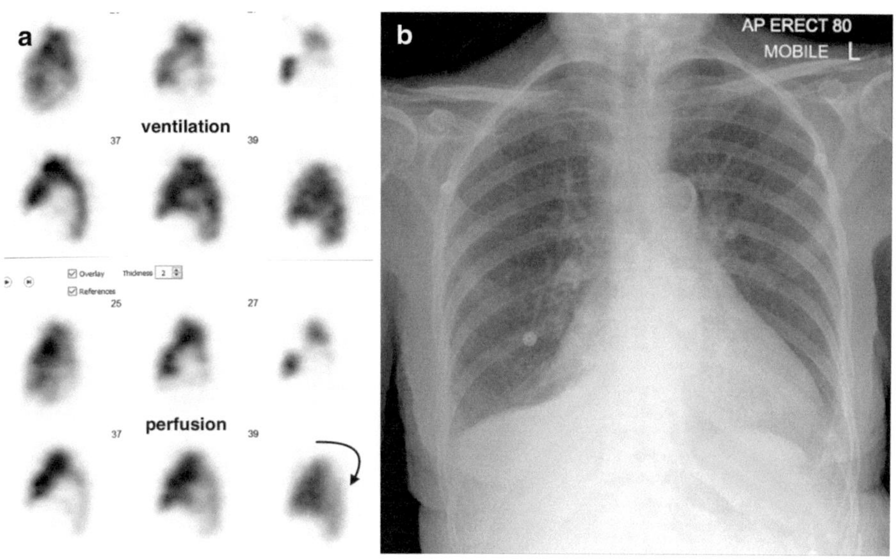

Fig. 23.12 Upper lobe diversion of pulmonary blood flow (**a**; curved arrow) occurs in patients with cardiovascular disease (**b**). Because it gives rise to ventilation/perfusion mismatching, it may be misinterpreted as pulmonary embolism

Further Reading

1. Alexander MS, Peters AM, Cleland JP, Lavender JP. Impaired left lower lobe ventilation in patients with cardiomegaly. An isotope study of mechanisms. Chest. 1992;101:1189–93.
2. Bajc M, Bauer RW, Schümichen C, et al. EANM guideline for ventilation/perfusion single-photon emission computed tomography (SPECT) for diagnosis of pulmonary embolism and beyond. Eur J Nucl Med Mol Imaging. 2019;46:2429–51.
3. Selwyn AP, Steiner R, Kivisaari FK, Forse G. Krypton-81m in the physiologic assessment of coronary arterial stenosis in man. Am J Cardiol. 1979;43:547–53.
4. Strickland NH, Hughes JM, Hart DA, Myers MJ, Lavender JP. Cause of regional ventilation-perfusion mismatching in patients with idiopathic pulmonary fibrosis: a combined CT and scintigraphic study. Am J Roentgenol. 1993;161:719–25.

Iodine-123 (Half-Life 13.2 h; Decays by Electron Capture to Te-123) and Iodine-131 (8.1 d, Beta Minus Emission, Xe-131)

24

24.1 Free Iodine

I-123 (159 keV) and I-131 (364 keV) are both used to image thyroid disease along similar lines to those described under pertechnetate (Tc-99mO_4) in Chap. 10. They have the additional role of imaging thyroid cancer, either in a diagnostic setting with I-123 and whole-body imaging for detection of metastases, or for therapy with I-131 in thyrotoxicosis or thyroid cancer. The thyroid has greater avidity for iodine than Tc-99mO_4, so normal ranges for thyroid uptake are higher.

24.2 I-123-Ioflupane ('DaT Scan') (MW 431 Da)

Dopamine is the neurotransmitter in the nerve terminals of the tracts from the midbrain that terminate in the basal ganglia. The secreted dopamine binds to dopamine transporters (DaT) located in the pre-synaptic nerve terminal and is returned to the nerve terminal for reuse. I-123-ioflupane binds to DaT and displays the integrity of the midbrain tracts. F-18-labelled DOPA (dihydroxyphenylalanine, a dopamine precursor) is the corresponding PET tracer for imaging basal ganglia. Dopaminergic function declines with age.

The shape of the corpus in normal DaT transaxial SPECT resembles a comma (Fig. 24.1) but typically in idiopathic Parkinson's disease (IPD) looks instead like a full stop (Fig. 24.2). There are variations in these typical pictures, including reduced accumulation in the caudate nuclei. Severe loss of dopaminergic function appears as reduced uptake throughout the corpora that may or may not be symmetrical (Fig. 24.3). Because of image scaling, background cerebral activity frequently looks very prominent in such patients. This is not because background activity is increased. Because only a tiny percentage of administered activity reaches the basal ganglia, reduced tracer accumulation in them has almost no impact on the whole-body tracer distribution. So, in your report, do not say 'background is increased' because it won't be.

A. M. Peters, M. Vadrucci, *Introduction to Nuclear Medicine for Trainees in Imaging and Imaging Sciences*, https://doi.org/10.1007/978-3-032-18364-4_24

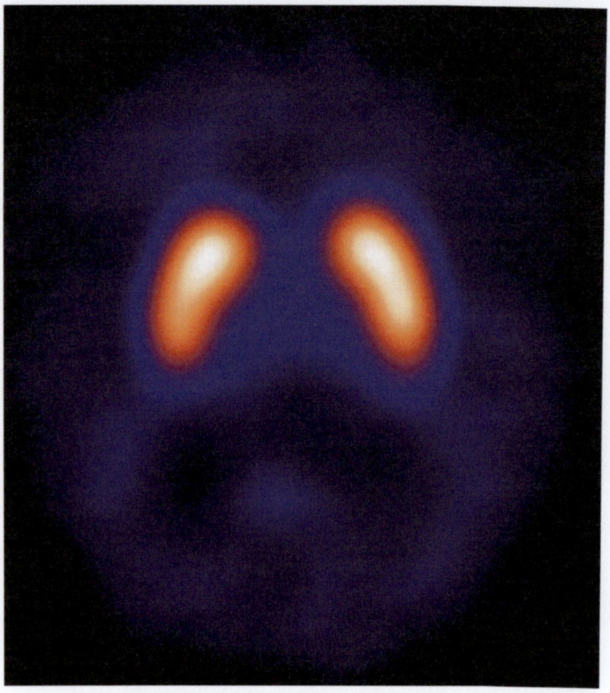

Fig. 24.1 Normal I-123-ioflupane ('DaT') SPECT. The corpus resembles a comma

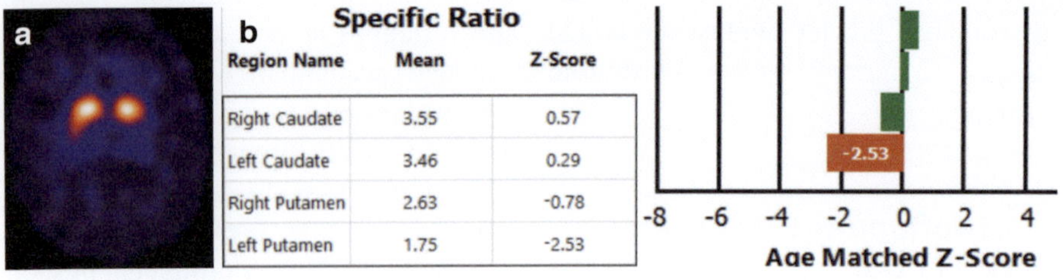

Region Name	Mean	Z-Score
Right Caudate	3.55	0.57
Left Caudate	3.46	0.29
Right Putamen	2.63	-0.78
Left Putamen	1.75	-2.53

Fig. 24.2 I-123-ioflupane SPECT in a patient with idiopathic Parkinson's disease showing a left corpus resembling a full stop and a normal right corpus resembling a comma (**a**). Quantification is based on z scores for each of the four elements of the basal ganglia (**b**). A score of less than −1.96, which is two standard deviations below the population mean for the patient's age, is considered abnormal, although some departments use a cut-off of 1.5

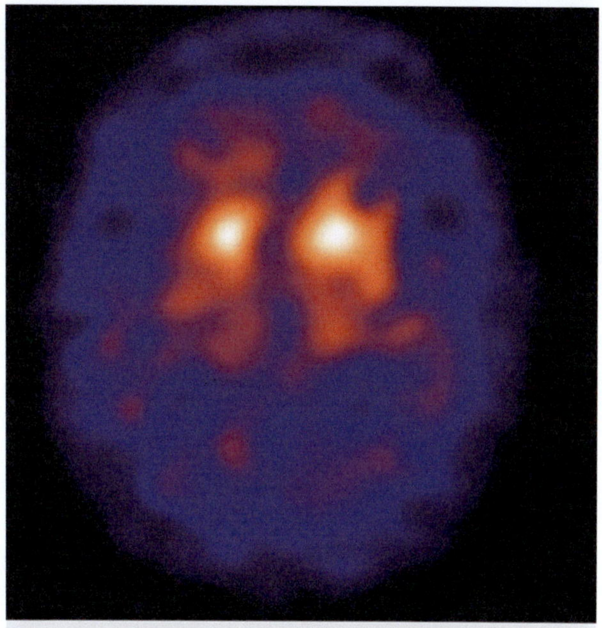

I-123-ioflupane SPECT

Specific Ratio

Region Name	Mean	Z-Score
Right Caudate	1.22	-3.74
Left Caudate	1.38	-3.61
Right Putamen	0.74	-4.35
Left Putamen	1.00	-3.91

Fig. 24.3 Abnormal I-123-ioflupane SPECT showing global, symmetrical and reduced tracer accumulation in the basal ganglia. Note that the brain background looks prominent, but this is not because it is increased but instead is the result of image scaling. Grossly abnormal findings such as these raise the likelihood of a Parkinson plus syndrome

DaT scintigraphy is performed either for extrapyramidal signs and symptoms or for dementia, especially from Lewy body disease (LBD). Corticobasal degeneration (CBD) is also associated with an abnormal scan, typically described as balanced loss. DaT scans, however, are not specific and serve to indicate dopaminergic dysfunction rather than diagnose its cause. There may, however, be clues. For example, unilateral reduced putaminal uptake suggests idiopathic Parkinson's disease (IPD) (Fig. 24.2), while the impression of a random distribution of abnormal uptake would suggest vascular Parkinsonism. Severe global dopaminergic dysfunction should raise a suspicion of a Parkinson plus syndrome, such as MSA or PSP (Fig. 24.3). Distinguishing between IPD and a Parkinson plus syndrome may be achieved with myocardial I-123-MIBG scintigraphy (see below).

Dopaminergic dysfunction with I-123-ioflupane is quantified by measuring the counts in all four elements of the basal ganglia as a ratio with the counts in a cerebral reference region, usually cerebellum. Whereas quantification in other systems in nuclear medicine is expressed in relation to a normal range, I-123-ioflupane uptake in a corpus ROI is expressed as a z score (Figs. 6.1 and 24.2). This is the number of standard deviations with which the corpus-to-background count ratio departs from the mean ratio derived from an aged-matched control population. An ROI z score of −1.96 indicates that the count ratio is 97.5% likely to be abnormally reduced. The other 2.5% is for the upper limit of normal, although an abnormally increased ratio is not recognised to be associated with pathology. The corresponding percentage for a z score of −1.5, which some departments use as the cut-off for normal, is 6.7%. Quantification of F-18-DOPA uses Patlak-Rutland analysis (Chap. 3) for measurement of tracer clearance into the basal ganglia.

24.2.1 Reporting a DaT Scan

Firstly, decide from the images alone whether the scan looks normal or abnormal, then check your impression from the quantification. Usually, the latter is concordant with the images. If the imaging is equivocal, the quantification takes on greater importance. If the overall interpretation remains uncertain, a repeat study in 12–18 months can be suggested. Alternatively, myocardial I-123-MIBG scintigraphy can be suggested. Absent myocardial uptake supports IPD or LBD. This is especially relevant to LBD which has a false-negative rate of about 20% with I-123-ioflupane. I-123-MIBG myocardial scintigraphy is usually normal in Parkinson plus syndromes (MSA and PSP) and in CBD.

24.3 I-123-Metaiodobenzylguanidine (MIBG) (MW 324 Da)

I-123-MIBG is an analogue of noradrenaline and accordingly accumulates in adrenergic tissue. Analogous to dopamine in the basal ganglia, noradrenaline secreted at sympathetic nerve terminals binds to a protein called noradrenaline transporter (NAT) and undergoes reuptake and storage in the pre-synaptic terminal for reuse. Chromaffin cells in the adrenal medulla and in paraganglia also express NAT and accumulate I-123-MIBG. I-123-MIBG is therefore used to image phaeochromocytoma and paraganglioma. Other neuroendocrine tumours also accumulate I-123-MIBG, including carcinoid and medullary thyroid cancer.

I-123-MIBG is a small molecule that undergoes glomerular filtration. Normal whole-body distribution of activity is liver (because of metabolism), intestine (biliary excretion), urine (urinary excretion), myocardium (adrenergic innervation), lungs (amine uptake by the pulmonary arterial endothelium) and salivary glands (adrenergic innervation; note how you have a dry mouth prior to public speaking) (Fig. 24.4). Avoid misinterpreting an accessory parotid as a lesion (Fig. 24.5). Imaging is conventionally performed at 4 and 24 h post-injection, although single imaging at 6 h is acceptable to avoid second-day attendance. This carries a minor risk of a false negative outcome. Thus, normal adrenal glands are seen at 24 h post-injection but not 6 h. The clearance of tracer from blood is rapid, yet localisation in target tissue, is clearer at 24 h (e.g. normal adrenals) because of a complex process of tracer redistribution.

Other indications for I-123-MIBG are management of neuroblastoma, which is a childhood malignancy arising from embryonic neural crest cells (Fig. 24.6), and autonomic neuropathy, especially the neuropathy of IPD, in which—unlike Parkinson-plus syndromes and CBD—there is reduced myocardial uptake (Fig. 24.7). As in IPD, there is reduced myocardial uptake in LBD.

Quantification of uptake is expressed as the ratio of activity in the myocardium to that in an ROI over the mediastinum (H-M ratio). Cut-off values reported in the literature for this ratio are variable but generally about 1.5. Lungs accumulate I-123-MIBG because of physiological uptake of amines in the pulmonary vascular endothelium (Fig. 24.7). (Radio-amine uptake was once used as a marker of lung function.) This may cause inaccuracy in the H-M ratio if the myocardial ROI includes any lung activity. There is also reduced myocardial accumulation in heart failure, giving rise to a potential false-positive for IPD.

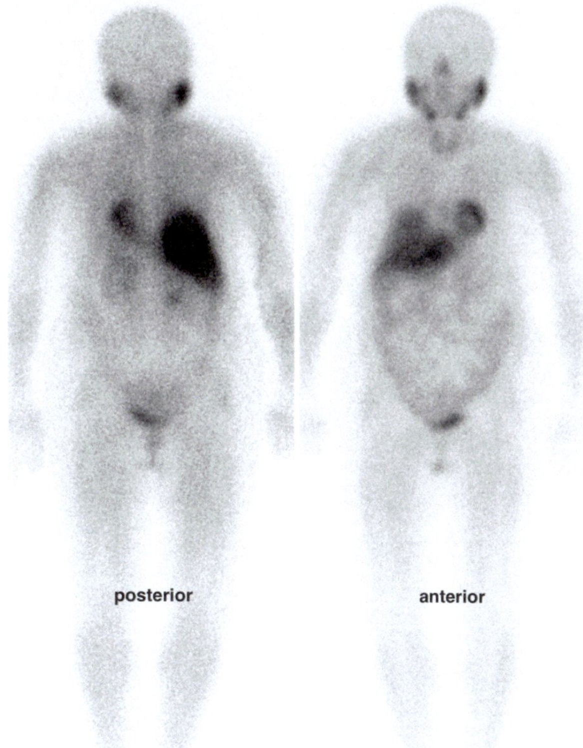

Fig. 24.4 Normal whole body I-123-MIBG scan 6 h post-injection. As a marker of the noradrenaline recycling receptor, tracer accumulation is seen in the salivary glands and myocardium. Hepatic activity reflects metabolism of the tracer. Thyroid activity is from free I-123. Intestinal and urinary activities are from hepatobiliary and renal excretion, respectively

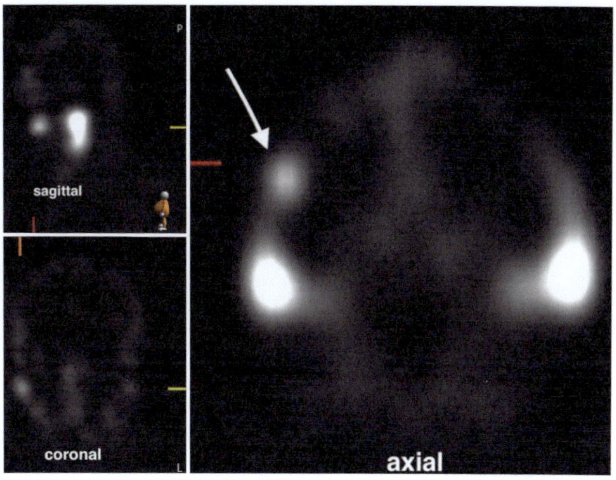

Fig. 24.5 An accessory parotid gland shown in this I-123-MIBG SPECT (arrow) is a normal variant and potential source of reporting error if not recognised as such

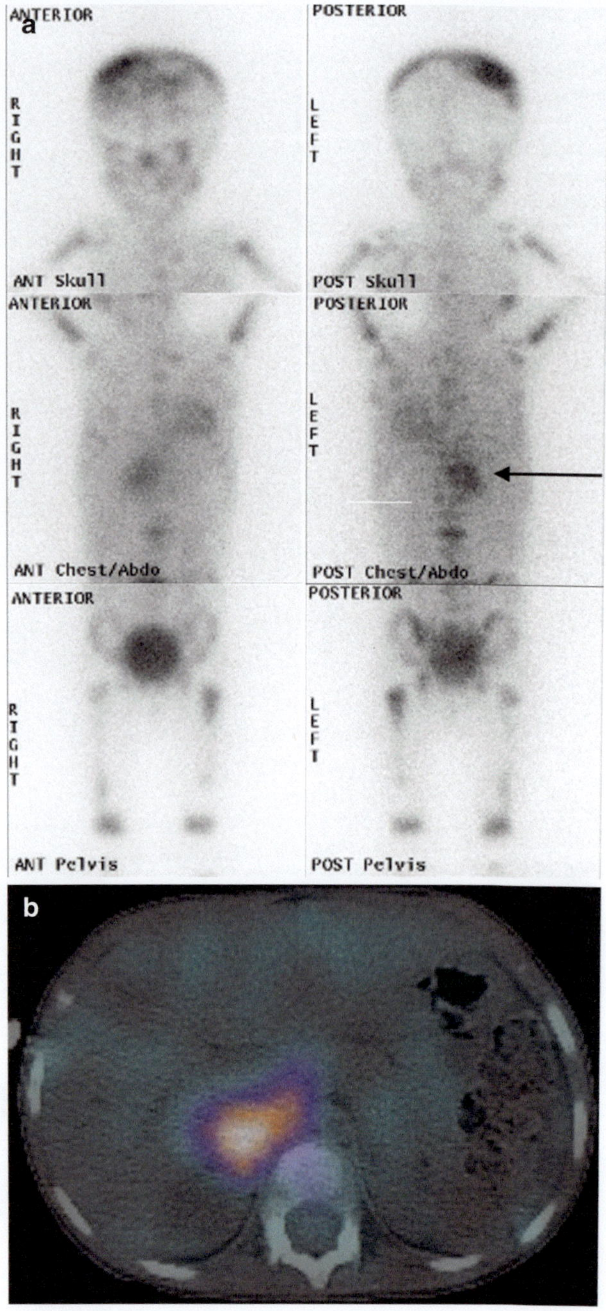

Fig. 24.6 (**a**) Neuroblastoma with skeletal involvement (arrow: soft tissue tumour). (**b**) SPECT/CT. Courtesy Lorenzo Biassoni, Hospital for Sick Children, London

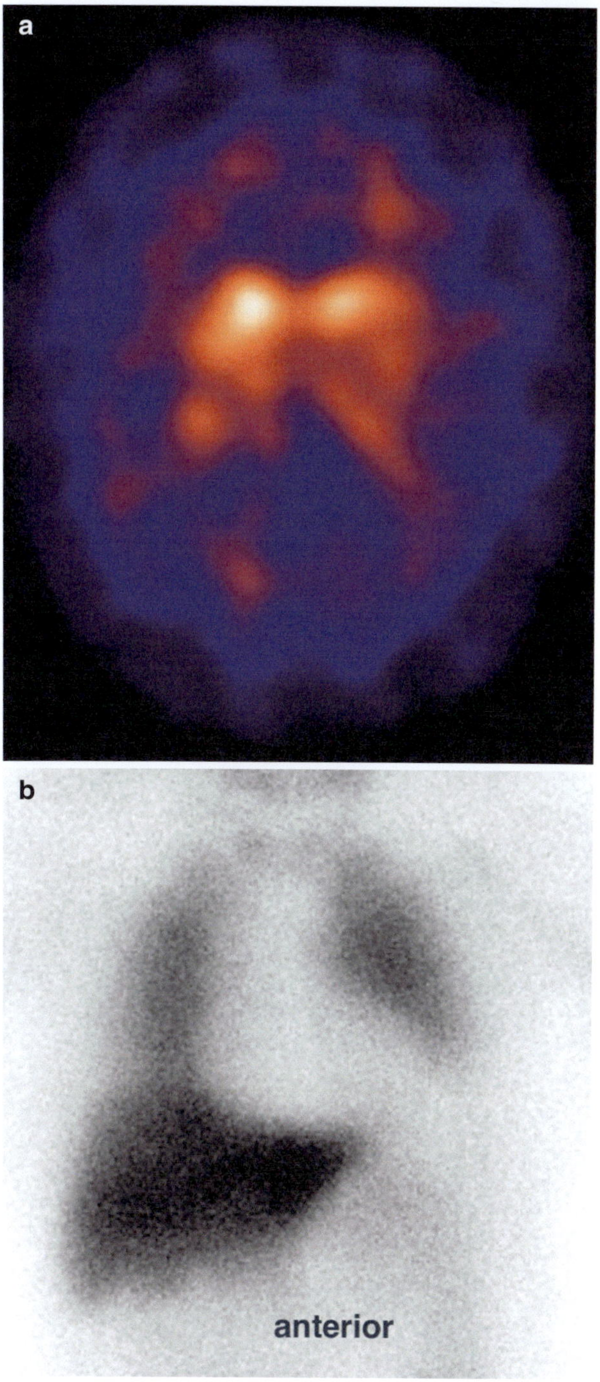

Fig. 24.7 Abnormal I-123-ioflupane SPECT in a patient with a Parkinsonian syndrome (**a**). The myocardial I-123-MIBG scan (**b**) shows absent tracer accumulation in the myocardium, favouring idiopathic Parkinson's disease. However, there is left ventricular dilatation so the absent uptake may instead be the result of heart failure, which can produce this picture. Note the prominent pulmonary tracer accumulation, which is physiological

24.3.1 Reporting an I-123-MIBG Scan

The role of I-123-MIBG in phaeochromocytoma and paraganglioma is to locate tumour and metastases in a patient with abnormal biochemistry (Figs. 24.8, 24.9 and 24.10) and abnormal CT. Hepatic uptake is usually quite prominent and on SPECT may appear heterogeneous. Homogeneous pulmonary activity may also be prominent but is normal (Fig. 24.7).

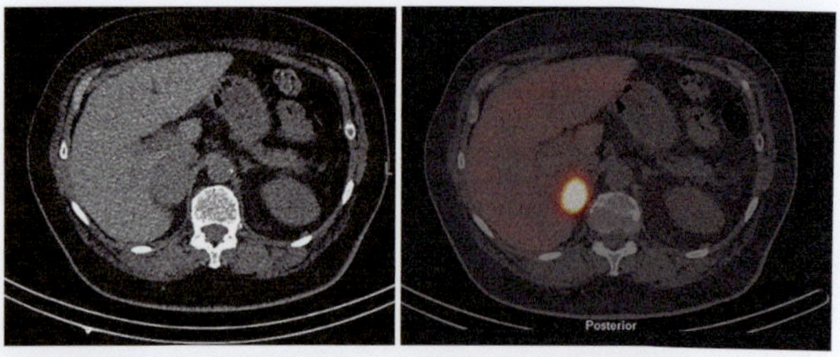

Fig. 24.8 CT (left panel) and I-123-MIBG SPECT/CT (right panel) showing a right-sided adrenal phaeochromocytoma

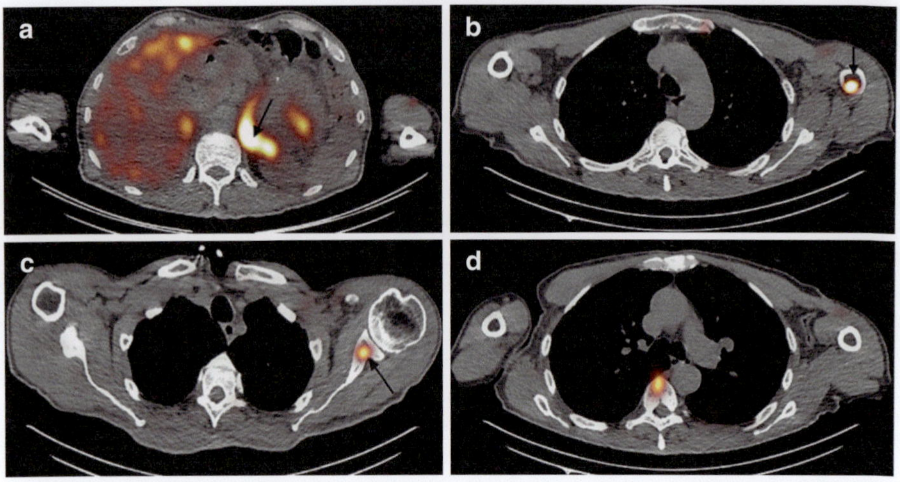

Fig. 24.9 I-123-MIBG SPECT/CT showing a left-sided phaeochromocytoma (**a**) with bone metastases in left humerus (**b**), left glenoid (**c**) and thoracic vertebra (**d**)

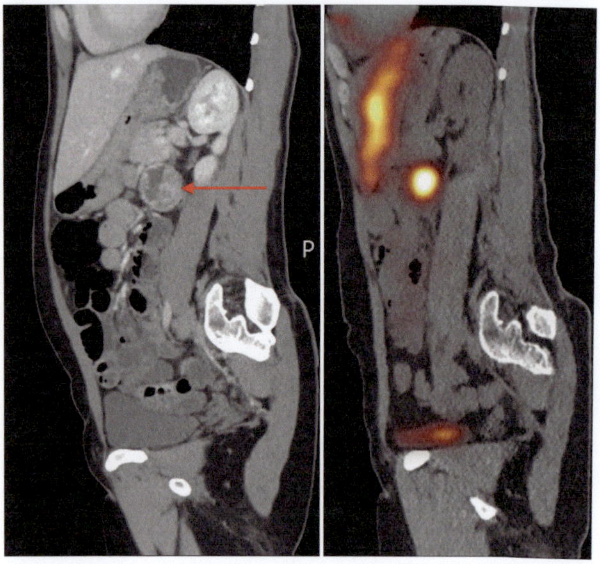

Fig. 24.10 Sagittal I-123-MIBG SPECT/CT showing a para-aortic paraganglioma (arrow)

24.4 I-123 Serum Amyloid P Component (MW 25 kDa)

SAP is a normal circulating protein involved in innate immunity against bacterial infections. It binds to amyloid fibrils and, labelled with I-123, is therefore an agent for imaging visceral amyloidosis (SAP scan). It has also been labelled with I-131 for whole-body counting and with I-125 for plasma clearance studies in amyloidosis. Plasma clearance halftime in healthy subjects is 24–30 h, but clearance is much faster in patients with heavy amyloid burden, who also show higher whole-body retention of tracer. In contrast to Tc-99 m-DPD (Chap. 15), I-123-SAP has not been successful for imaging myocardial amyloidosis nor brain amyloidosis because of its high molecular weight and therefore inability to penetrate the blood-brain barrier.

Further Reading

1. Blake GM, Lewington VJ, Zivanovic MA, Ackery DM. Glomerular filtration rate and the kinetics of ^{123}I-metaiodobenzylguanidine. Eur J Nucl Med. 1989;15:618–23.
2. Booij J, Busemann Sokole E, Stabin MG, Janssen AG, de Bruin K, van Royen EA. Human biodistribution and dosimetry of [123I]FP-CIT: a potent radioligand for imaging of dopamine transporters. Eur J Nucl Med. 1998;25:24–30.
3. Catalan M, Dore F, Polverino P, et al. ^{123}I-Metaiodobenzylguanidine myocardial scintigraphy in discriminating degenerative Parkinsonisms. Mov Disord Clin Pract. 2021;8:717–24.
4. Sayed RH, Hawkins PN, Lachmann HJ. Emerging treatments for amyloidosis. Kidney Int. 2015;87:516–26.

25 Selenium-75 (Half-Life 120 d; Decays by Electron Capture to As-75; 136, 265 and 401 keV)

25.1 Se-75-Homocholic Acid Taurine (MW 595 Da)

Se-75-HCAT is a bile acid analogue used for diagnosing bile acid diarrhoea (BAD). BAD results from excessive bile acid entry into the colon. It is common and frequently misdiagnosed as diarrhoea-predominant irritable bowel syndrome (IBS). It is subdivided into three types: type 1 BAD results from disease in or previous resection of the terminal ileum; type 2 is idiopathic BAD arising in otherwise healthy individuals and type 3 occurs in post-surgical patients, especially after cholecystectomy and vagotomy.

Following oral administration and terminal ileal absorption, Se-75-HCAT enters the whole-body bile acid pool and undergoes enterohepatic recirculation. It is slowly lost from the body via faecal excretion. To measure this loss, whole body counting using an uncollimated gamma camera is performed 1–3 h after ingestion and again at 7 days. Without its collimator, a gamma camera cannot form an image but becomes a highly sensitive radiation detector. Counts are recorded from the patient first facing the camera and then with back to it. As in Tc-99m-DMSA scintigraphy, the geometric mean ($\sqrt{[x \times y]}$) is calculated from the two counts and the 7-day count expressed as a percentage of the first day count to give whole-body retention (WBR). WBR values of 0–5%, 5–10% and 10–15% are respectively diagnosed as severe, moderate and mild BAD.

Enterohepatic bile acid recirculation is illustrated in Fig. 25.1. About 95% is reabsorbed on each pass through the terminal ileum. A further 1% is absorbed in the colon, so ~4% is lost into the faeces per cycle. Recycling frequency is 4–6 per day. For a recycling frequency of 5 per day, 20% of Se-75-HCAT would be lost per day giving an exponential decline in whole body Se-75-HCAT content with a rate constant of 0.2 day^{-1}. From Eq. 1.4, it can be calculated that WBR at 7 days would be 25%. When ileal reabsorption is impaired or recycling rate is increased, WBR at 7 days will be reduced (Fig. 25.2). Thus, a recycling frequency of 8 per day would give a WBR of 10.6% for a normal 96% reabsorption per cycle.

Impaired retention in type 1 BAD is readily attributed to bile acid malabsorption in diseased ileum. In type 2, however, patients are generally well and, as a group, no structural or functional abnormalities in the terminal ileum have been demonstrated, raising the probability that impaired retention may be the result of increased recycling rate. This notion is supported, for example, by the high prevalence of reduced WBR and BAD seen following cholecystectomy, which, in the absence of gall bladder storage, increases recycling rate. Of the four segments of the bile acid journey, illustrated in Fig. 25.1, the longest is ampulla to terminal ileum. Patients

A. M. Peters, M. Vadrucci, *Introduction to Nuclear Medicine for Trainees in Imaging and Imaging Sciences*, https://doi.org/10.1007/978-3-032-18364-4_25

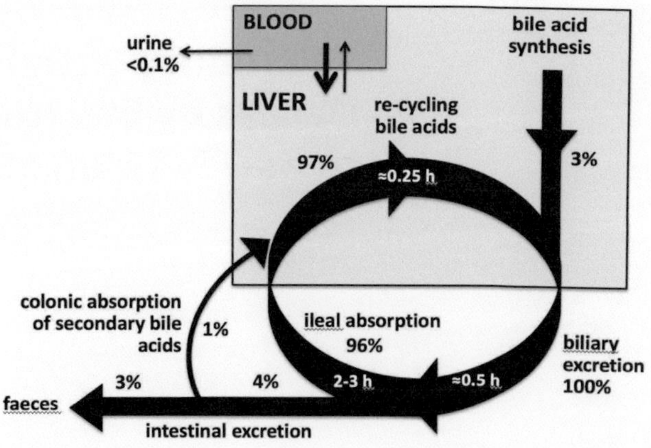

Fig. 25.1 Diagram summarising bile acid recycling. (From Peters and Walters [2]). Ileal absorption is shown as 96% in this diagram

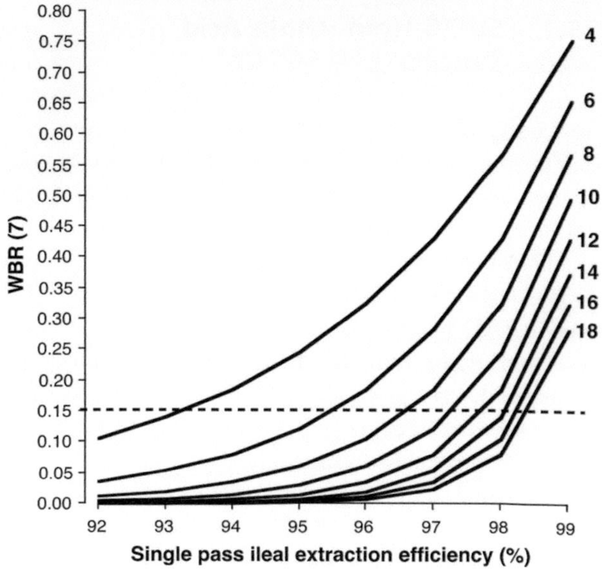

Fig. 25.2 Whole body retention of Se-75-HCAT as a function of bile acid recycling frequency and single pass ileal extraction efficiency. (Reprinted from Peters and Walters [2])

with rapid intestinal transit, therefore, such as those with autonomic neuropathy, are likely to have BAD. Moreover, IBS and BAD may overlap insofar as IBS causes increased intestinal transit which in turn causes increased bile acid recycling rate.

Enterocytes in the terminal ileum sense intraluminal bile acid concentration and, in response, secrete a hormone called FGF19 which passes to the liver via the portal vein and inhibits the rate-limiting enzyme for bile acid synthesis. To explain why BAD should occur despite normal ileal integrity and function, it has been proposed that it is the result of a breakdown in this negative feedback mechanism, resulting in an increased rate of hepatic bile acid synthesis. This would deposit more bile acid into the colon, since, at steady state, secretion rate must balance excretion rate. It would not, however, affect WBR unless the elevated secretion rate overwhelmed ileal tracer absorption capacity. Whether increased bile acid secretion reduces ileal bile acid extraction efficiency remains an unresolved issue leaving open the possibility that normal WBR does not exclude BAD.

Error in whole body counting may arise when a radioactive patient enters the vicinity of the uncollimated gamma camera. Such is the sensitivity of an uncollimated camera, this could occur in an adjacent room. Some departments only perform the counting when there are no other patients in the department. Se-75-HCAT in the distal colon is no longer in the bile acid pool and may overestimate WBR. The patient may not stand in the same place at 7 days, giving rise to geometric counting errors. Se-75-HCAT concentration can be assayed in blood. Taking two blood samples is a potential alternative to whole-body counting. The first sample would need to be taken after complete mixing of tracer throughout the bile acid pool, but the time required for this, probably a few days, has not been established for Se-75-HCAT.

Further Reading

1. Notghi A, James G, O'Brien J, et al. British nuclear medicine society SeHCAT guidelines. Nucl Med Commun. 2024;45:564–72.
2. Peters AM, Walters JRF. Recycling rate of bile acids in the enterohepatic re-circulation as a major determinant of whole body ^{75}SeHCAT retention. Eur J Nucl Med Mol Imaging. 2013;40:1618–21.

Indium-111 (Half-Life 2.8 d; Decays by Electron Capture to Cd-111; 172 keV and 245 keV)

26

26.1 In-111-DTPA (MW 545 Da)

DTPA chelates In-111 as well as Tc-99mO_4 (Chap. 11). In-111-DTPA has similar kinetics to Tc-99m-DTPA but has limited use in routine nuclear medicine and preferred to Tc-99m-DTPA only when its longer physical half-life offers an advantage, such as imaging the circulation of CSF following intrathecal injection. In-111 sometimes finds a role in dual isotope studies when the other radiopharmaceutical is labelled with Tc-99m, usually confined to research studies. For example, In-111-labelled polyclonal human immunoglobulin injected into the web-space of the hand was used alongside Tc-99m-nanocolloid injected into the breast in work aimed at a better understanding of breast cancer-related lymphoedema.

26.2 In-111-Labelled Proteins

26.2.1 In-111-Human Polyclonal Immunoglobulin (HIG)

In-111-HIG is efficiently extracted in lymph nodes and can be used for lymphoscintigraphy. It has also been used to image inflammation. The underlying mechanism is increased endothelial permeability, which allows the macromolecule to diffuse into the interstitial space. No mechanism, however, has been identified that traps it and keeps it from diffusing back into the circulation.

26.2.2 In-111-Labelled Monoclonal Antibodies

Leucocyte migration from blood into the extravascular space is orchestrated by proteins called selectins, which belong to a superfamily of proteins called adhesion molecules. These molecules comprise cell surface proteins that mediate cell-to-cell interactions. There are three selectins of importance—E-selectin, expressed on the intraluminal surface of activated endothelial cells; P-selectin, expressed on endothelial cells and the surface of activated platelets; and L-selectin, expressed on leucocytes and shed during extravascular migration. E-selectin is activated by cytokines and expressed during inflammation. Its function is to induce 'rolling' of leucocytes along the endothelial surface prior to extravascular migration.

A. M. Peters, M. Vadrucci, *Introduction to Nuclear Medicine for Trainees in Imaging and Imaging Sciences*, https://doi.org/10.1007/978-3-032-18364-4_26

Radiolabelled monoclonal antibodies raised against adhesion molecules have been explored as imaging probes. An example is anti-E-selectin, code-named 1.2B6, which, labelled with In-111, successfully images a range of inflammatory diseases including inflammatory bowel disease, rheumatoid arthritis and orthopaedic infection. The antibody-antigen complex is internalised in the endothelial cell so that the labelling of target tissue is stable. Other radiolabelled antibodies against vascular adhesion molecules were found to be shed when bound to antigen and therefore of little use.

An In-111-labelled MAB, code-named P256, binds to the platelet fibrinogen receptor and gives images of thrombus formation. It never gained clinical use, however, because it binds to circulating platelets and therefore targets thrombus as it forms rather than pre-formed thrombus. Platelets radiolabelled in vitro with either Tc-99m or In-111 also have this drawback, and, after early clinical activity, were dropped for this application.

26.3 In-111-Octreotide (MW 1019 Da)

Somatostatin (SMS) is a hormone secreted by the brain, gastrointestinal tract, and pancreas that displays a wide range of anti-growth properties, including inhibition of growth hormone secretion by the pituitary, and of the actions of insulin and growth hormone. Octreotide is a peptide analogue of SMS used for treating the symptoms of neuroendocrine tumours such as carcinoid syndrome. SMS is cleared from blood within a few minutes and is not therefore viable as a therapeutic agent. Octreotide, in contrast, has a clearance half-time of 90 min and is therefore suitable for therapy. Octreotide was labelled with In-111 in the 1990s and developed for imaging neuroendocrine tumours that express SMS receptors (Fig. 26.1). More recently, Tc-99m-labelled SMS analogues have been introduced (Fig. 26.2). However, the optimal SMS analogues for imaging are the Ga-68-labelled peptides (Chap. 29). There are 5 receptors for SMS, all widely distributed in the body and variably expressed by a range of neuroendocrine tumours. The effect of an SMS analogue, whether for treatment or imaging, depends on the SMS receptors to which it binds, and the receptors expressed by the tumour.

The biodistribution of labelled SMS peptides includes the pituitary, thyroid, liver, spleen, kidney parenchyma, gastrointestinal tract and urine. The pituitary, thyroid and especially the spleen express SMS receptors. In normal liver, SMS receptors are expressed in bile ducts but not hepatocytes, pointing to biliary excretion as the source of gut activity. In cirrhosis, hepatocytes, interestingly, *do* express SMS receptors. The spleen is also interesting because although one might expect SMS receptors to be expressed in the lymphoid tissue, the strongest expression is in the red pulp, leading to speculation that SMS may play a role in intrasplenic blood cell trafficking.

Following binding of an SMS peptide to its receptor, the receptor-peptide complex is internalised in the cell. Tumour tracer accumulation therefore remains unchanged for many hours after injection.

As a small peptide, an SMS analogue undergoes glomerular filtration followed by tubular reabsorption, explaining prominent renal uptake. Used in doses for radiotherapy, this peptide reabsorption is potentially reno-toxic. Intravenous infusion of unlabelled amino acids competitively blocks tubular radio-peptide uptake and is used to prevent tubular injury in patients receiving such therapy.

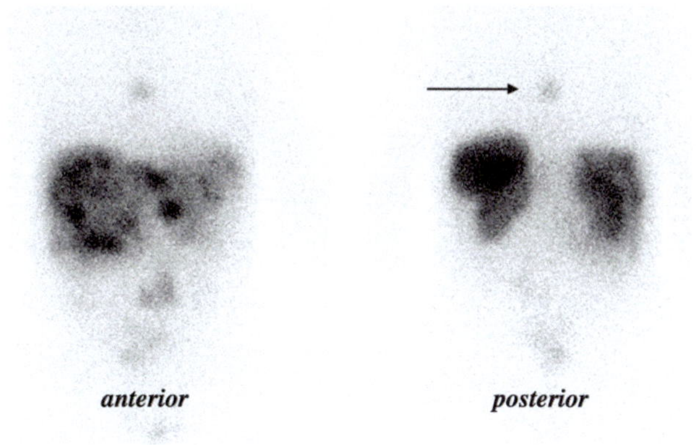

Fig. 26.1 In-111-octreotide scan in patient with metastases from carcinoid. Note intrathoracic deposit (arrow). The spleen expresses somatostatin receptors and is therefore physiologically prominent, as it is with Ga-68-dotatate. Renal parenchymal activity is the result of tubular reabsorption of the labelled peptide following glomerular filtration. Abdominal activity arises from hepatobiliary excretion

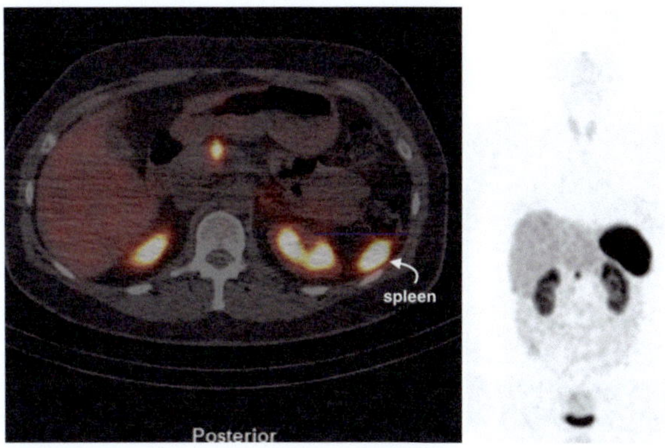

Fig. 26.2 Tc-99m-labelled octreotide (Tektrotyd) scan showing a neuroendocrine tumour in the pancreas. Pituitary and thyroid glands express somatostatin (SMS) receptors and are faintly visible. Kidneys (by reabsorbing filtered tracer) and especially spleen (which expresses abundant SMS receptors) are prominent

26.4 In-111-Labelled Leucocytes

Labelling autologous leucocytes with In-111 for imaging infection and inflammation—the 'white cell scan'—was developed in the early 1980s. To label leucocytes with In-111 (or Tc-99m-HMPAO, see below), a peripheral venous blood sample of 50 mL is obtained from which the 'buffy coat' is collected by gentle centrifugation. The buffy coat, which is rich in leucocytes, is exposed in vitro for 15 min to In-111 that has been complexed to a lipophilic chelating agent such as oxine or tropolone. Being lipophilic, the complex crosses the blood cell membrane and indiscriminately labels all blood cells in the sample. In a buffy coat, most of the cells are granulocytes and lymphocytes, but the sample also contains variable numbers of platelets and red cells which also become labelled. By centrifugation, the labelled cells are 'washed' with saline containing some autologous plasma and returned to the patient via an intravenous injection. Once inside the labelled cell, the In-111 becomes firmly bound to intracellular proteins. The labelling is therefore stable with negligible isotope elution. Inclusion of the autologous plasma in the wash protects the cells from damage—so-called 'collection injury' (Fig. 26.3).

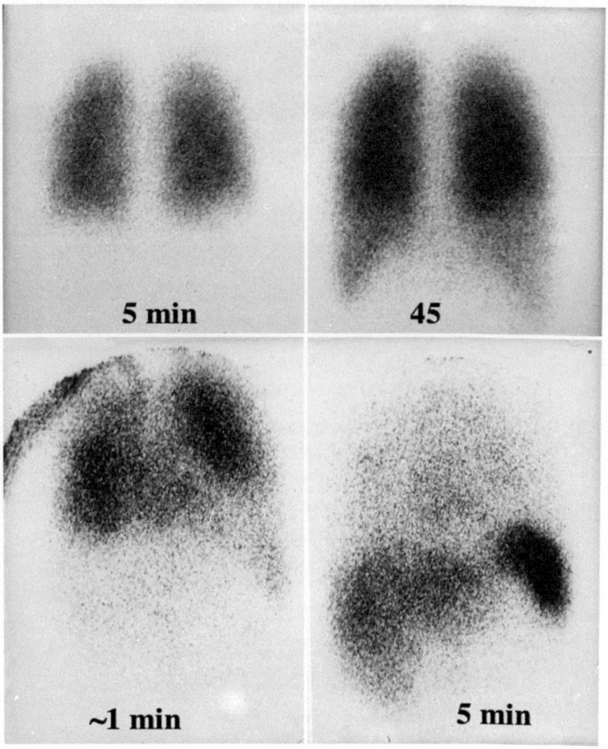

Fig. 26.3 Leucocyte 'collection' injury. Effect on first pass lung transit of in vitro labelling of cells suspended in autologous plasma (lower panels) compared with saline (upper panels). Isolation of leucocytes from plasma reduces their deformability and renders them ineffective for imaging inflammation. Instead, they undergo premature removal into the reticuloendothelial system, especially the liver

Lymphocytes are radiosensitive and do not survive radiolabelling. Monocytes and basophils are too few to accumulate significant In-111. Depending on their numbers in peripheral blood, eosinophils take up a small proportion of In-111. The white cell scan is therefore essentially a neutrophil scan and therefore only positive in pathology involving neutrophil migration.

The physical half-life of In-111 of 2.8 days is suitable for imaging and quantifying blood cell traffic. Thus, following release from bone marrow, neutrophils display a survival in blood that is exponential—in keeping with random physiological destruction—with a mean lifespan of about 10 h. This contrasts with platelets and red cells both of which display survivals that are linear and consistent with age-related destruction, 9 days for platelets and 120 days for red cells. Neutrophil migration into inflamed tissue is detectable in a white cell scan within a few hours of injection and is ongoing up to 24 h, by which time all the labelled neutrophils have left the circulation.

In-111-labelled neutrophil studies have transformed our understanding of physiological neutrophil kinetics, which is important for the interpretation of the scan. It had been known that neutrophils in blood are equally distributed and exchange between marginating and circulating compartments. The marginating compartment was thought to comprise neutrophils rolling along endothelial surfaces throughout the body, functioning in a kind of protective surveillance against infection, but it is now known from imaging that the marginating pool resides in the liver, spleen and bone marrow, and to a lesser extent in the lungs. Margination on endothelium elsewhere is pathological. Neutrophils have mean transit times through spleen and bone marrow of about 10 min, and through the liver of about 2 min. Such slow transit is known as cell pooling—not sequestration, which implies an element of irreversibility. Interestingly, despite their contrasting sizes, platelets and neutrophils display almost identical mean transit times through the spleen, which remains unexplained.

Following i.v. injection, In-111-labelled leucocytes mix between the circulating and marginating compartments. Imaging at 40–45 min

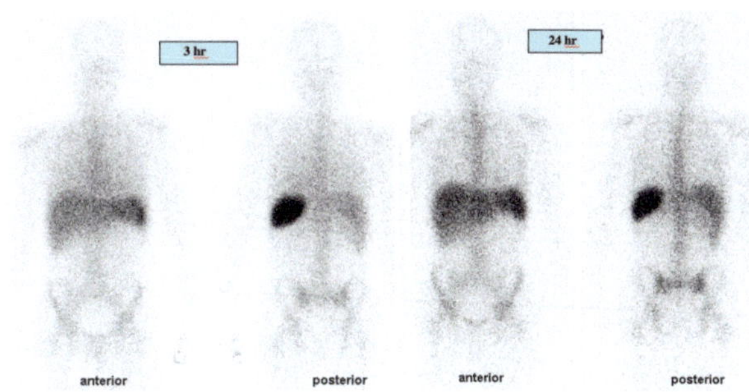

Fig. 26.4 Normal In-111-leucocyte scan at 3 and 24 h post-injection. The cells initially 'pool' in liver, spleen and bone marrow and, then, over the course of a mean intravascular residence time of 10 h, they undergo physiological destruction in the same organs

post-injection shows prominent activity in liver, spleen and marrow (Fig. 26.4). The lungs are also moderately prominent. Blood pool is clearly visible up to about 3 h post-injection but disappears by 24 h, as the neutrophils undergo random physiological destruction in the liver, spleen and bone marrow. A blood pool signal that is still visible 24 h post-injection indicates the presence of large numbers of labelled red cells or platelets, both of which have much longer intravascular life spans than neutrophils, and makes the scan unreliable.

26.4.1 Reporting an In-111-Leucocyte Scan

Firstly, verify that the indication is appropriate. Pyrexia of unknown origin (PUO) is not a valid indication as the majority of causes of PUO do not involve neutrophil migration. As septic inflammatory disease progresses from acute to chronic, the migrating cell population changes from neutrophil- to mononuclear-predominant, and the white cell scan is less likely to be positive. Secondly, if the peripheral blood neutrophil count is not raised, it not only makes septic pathology less likely but also results in excessive In-111 accumulating in red cells and platelets rather than neutrophils during the labelling procedure. Purified neutrophil preparations have been used in research but are not available in most routine cell labelling services.

Imaging is usually performed at 3 and 24 h post-injection. Imaging at 3 h should show a physiological distribution of activity—predominantly spleen and bone marrow with less prominent hepatic activity (Fig. 26.4). Early lung activity is a useful marker of post-collection neutrophil integrity, being markedly increased in the presence of cell damage (Fig. 26.3). Heavy liver uptake also indicates cell damage. Neutrophils are physiologically destroyed in the liver, spleen and marrow so that the pooling signal is gradually replaced by one that shows neutrophil destruction sites. In other words, the normal distribution does not change much over time.

Indications for In-111-leucocytes at the time of their introduction were abdominal abscess (Fig. 26.5), inflammatory bowel disease (Fig. 26.6), vasculitis (Fig. 26.7) and musculoskeletal infection (Fig. 26.8). In-111-leucocytes are particularly useful for diagnosing abdominal abscesses that communicate with bowel. These are difficult to diagnose with other imaging techniques because the abscess decompresses spontaneously by draining into bowel lumen. In IBD, imaging shows how neutrophils migrate into bowel wall and then into bowel lumen and are excreted in the faeces.

In-111-leucocytes provide an effective platform for research studies, showing for example the blockade of neutrophil migration into rheumatoid joints by anti-TNFα and effectiveness of anti-inflammatory therapies for IBD, COPD and

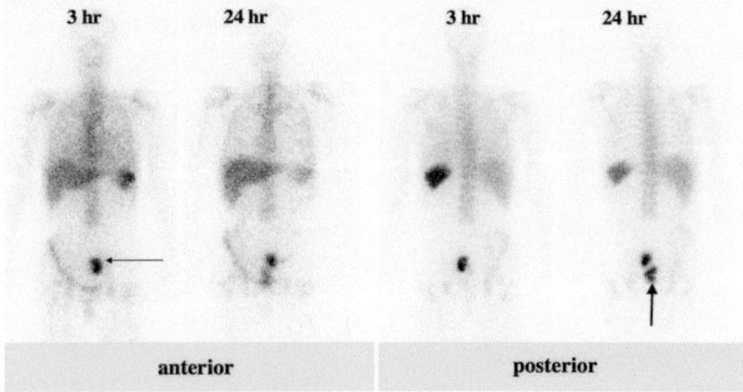

Fig. 26.5 Pelvic abscess (horizontal arrow) in communication with bowel lumen. At 24 h post-injection, activity is visible in the rectum (vertical arrow). Because of spontaneous decompression, these abscesses are difficult to identify and carry an unfavourable prognosis. Note loss of bone marrow uptake in the left hemipelvis as a result of previous radiotherapy

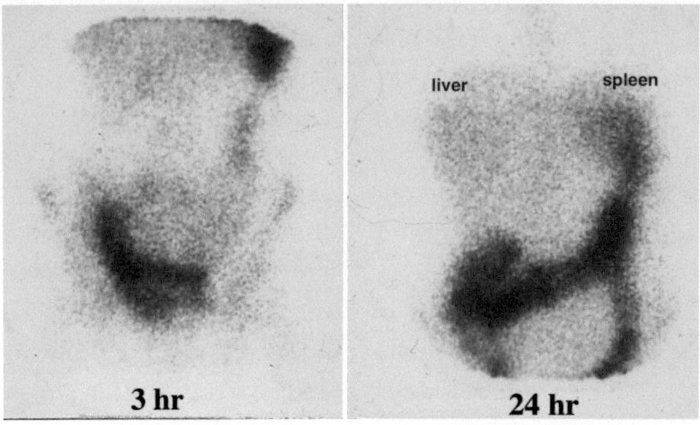

Fig. 26.6 In inflammatory bowel disease (in this case, Crohn's disease), In-111-labelled neutrophils migrate into the inflamed bowel wall and then into the lumen and are excreted in the faeces. This allows quantification of disease activity either by faecal collection or preferably whole body counting

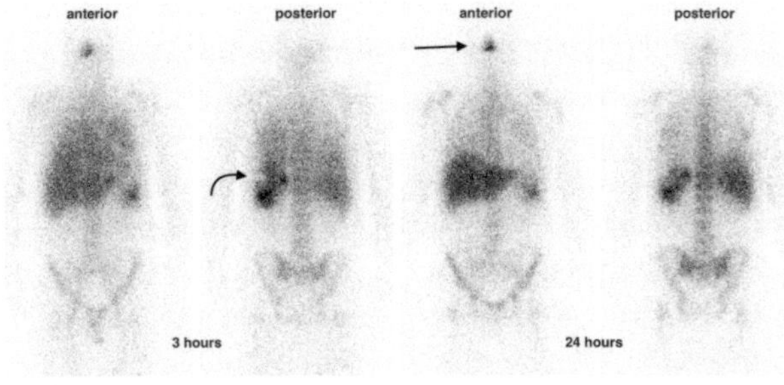

Fig. 26.7 In-111-leucocyte scan in the renamed condition, granulomatosis with polyangiitis. Note nasal activity (straight arrow) and splenic infarct (curved arrow). There is prominent lung activity at 3 h because of neutrophil priming. This is a state in which neutrophils lose deformability as a result of in vivo exposure to systemic inflammatory cytokines. They undergo de-priming in the lungs and re-enter the circulation

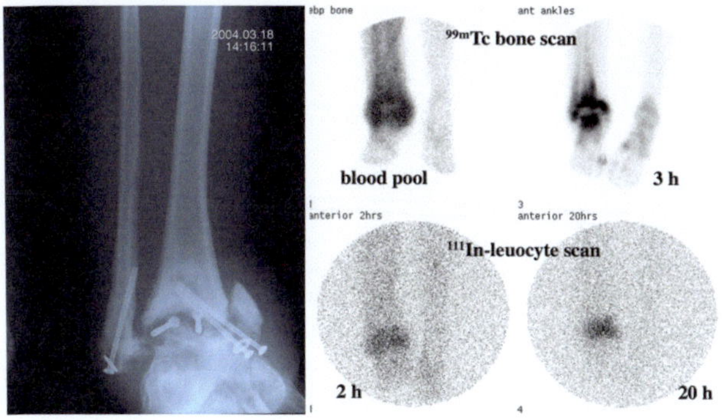

Fig. 26.8 In-111-leucocyte scan in a patient with infected ankle following fracture and surgical fixation. The Tc-99m-MDP bone scan shows increased vascularity on early blood pool imaging and markedly increased tracer accumulation on delayed imaging. In-111-leucocyte scan shows increased accumulation at 3 and 24 h post-injection, confirming infection. The bone scan in orthopaedic bone infection is non-specific. It is only useful if normal, when it excludes infection (Chap. 15)

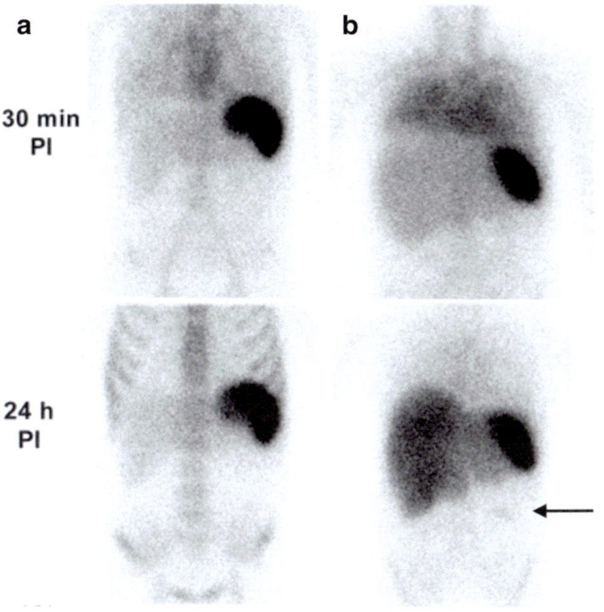

Fig. 26.9 In-111-leucocyte scan in severe alcoholic hepatitis (**b**). The malfunctioning inflamed liver is unable to pool neutrophils, and liver activity is abnormally low at 30 min post-injection. Hepatic uptake at 24 h, however, increases up to fourfold because of intrahepatic neutrophil migration. Normally, intrahepatic neutrophil pooling and destruction are balanced, giving no significant increase between 30 min and 24 h (**a**). Note the intense pooling in the lungs (b, upper panel) as a result of neutrophil priming. There is also faint gut activity (arrow), the origin of which is unclear. (Reprinted from Potts et al. [5])

more recently severe alcoholic hepatitis in which there is prominent neutrophil migration into the liver (Fig. 26.9).

Nowadays, the main indication for In-111-labelled leucocytes is musculoskeletal infection for which they remain the best option. Bone marrow uptake must be imaged in these studies because physiological marrow activity can be misinterpreted as skeletal infection (Fig. 26.10). Physiological marrow uptake should be imaged with Tc-99m-nanocolloid the day before In-111-leucocytes, even for suspected infection in the

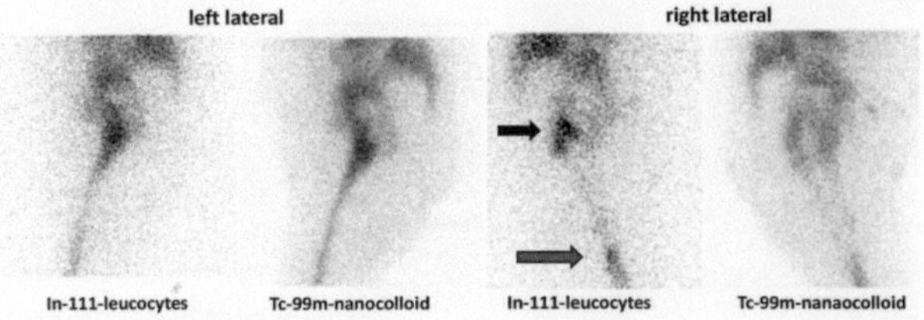

Fig. 26.10 In-111-labelled leucocyte/Tc-99m-nanocolloid scintigraphy (lateral projections) in an infected right total hip replacement. The Tc-99m-nanocolloid scan, performed the day before administration of In-111-leucocytes, shows bone marrow distribution. It is discordant in the 24-h In-111-leucocyte scan because, unlike the leucocytes, Tc-99m-nanocolloid is not taken up at the site of infection (arrows). There is concordance in the left hip and femur with normal accumulation of both tracers in bone marrow

peripheral skeleton because marrow anywhere in the skeleton is readily activated by disease or metalwork.

26.5 Tc-99m-Labelled Leucocytes

In the mid-1980s, Tc-99m-HMPAO was introduced for imaging cerebral blood flow. As a highly lipophilic chelate, it efficiently labels blood cells in vitro. Once inside the cell, the Tc-99m, like an In-111 chelate, is trapped, although its rate of escape (elution) is faster than that of In-111 and the labelling therefore less stable. Tc-99m provides a much higher photon flux than In-111, so Tc-99m-HMPAO-labelled leucocytes give images of higher resolution with a lower radiation exposure (Fig. 26.11). The eluted activity, however, is excreted in urine and bile (Fig. 26.12), giving rise to complications for imaging the abdomen.

Tc-99m-HMPAO leucocyte scanning was used to image IBD but has now become nearly obsolete for this indication following the introduction of new diagnostic methods. It remains, however, a good method for localising disease activity in IBD (Fig. 26.11). Activity localises in inflamed bowel within 60 min of injection, so the normal bowel excretion is not a problem. Tc-99m-HMPAO-leucocytes continue to be used to image musculoskeletal (MSK) infection but with less impressive results because Tc-99m-HMPAO has an affinity for eosinophils that is 20-fold greater than for neutrophils. Eosinophils play a significant role in IBD but not in MSK infection. In-111-leucocytes *are* effective in MSK infection, but their reputation has been damaged by the inappropriate use of Tc-99m-HMPAO leucocytes. FDG PET/CT has consequently almost replaced white cell scanning for MSK infection, despite being non-specific and inferior to In-111-leucocytes.

26.5.1 Reporting a Tc-99m-Leucocyte Scan

For Tc-99m-HMPAO, the main indication is IBD. Imaging is at 1 and 3 h post-injection. The physiological distribution is the same as for In-111-leucocytes. However, imaging the abdomen beyond 3 h post-injection is complicated by excreted urinary and bowel activity and therefore usually unhelpful.

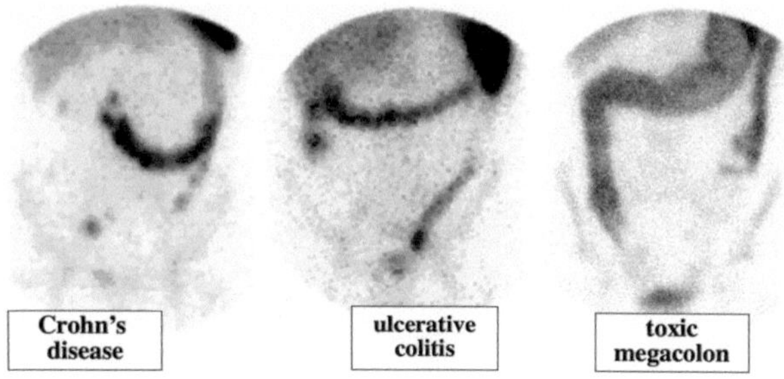

Fig. 26.11 Tc-99m-HMPAO-labelled leucocytes replaced In-111-leucocytes for imaging inflammatory bowel disease but have now themselves been largely replaced by other diagnostic techniques. They are, however, useful for localising disease activity as shown in these three images, acquired 2-3 h after injection. Note the skip lesions in Crohn's disease

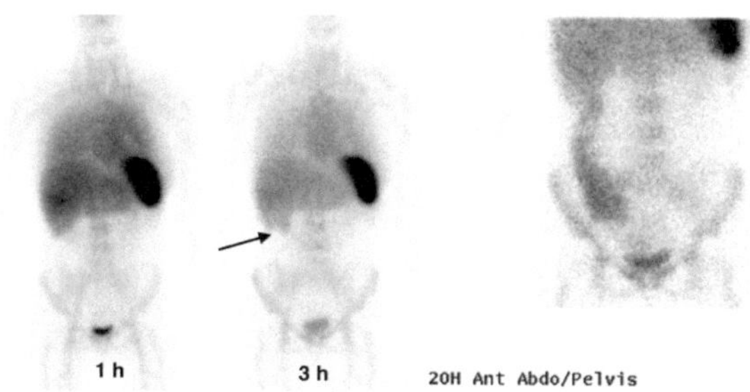

Fig. 26.12 Non-specific bowel activity in Tc-99m-HMPAO-leucocyte scintigraphy. No evidence of disease. Bowel activity is the result of biliary excretion of activity eluting from the labelled cells (arrow: gallbladder). (Courtesy Alexander Gordon, King's College Hospital, London)

26.6 In-111-Labelled Platelets

Platelets are efficiently labelled with In-111 and their Isolation from blood is easier than isolation of leucocytes. Platelets have an age-dependent lifespan of 9 days, so the time-concentration profile of In-111-labelled platelets in blood is linear. In-111-labelled platelets are used to measure platelet lifespan in patients with a low platelet count, usually from idiopathic thrombocytopaenic purpura (ITP), and to confirm the spleen as the major site of premature platelet destruction prior to splenectomy. A normal scan shows blood pool activity, prominent spleen and faint liver (Fig. 26.13), while in ITP either the spleen becomes more prominent over time or activity localises in the liver. Deep vein thrombosis can be imaged with labelled platelets, but this application has not taken hold because thrombosis needs to be active to accumulate platelets. Platelets can also be readily labelled with Tc-99m-HMPAO but have found no routine clinical application.

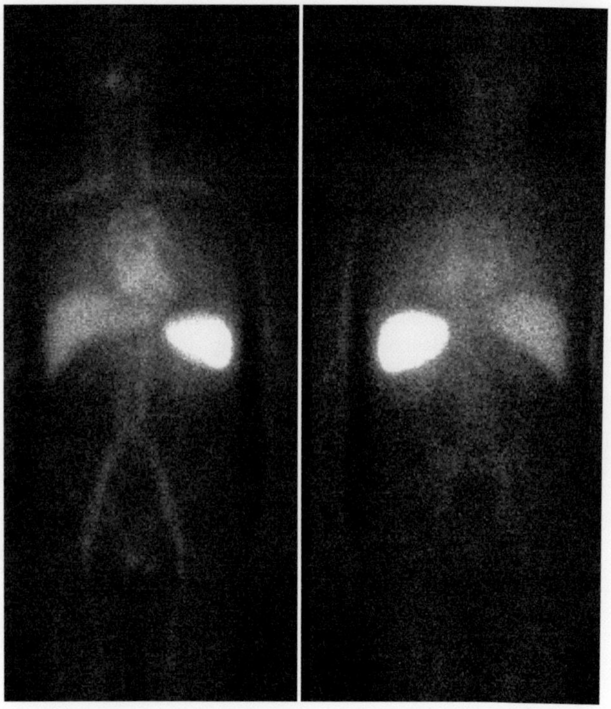

Fig. 26.13 Normal distribution of In-111-labelled platelets at 30 min post-injection, which is almost exclusively between blood and spleen. Most of the hepatic activity is blood pool signal. Platelets pool in the spleen with a mean transit time of 10 min, similar to the mean intrasplenic transit time of granulocytes. This is despite their markedly disparate sizes, suggesting a possible form of loose cell adhesion. (Courtesy Thomas Gruning, Derriford Hospital, Plymouth)

Further Reading

1. Bhatti M, Chapman P, Peters M, Haskard D, Hodgson HJ. Visualising E-selectin in the detection and evaluation of inflammatory bowel disease. Gut. 1998;43:40–7.
2. Dhawan RT, Peters AM. Withdrawal of indium-111: implications for white-cell imaging. The nuclear medicine community must act. Nucl Med Commun. 2014:789–91.
3. Peters AM. The utility of [99mTc]HMPAO-leukocytes for imaging infection. Semin Nucl Med. 1994;24:110–27.
4. Peters AM, Saverymuttu SH, Wonke B, Lewis SM, Lavender JP. The interpretation of platelet kinetic studies for the identification of sites of abnormal platelet destruction. Br J Haematol. 1984;57:637–49.
5. Potts JR, et al. In vivo imaging of hepatic neutrophil migration in severe alcoholic hepatitis with ^{111}In-radiolabelled leucocytes. Biosci Rep. 2018;38(4):BSR20180466. https://doi.org/10.1042/BSR20180466.

27 Radionuclides of Historical Interest

27.1 Thallium-201 (Half-Life 73 h; Decays by Electron Capture to Hg-201; 68–81 keV X-Rays)

Tl-201 is a low-energy potassium analogue. Before Tc-99m-MIBI and Tc-99m-tetrafosmin, Tl-201 was used for myocardial perfusion scintigraphy. Like Tc-99-MIBI, it was also used for imaging tumours, especially parathyroid adenomas. As a potassium analogue, it rapidly accumulates in all tissues following i.v. injection and has an early whole-body distribution that approximates the distribution of cardiac output, i.e., it is a chemical microsphere. Over time, Tl-201 redistributes throughout the body and equilibrates with native potassium to give an image of whole-body tissue potassium distribution. So, for myocardial perfusion scintigraphy, immediate imaging portrays the distribution of myocardial blood flow, whilst delayed imaging portrays the distribution of viable tissue. Thus, a defect on early post-stress imaging that remains a defect on delayed imaging is interpreted as a myocardial infarct, whereas one that 'fills in' on delayed imaging is interpreted as stress-induced myocardial ischaemia. Equilibration with potassium takes a surprisingly long time—about 24 h. Hibernating myocardium was discovered from very delayed Tl-201 imaging which showed that a non-functioning ischaemic territory of myocardium was nevertheless viable and could regain function following revascularisation.

27.2 Chromium-51 (Half-Life 28 days; Decays by Electron Capture to V-51; 320 keV)

Cr-51-EDTA is preferable to Tc-99m-DTPA for measuring GFR because it displays less binding to plasma protein, although it is low with both. However, it has been withdrawn so that GFR is now routinely measured with Tc-99m-DTPA in UK. In Europe, the contrast medium iohexol is favoured, while in the USA it is iodine-125-iothalamate.

In early years of nuclear medicine, Cr-51 was used to label blood cells, especially red cells for the measurement of blood volume and red cell life span in haemolytic anaemias. Because the labelling is not sufficiently stable over an extended period, blood sampling for measurement of life span, the normal of which is 120 days, is terminated after a few weeks and life span estimated from forward extrapolation of the time-blood concentration curve, unless lifespan is ultra-short and all the labelled cells have already left the circulation. When red cell lifespan is expected only to be a few days, In-111-labelled

A. M. Peters, M. Vadrucci, *Introduction to Nuclear Medicine for Trainees in Imaging and Imaging Sciences*, https://doi.org/10.1007/978-3-032-18364-4_27

red cells are an option for its measurement. This also allows for the detection (rather than localisation) of GI bleeding by counting the faeces.

Cr-51 was also used to measure neutrophil mean residence time in blood. This is remarkably short at 10 h meaning that the entire neutrophil population is replaced twice a day. The spleen is particularly active in physiological neutrophil destruction. Indeed, it has been estimated that there is a permanent arterio-venous neutrophil gradient of ~3% across the spleen and suggested that such an active intrasplenic environment of apoptosis explains why carcinoma secondaries are rarely seen in the spleen.

27.3 Gallium-67 (Half-Life 3.3 days; Decays by Electron Capture to Zn-67; 93, 185 and 300 keV)

Ga-67-citrate (MW 256 Da) was introduced in the early 1970s to image tumours, although imaging inflammation became its main use. Following i.v. injection, it forms a metal-protein complex with circulating transferrin, which, as a macromolecule, diffuses into the interstitial space at sites of inflammation and neoplasms where capillary endothelial permeability is increased and binds to transferrin receptors on extravascular macrophages. Its main disadvantage for imaging abdominal inflammation is intestinal excretion. This necessitates delayed imaging, for example 72 h, when the intestinal activity has cleared (Fig. 27.1). It is, however, effective for imaging intrathoracic disease (Figs. 27.2 and 27.3). It is also useful for orthopaedic inflammation in the limbs because the 72-h limitation does not apply, and imaging can take place within several hours of administration. Like labelled leucocytes, it shows physiological bone marrow uptake (Fig 27.1) and imaging needs to be correlated with a contemporaneous bone scan. Because it targets a wide range of diseases that cause fever, it found most use in localising pathology (rather than diagnosing it) in fever of unknown origin. Using Ga-68 instead to improve image resolution is not feasible because the physical half-life is too short.

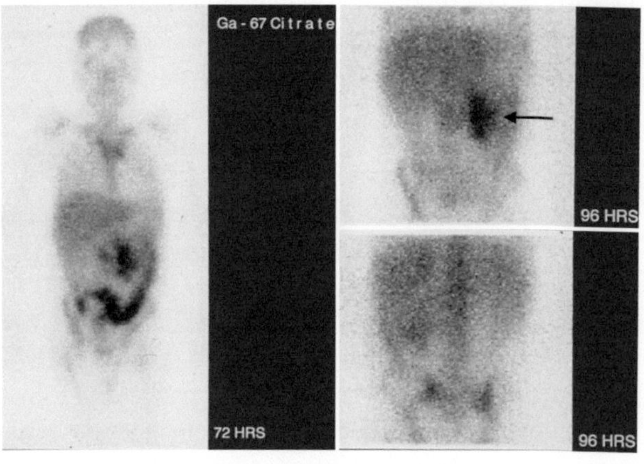

Fig. 27.1 Ga-67-citrate scan in a patient with abdominal abscess (arrow). Normal intestinal activity persisted until 72 h post-injection

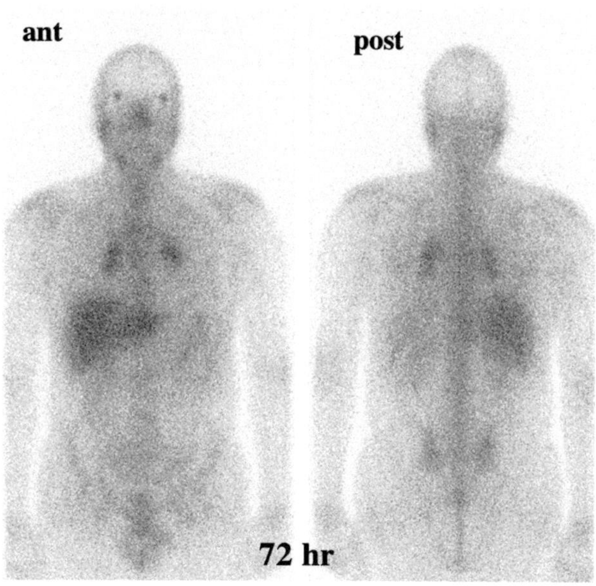

Fig. 27.2 Bilateral hilar Ga-67-citrate accumulation in a patient with sarcoidosis. In this case, there is minimal intestinal activity, emphasising its variability

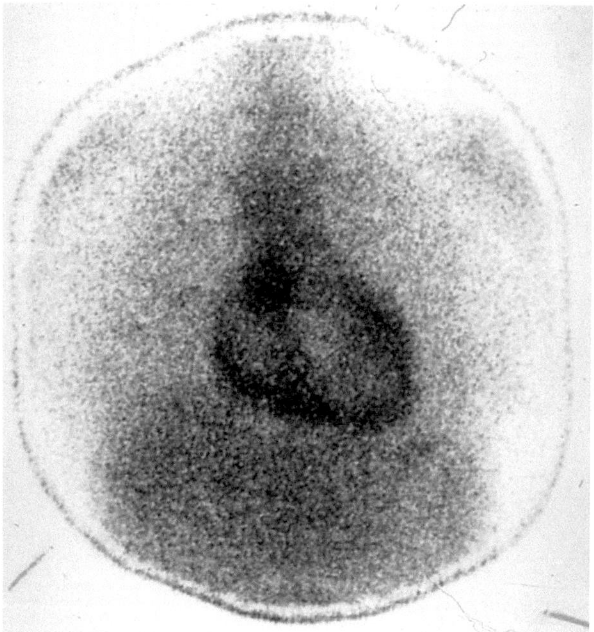

Fig. 27.3 Ga-67-citrate accumulation in pericarditis

Further Reading

1. Lavender JP, Lowe J, Barker JR, Burn JI, Chaudhri MA. Gallium 67 citrate scanning in neoplastic and inflammatory lesions. Br J Radiol. 1971;44:361–6.
2. Sapirstein LA. Fractionation of the cardiac output of rats with isotopic potassium. Circ Res. 1956;4:689–92.

Part VI

Positron Emission Tomography (PET)

In the last few years, PET has mushroomed in use, especially in the form of hybrid imaging which co-registers PET and CT. F-18 and Ga-68 are the radionuclides in most abundant use, especially F-18-FDG which is widely used to image cancer, the myocardium, brain and inflammation. Ga-68 has a narrower spectrum of use, largely confined to prostate cancer as Ga-68-PSMA and neuroendocrine tumours as Ga-DOTATATE.

28 Compounds of Fluorine-18 (Half-Life 110 min)

28.1 Sodium Fluoride-18 (MW 42 Da)

NaF-18 is taken up by bone by binding directly into the hydroxyapatite crystals, that constitute the main mineral component of the skeleton. Like Tc-99m-diphosphonates, NaF-18 portrays bone turnover, thereby giving bone PET/CT (Figs. 28.1 and 28.2). NaF-18 has a high extraction efficiency in bone and therefore a plasma clearance that reflects blood flow of the entire skeleton. As a PET tracer, it can be used to measure bone perfusion, which is surprisingly high—about 150 ml/min/100 ml in vertebrae. Also like the diphosphonates, NaF-18 accumulates in pathological tissue and for example provides high-resolution PET/CT images of calcification in coronary atherosclerosis.

A. M. Peters, M. Vadrucci, *Introduction to Nuclear Medicine for Trainees in Imaging and Imaging Sciences*, https://doi.org/10.1007/978-3-032-18364-4_28

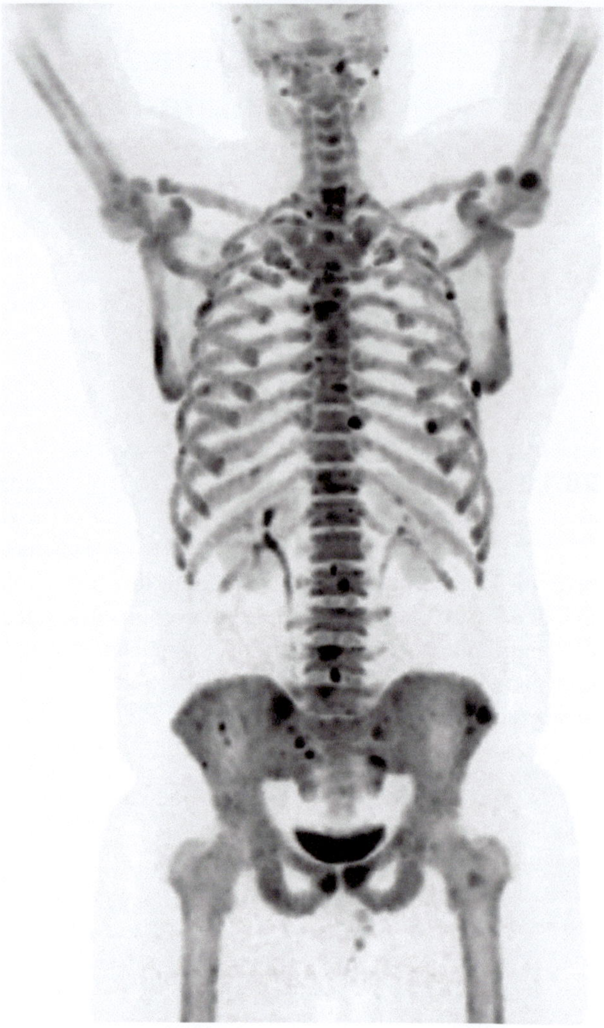

Fig. 28.1 MIP showing multiple foci of NaF-18 accumulation in the skeleton consistent with multiple bone metastases. Note also inflammatory osteoblastic activity at the symphysis pubis

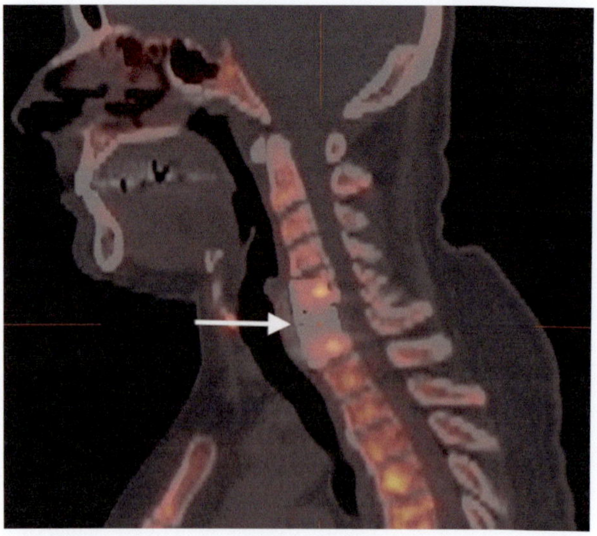

Fig. 28.2 Patient with previous bone lymphoma showing absent fluoride uptake in treated C6 lesion

28.2 F-18-Fluorodeoxyglucose (FDG) (MW 181 Da)

FDG is widely used to image cancer and inflammatory disease. FDG is recognised by the hexokinases of all tissues and taken up as though it was glucose. However, the relative clearance rates of FDG and glucose vary across tissues, their ratio in a tissue being described as the 'lumped constant'. In some tissues, clearance rates are identical, in which case the lumped constant is unity. All cells take up glucose and therefore accumulate FDG broadly in proportion to their metabolic activity. Cancers have a metabolism that is inefficient as well as increased and are therefore conspicuous in FDG PET scans. Inflammatory cells are also metabolically active so that inflammation also gives positive images on PET/CT.

Brain uses glucose exclusively for energy requirements and is the most active normal organ in an FDG PET scan. This is followed by myocardium, although uptake depends on its metabolic status. Thus, following prolonged fasting, the myocardium uses more fatty acids and less glucose, a metabolic situation that is exploited to image myocardial inflammation, especially sarcoidosis.

In general, FDG kinetics are summarised in the compartmental model shown in Figs. 3.3 and 3.8. FDG enters the cell from blood along the pathway K_1. Inside the cell, it either undergoes phosphorylation to FDG-6-phosphate (FDG-6-P) along pathway k_3 or diffuses back into blood along pathway k_2. K_1 is written in upper case because it represents tissue perfusion while the other k values are in lower case to distinguish them as rate constants.

In the cells of all tissues including cancers but apart from liver and kidney, FDG is trapped after it is phosphorylated because firstly FDG-6-P is not recognised by the enzymes of glycolysis and secondly there is no glucose-6-phosphatase to dephosphorylate FDG-6-P. In the liver, FDG-6-P cannot be utilised by enzymes of glycogen synthesis, but k_4 is active because of the presence of glucose-6-phosphatase which the liver needs to maintain a normal blood glucose level during fasting. For the same reason, k_2 is high in the liver allowing glucose and FDG to exchange quite freely between hepatocytes and blood. In fact, the values of k_2 and k_3 in the liver are such that of every 200 molecules of FDG that enter the hepatocyte, only one is phosphorylated while 199 return to blood.

Volume of distribution of FDG in a tissue is the concentration ratio of unphosphorylated FDG between cells and plasma. It is unitless but sometimes displayed with units of ml/ml. In the liver, it approaches unity but is lower in other tissues. Because of its high blood volume (25% of total volume) and high FDG distribution volume, the liver is essentially a blood pool region in FDG PET at 60 min post-injection, when imaging is usually undertaken. Thus, about 75% of the intrahepatic activity arises from blood pool and about 25% from FDG-6-P.

Glucose transporters (GLUTs) translocate glucose into the cell from blood, and hexokinase mediates its phosphorylation to glucose-6-phosphate. In general, tissue hexokinases are saturable at relatively low blood glucose levels (BGL), including hexokinases of cancers, which means that FDG must compete with glucose for uptake. Thus, BGL needs to be checked in cancer patients immediately before they have a PET scan. If it is greater than about 12 mmol/l, rescheduling the patient must be considered. Again, the liver is an exception because of its role in glucose homeostasis. Thus, hepatic hexokinase, called glucokinase, is not saturable at physiological BGL, so the liver phosphorylates whatever glucose and FDG comes its way and utilises glucose for the synthesis of glycogen.

The blood FDG clearance curve is multiexponential. Early mixing between blood and interstitial space is followed by clearance into tissues. About 50% of administered activity remains in blood at 60 min post-injection and about 25% at 120 min. Imaging can therefore be continued beyond 60 min, if the need arises, leading to higher tissue SUV values. Late imaging, allowing extra time for blood FDG clearance, is an option when the patient has a high BGL.

Uptake of positron-emitters is quantified as the standard uptake value (SUV), which is defined as follows

$$\text{SUV} = \text{concentration of tracer in tissue} \times [\text{weight / administered activity}] \quad (28.1)$$

SUV can be based on the single 'hottest' pixel (SUVmax) or on the average pixel activities throughout the volume of interest (SUVmean).

Rather than SUV for grading, the count rate in a tumour can be expressed in relation to uptake in a physiological reference tissue, usually the liver, as in the Deauville criteria for the staging of lymphoma. Use of the liver however ignores the ways in which hepatic glucose kinetics differ from those of other tissues, especially the brain, the kinetics of which resemble those of tumours. At 60 min post-injection, brain SUV shows an inverse exponential relationship with BGL with an exponential constant similar to that estimated from the effect that BGL has on tumour FDG accumulation. Liver SUV in contrast shows a weak relationship with BGL, which, for two reasons, is positive. Firstly, high BGL tends to increase intravascular activity by reducing whole body FDG clearance, thereby increasing the hepatic blood pool signal and making more FDG available for phosphorylation. Secondly, high BGL stimulates the pancreas to secrete insulin, which upregulates hepatic glucokinase.

As small diffusible molecules not bound to plasma protein, glucose and FDG are freely filtered at the glomerulus. However, FDG is not reabsorbed by the renal tubule and is instead excreted unchanged in urine. The transporter responsible for tubular reabsorption of glucose is the sodium glucose transporter which reabsorbs glucose along with sodium. So, unlike hexokinases, this transporter does not recognise FDG. The kidney contains gluose-6-phosphatase to dephosphorylate reabsorbed filtered glucose and return it to the circulation.

28.2.1 Patient Preparation

To perform an FDG PET-CT scan, the patient needs to be in a complete fasted state for at least 4 h because physiological high insulin levels in the post-prandial state may alter the biodistribution of the tracer by driving FDG into skeletal muscles (Fig. 28.3). Insulin-dependent diabetic patients should be scheduled for appointment at least 4 h after their last insulin injection, or at least 6 h if long-acting. Patients on a continuous insulin infusion pump may have the scan as long as they have fasted and the infusion is kept constant during the 60 min period of tracer accumulation and subsequent imaging. Patients on oral diabetic medications may have the scan normally, keeping in mind that metformin is known to cause diffuse bowel activity as a result of upregulation of the GLUT receptors in the intestinal mucosa (Fig. 28.4). The presence of high fasting blood glucose levels in poorly controlled diabetics is not an absolute contraindication for the scan as it does not impact the diagnostic yield of the study. Nevertheless, delaying the scan for a few hours if possible, or further hydration, can be attempted to lower the blood sugar levels before proceeding.

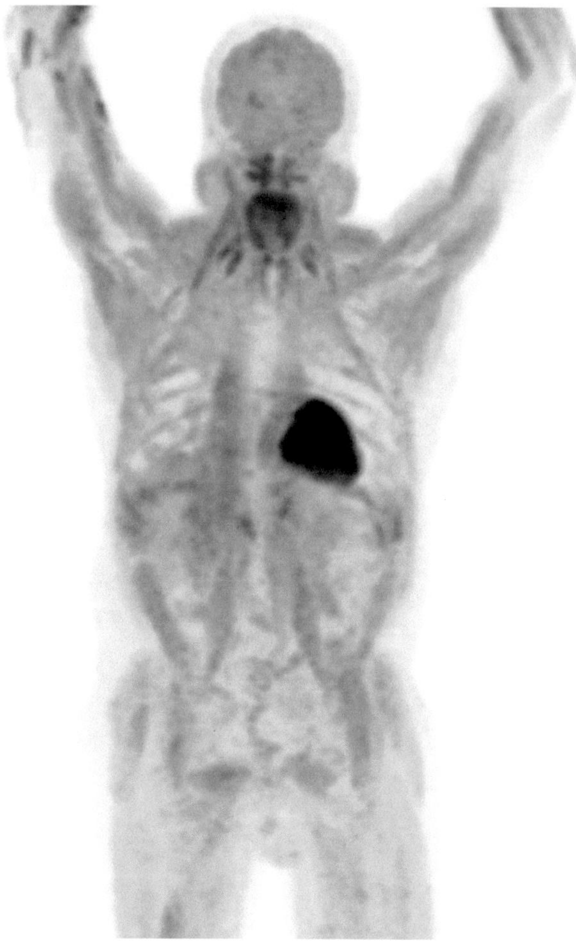

Fig. 28.3 F-18-FDG PET-CT scan showing diffuse increased muscle uptake with reduction of the physiological visceral activity, e.g. liver, kidneys, due to inadequate fasting period prior to the scan

Patients should avoid strenuous exercise the day before the exam to minimise muscular activation (Fig. 28.5). Following tracer administration, the patient should be kept warm, especially during the colder months, to minimise physiological activation of brown fat (Fig. 28.6). When studying pathology in the head and neck, it is useful to recommend patients not to talk during the uptake phase in order to reduce the risk of physiological functional uptake in the tongue and vocal cords (Fig. 28.7) that can make interpretation difficult and mask underlying lesions.

To answer specific questions about inflammatory cardiac pathology, such as sarcoidosis or infective endocarditis, it is important to suppress physiological myocardial tracer accumulation. This is achieved by giving a low carbohydrate, high protein diet over the 18–24 h prior to the scan, which induces a metabolic switch to β-oxidation (Fig. 28.8).

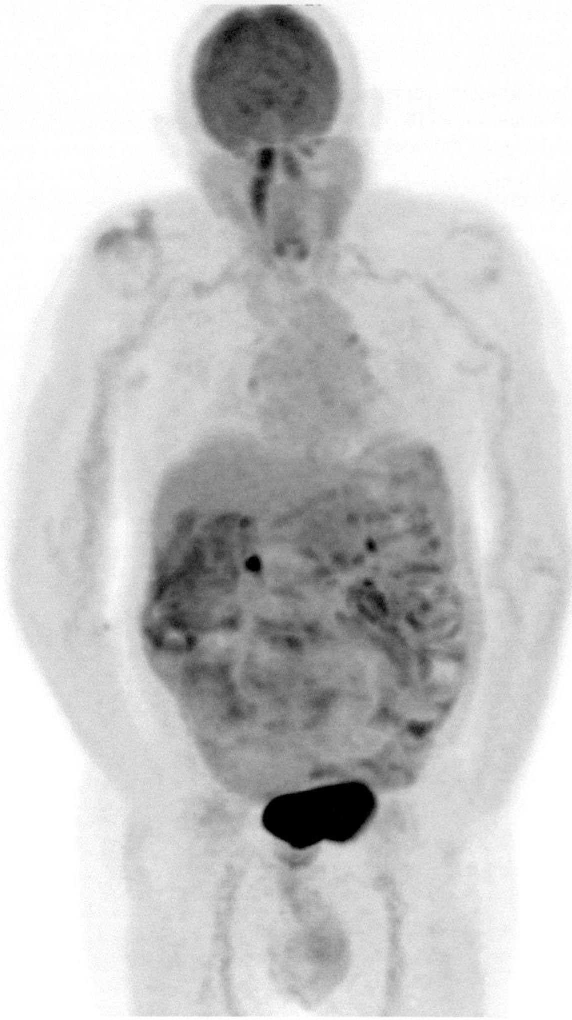

Fig. 28.4 F-18-FDG PET-CT scan in a diabetic patient receiving metformin showing diffuse bowel uptake caused by the medication. Note also asymmetrical activation of the neck muscles due to posture

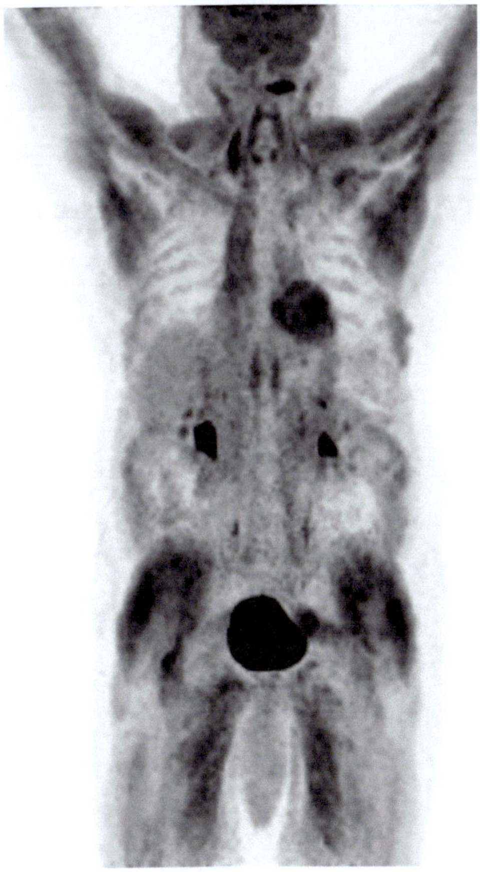

Fig. 28.5 Widespread skeletal muscle tracer accumulation in a patient who undertook strenuous exercise a few hours before injection of F-18-FDG

28.2.2 Reporting an F-18-FDG PET/CT Study

The standard PET-CT acquisition protocol is a base of skull (or vertex) to thigh acquisition 50–60 min after tracer administration The lower limbs should be included with pathologies such as acral melanoma, multiple myeloma, myositis or orthopaedic inflammation in the extremities.

Typical 60 min physiological biodistribution of FDG comprises predominantly liver, brain and myocardium (if no specific cardiac preparation) (Fig. 28.9). Urinary activity is also seen because filtered FDG is not reabsorbed, as explained above. To reliably report FDG PET-CT, it is necessary to recognise a wide range of normal variants. Lymphoid tissue in the Waldeyer's ring and ileocaecal area may show variable physiological uptake, especially in young patients. There may be variable degrees of skeletal muscle uptake due to strain during the uptake phase or in the hours before. Physiological small and large bowel activity may vary significantly between patients and in the same patient over time as a result of several factors such as medications, peristalsis and tracer excretion, and should not be misinterpreted for disease unless clearly focal. Uptake in the ovaries and uterus may vary according to the menstrual cycle in pre-menopausal

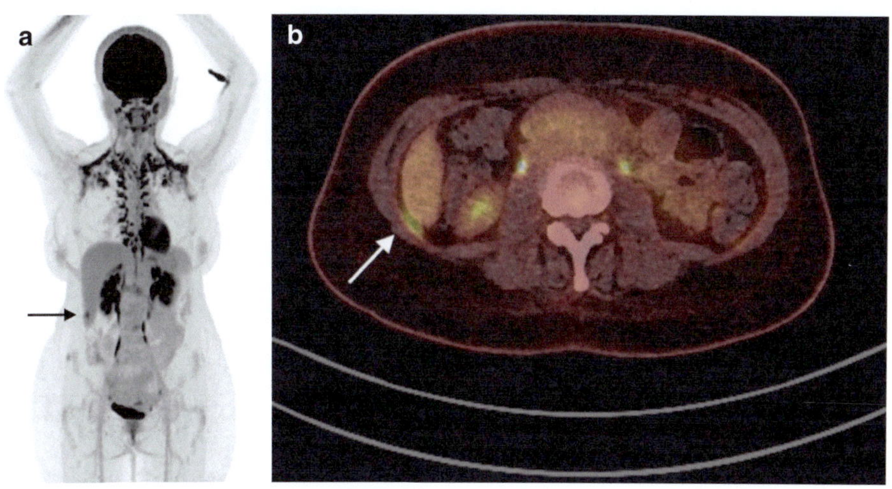

Fig. 28.6 F-18-FDG MIP showing typical symmetrical distribution of activated brown fat in the neck, supraclavicular fossae and paravertebral spaces (**a**). Also note tracer accumulation with no structural correlate in the subhepatic space (arrow), an uncommon but recognised site of brown fat (**b**)

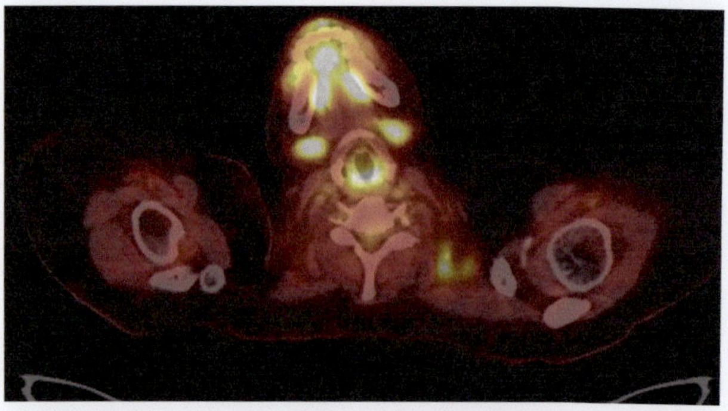

Fig. 28.7 F-18-FDG PET-CT scan showing intense symmetrical vocal cord and tongue activity due to phonation during the 60 min post-injection period

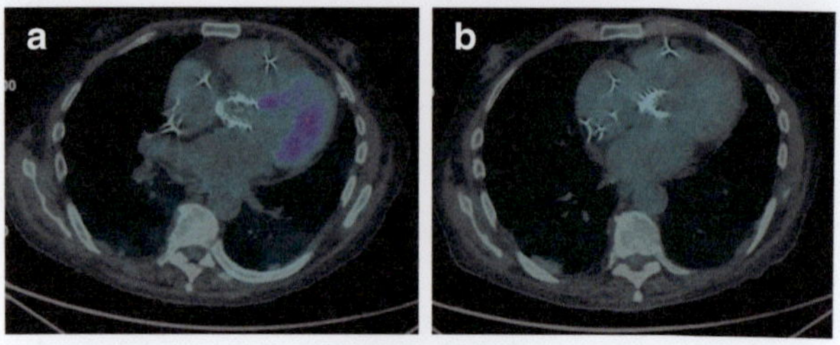

Fig. 28.8 Axial images showing physiological uptake of F-18-FDG in the left ventricle (**a**) and complete suppression on the repeat study after implementation of a low-carbohydrate diet (**b**)

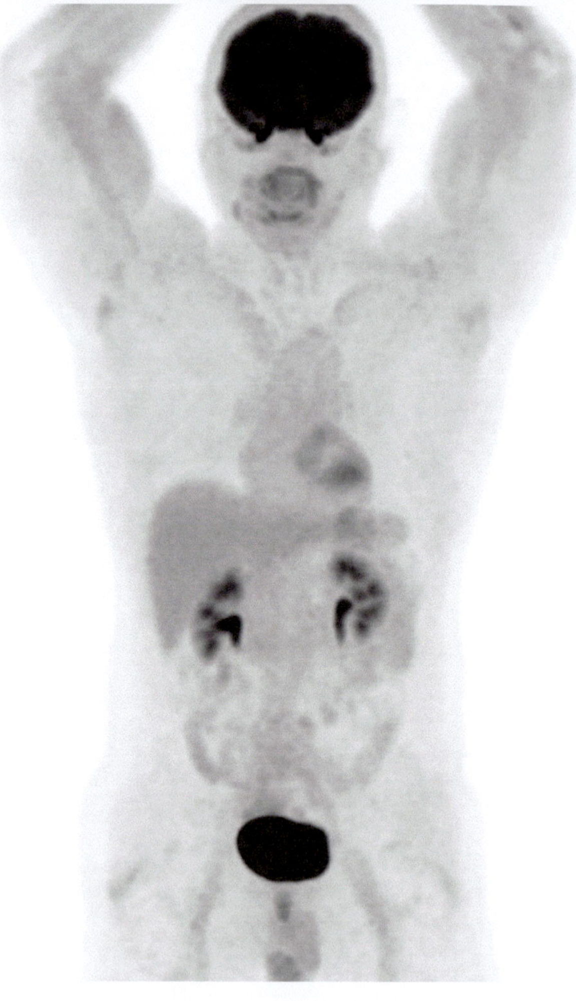

Fig. 28.9 Typical normal biodistribution of F-18-FDG in a male patient. Note activity in the tonsils and testes

patients and is often asymmetrical. Following the menopause, however, it should be regarded as abnormal. Physiological uptake in the testes is symmetrical and tends to decrease with age.

Increased FDG uptake is seen as an incidental finding in many benign lesions, the most common of which are thyroid nodules, colonic polyps and adrenal adenomas. Increased uptake resulting from inflammation may be seen over extended periods at surgical sites or following radiotherapy, and mimic residual disease.

When reporting an oncological scan, make note of the site and SUVmax of the main lesions and always use the CT component and prior imaging for anatomical correlation. Suggest a biopsy site when appropriate by indicating the 'hottest' accessible lesion. When assessing response to treatment, always give the variation in size and FDG uptake in the index lesions if a prior PET is available. Response assessment in lymphoma uses a clinically validated 5-point visual scale known as the Deauville criteria (Fig. 28.10), where any uptake below the liver background is considered a complete response.

Even PET reporters with more experience will often encounter diagnostic uncertainty in their practice. Recommend appropriate further radiological investigations or multidisciplinary team review for indeterminate lesions that can potentially change the management, for example a potential solitary bone lesion in a patient with localised breast cancer. Another common confusing clinical scenario is that of activity in lymph nodes that may be reactive or pathological and can potentially change the stage of the tumour. Review of the CT component can help in identifying typical characteristics of benign lymph nodes, e.g. oval shape and a visible fatty hilum. Knowledge of the typical pattern of nodal spread of the cancer being studied can also help interpretation, but ultimately a degree of uncertainty is often unavoidable especially with respect to small lesions.

The challenge interpreting non-oncological FDG PET-CT studies, for example vasculitis (Fig. 28.11) or fever of unknown origin, arises mainly from medications, especially steroids or other immunosuppressants, that may lead to false negative results. Hence, wherever possible, the scan should be performed before initiating such treatments.

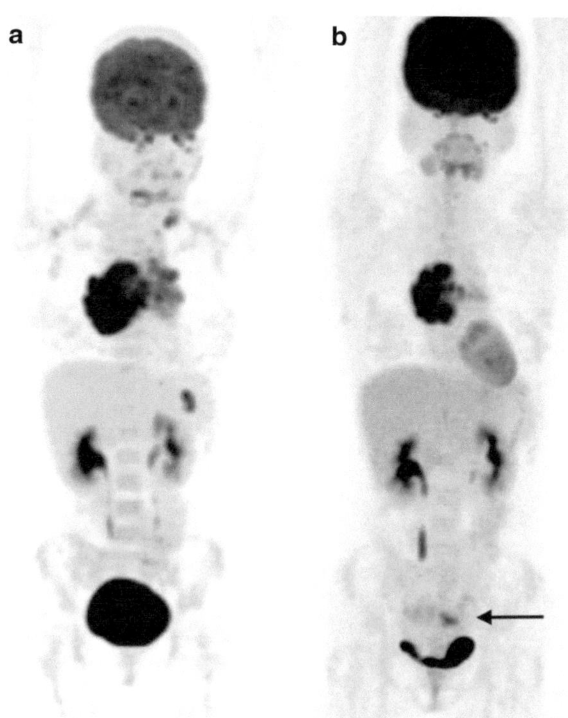

Fig. 28.10 F-18-FDG PET-CT in a patient with mediastinal lymphoma before (**a**) and after (**b**) treatment. The mass has reduced in size, but uptake remains visually higher than the liver in keeping with a Deauville 5 response. Note also physiological left ovarian uptake on the post-treatment scan (arrow)

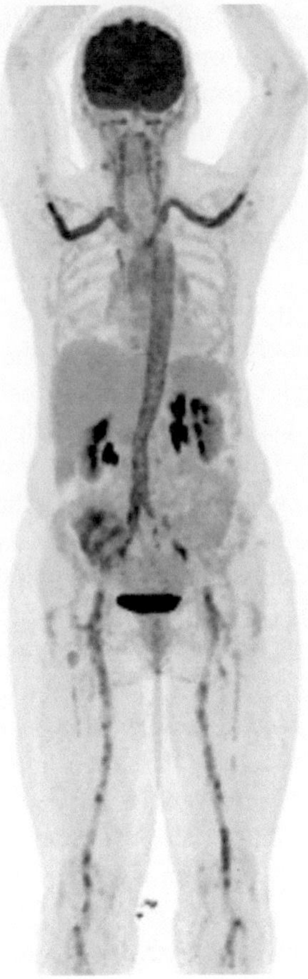

Fig. 28.11 F-18-FDG PET-CT scan showing florid large vessel vasculitis involving aorta and major arteries. Note also physiological ileocaecal activity in the right iliac fossa

28.3 F-18-Choline (MW 121 Da)

Choline is an essential nutrient involved in many physiological processes, such as the synthesis of the neurotransmitter acetylcholine and the metabolism of lipids. Prostate cancer often has increased metabolism of choline, which is an essential component of the phospholipids in the cell membrane. Choline labelled with F-18 is therefore used as a PET agent for imaging prostate cancer, although its use has declined due to the higher sensitivity and specificity of PSMA PET (see below). Nevertheless, its clinical use as a prostate cancer imaging agent in the early 2010s led to the serendipitous discovery that hyperfunctioning parathyroid tissue, such as adenomas, may also demonstrate increased choline metabolism. Parathyroid hormone is linked to upregulation of choline kinase in proliferating parathyroid cells. As a result, F-18-choline is increasingly used in the preoperative detection of parathyroid adenomas (Fig. 28.12) in normal and ectopic locations, with the benefit of higher PET spatial resolution and overall improved detection rate when compared to conventional scintigraphy with Tc-99m-sestamibi (Chap. 16).

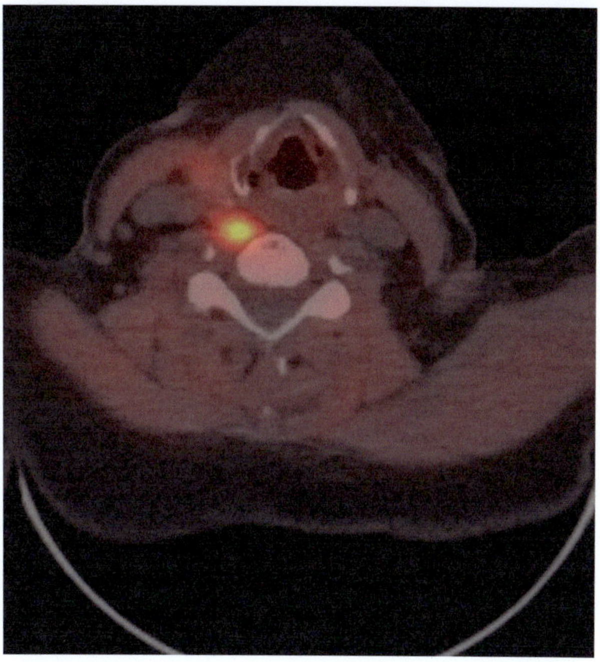

Fig. 28.12 Nodule posterior to the right lobe of the thyroid demonstrating intense F-18-choline uptake in keeping with a right-sided parathyroid adenoma

28.4 F-18-Amyloid Agents (e.g. Florbetaben MW 358 Da)

The challenge facing imaging agents for imaging brain plaque is restricted transport across the blood-brain barrier (BBB). Small molecular weight agents such as F-18-florbetaben, which has a MW of 358 Da and is the most widely used tracer for amyloid in Europe, are therefore attractive. After crossing the BBB, F-18-florbetaben binds irreversibly to areas of the cortex that contain aggregates of β-amyloid, the protein considered to be the main component of the neuronal plaques that are the hallmark of Alzheimer's disease (Figs. 28.13 and 28.14).

Florbetaben distributes rapidly in the brain after i.v. injection and clears within the first 60 min from the cerebellum while it is retained in normal white matter as well as in amyloid plaques. It is highly protein-bound in plasma but crosses the blood brain barrier because it is lipophilic. It is mainly excreted through the gallbladder and in smaller part through urine.

The presence of β-amyloid aggregates in the brain, as detected by these tracers, is a necessary but not sufficient condition for the diagnosis of Alzheimer's disease.

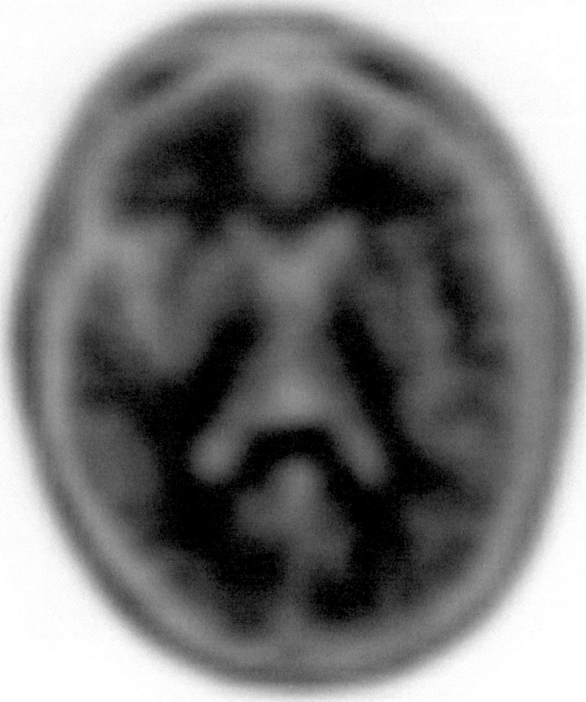

Fig. 28.13 Normal F-18-Florbetaben image of the brain showing preserved grey-white matter differentiation and higher uptake in white matter

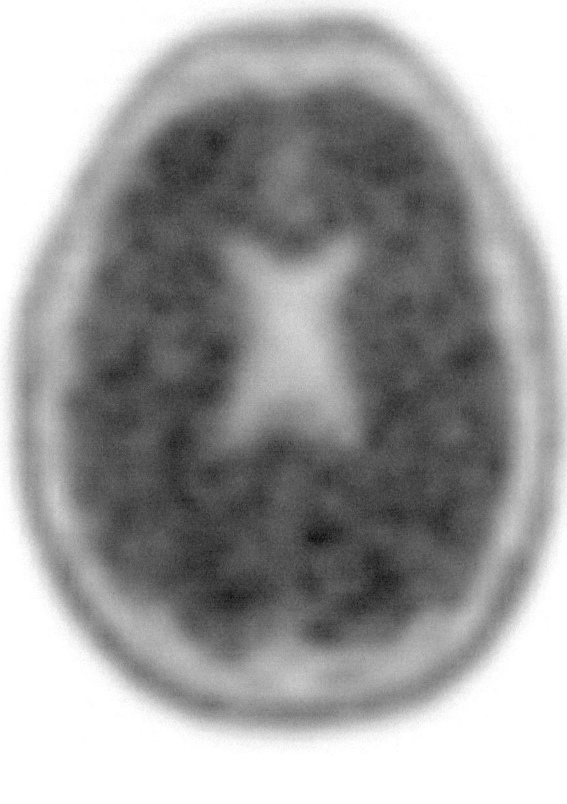

Fig. 28.14 Abnormal F-18-florbetaben brain study showing loss of the normal grey-white matter differentiation and similar levels of uptake in white and grey matter

Further Reading

1. Boellaard R, Herrmann K, Barrington SF, et al. [18F] FDG PET/CT: EANM procedure guidelines for tumour imaging: version 3.0. EANM J. 2025;1:100006.
2. Glaudemans AW, de Vries EF, Galli F, Dierckx RA, Slart RH, Signore A. The use of (18)F-FDG-PET/CT for diagnosis and treatment monitoring of inflammatory and infectious diseases. Clin Dev Immunol. 2013;2013:623036.
3. Kirienko M, Gelardi F, Fiz F, Bauckneht M, et al. Personalised PET imaging in oncology: an umbrella review of meta-analyses to guide the appropriate radiopharmaceutical choice and indication. Eur J Nucl Med Mol Imaging. 2024;52:208–24.

Compounds of Gallium 68 (Half-Life 68 min; Decays 89% by Positron Emission and 11% by Electron Capture to Zinc-68)

29

29.1 Ga-68-PSMA (MW 1011 Da)

PSMA (prostate-specific membrane antigen) is a type II transmembrane protein that is present in all prostatic tissues but overexpressed in most prostatic cancers. Its denomination is somewhat of a misnomer as PSMA expression is also physiologically found in many tissues including bowel, tubular system of the kidneys, salivary and lacrimal glands, liver and spleen (Fig. 29.1). It plays a role in glutamate metabolism in the neurotransmitter system and in folate metabolism in the digestive tract, but its function in the prostate cells is not well understood.

Nevertheless, its elevated expression in prostate cancer cells makes it a well-suited target for imaging this disease. PSMA was first labelled in the early 2000s with C-11, a positron-emitting isotope with a short half-life of approximately 20 min, and shortly after with Ga-68. It is now widely employed in clinical practice for staging, restaging and response assessment of prostate cancer. More, recently PSMA compounds labelled with F-18 were introduced. It is estimated that approximately 10% of prostate tumours do not overexpress PSMA and cannot, therefore, be imaged with this tracer.

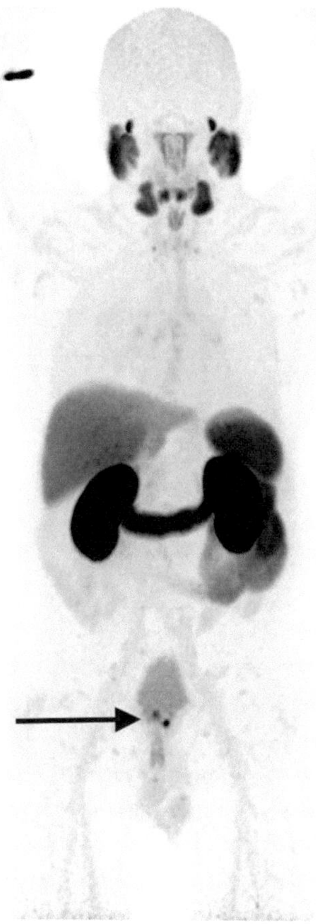

Fig. 29.1 Biodistribution of Ga-68-PSMA in a patient with prostate cancer confined to the prostate (arrow)

A. M. Peters, M. Vadrucci, *Introduction to Nuclear Medicine for Trainees in Imaging and Imaging Sciences*, https://doi.org/10.1007/978-3-032-18364-4_29

Standard whole-body PET acquisition is performed 50–60 min after tracer administration with a recommended activity of 1.8–2.2 MBq/kg, although this may vary according to local protocols and PET camera sensitivity. PSMA can also be labelled with lutetium-177 for theragnostic applications.

29.1.1 Reporting a PSMA PET-CT Study

Detecting the primary tumour in staging is usually straightforward as the target-to-background ratio is in most cases very high. Note whether the uptake is unifocal or multifocal, or if it reaches the seminal vesicles. On follow-up after prostatectomy, assessment of the prostatic bed may be impaired by urinary activity in the bladder. Dynamic image acquisition over the pelvis immediately following tracer injection, before activity has reached the bladder, may therefore be helpful to obviate this issue (Fig. 29.2).

Nodal staging is more difficult because of reactive lymph nodes, but these are usually low grade compared to the primary. Note that external iliac and inguinal lymph nodes almost always display isolated and low-grade reactivity in prostate cancer. Always compare the PET images with the underlying CT component to avoid misinterpreting physiological urinary activity in the ureters. Reporting of positive lymph nodes is not based on size criteria because very small lymph nodes can be detected with PSMA.

Bone is the most common site of metastatic spread in prostate cancer. Detection of metastases in other organs may be hindered by the physiological background activity, for example in the liver, and the reporter needs to adjust the PET colour scale accordingly when assessing different organs. Many benign and malignant conditions not related to prostate cancer have been incidentally identified on PSMA PET, including lung, renal, and liver malignancies, multiple myeloma, liver haemangiomas and Paget's disease (Fig. 29.3). Further corroboration of the PET findings with other imaging or histology should therefore be sought in equivocal cases. Some PSMA compounds labelled with F-18 are known to cause focal unexplained bone uptake (UBU), more commonly in ribs and pelvis (Fig. 29.4). These areas do not have a structural correlate on CT and require careful interpretation to avoid overstaging.

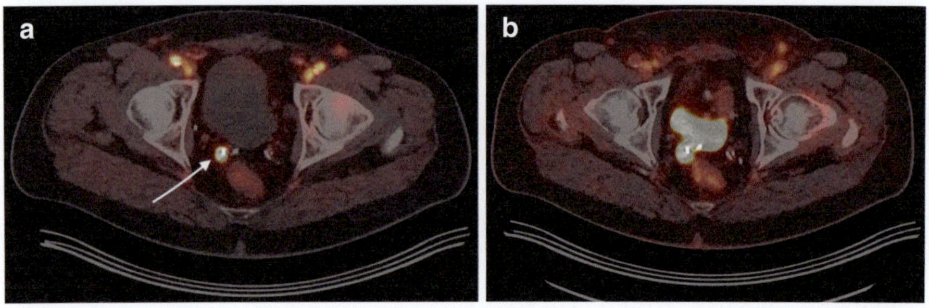

Fig. 29.2 An early frame from the dynamic sequence of images shows accumulation of Ga-68-PSMA in the right prostatectomy bed consistent with recurrent prostate cancer (**a**). On late images (right), this is partially obscured by the activity reaching the adjacent urinary bladder (**b**)

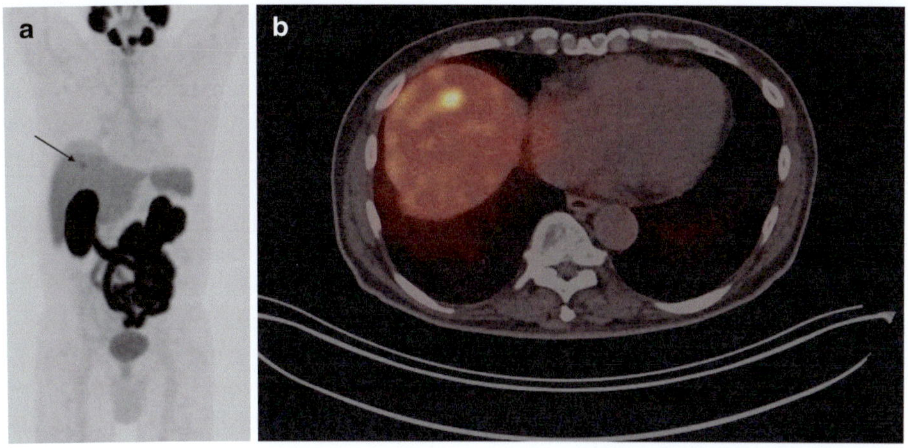

Fig. 29.3 Ga-68-PSMA MIP (**a**) and axial image (**b**) showing faint focus in the liver at a site of a known haemangioma (arrow)

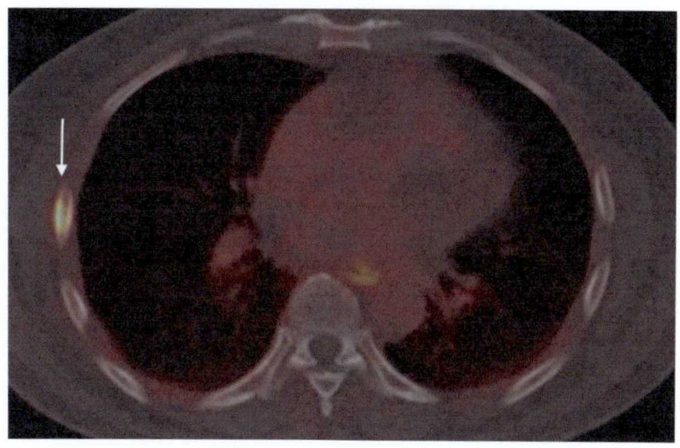

Fig. 29.4 Faint focus of uptake in a rib (arrow) in an otherwise normal F-18-PMSA scan was interpreted as likely benign

29.2 Ga-68 DOTA (TATE, NOC, NOC; MW 1500 Da)

Somatostatin receptor (SSTR) analogues labelled with Ga-68 are used for imaging neuroendocrine tumours. The biodistribution resembles that of octreotide compounds labelled with In-111 and Tc-99m, but Ga-68 provides higher spatial resolution and better reporting confidence, thanks to the use of a PET scanner rather than a gamma camera. As with PSMA, pairing with lutetium-177 is available for radionuclide therapy.

29.2.1 Reporting a Ga-68-DOTA PET/CT Study

As with every tracer in nuclear medicine, it is important to understand the physiological distribution of SSTR tracers in the body when reporting a scan. SSTRs are expressed normally in high numbers in the pituitary gland, adrenals, spleen and accessory spleens, which always demonstrate high uptake (Fig. 29.5). Ga-68-DOTATATE is a hydrophilic compound that is partially reabsorbed by the distal renal tubules leading to high

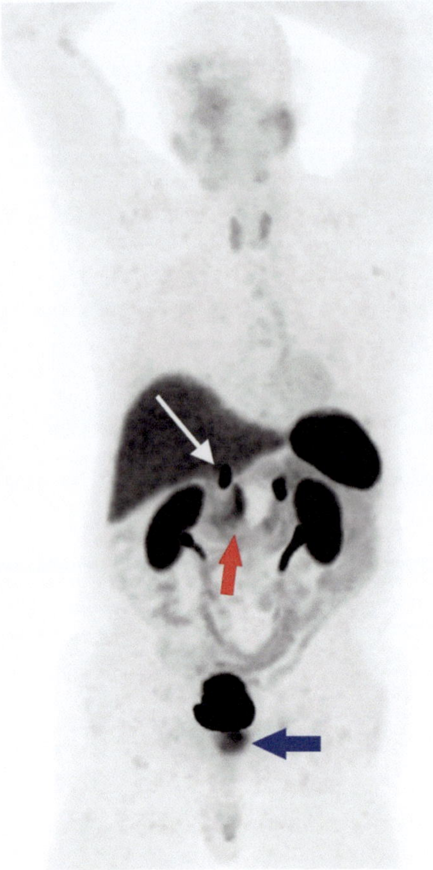

Fig. 29.5 Normal Ga-68-DOTATATE scan. Note physiological uptake in the uncinate process of the pancreas (red arrow), prostate (blue arrow) and adrenals (white arrow—right adrenal)

activity in the renal cortex and urinary collecting system. The thyroid, liver and prostate gland may also demonstrate variable low to moderate physiological uptake in a homogeneous pattern.

Of note, the uncinate process has a physiologically higher concentration of SSTRs compared to the rest of the pancreas. This is usually of moderate grade in a non-diffuse pattern and should not be confused for pathology. Correlation with anatomical imaging such as MRI or dedicated CT is essential to avoid misinterpretation.

The intensity of tracer uptake in tumours is proportional to the expression of SSTRs within the lesion. In high-grade undifferentiated disease, therefore, tracer accumulation tends to be low or non-existent (Fig. 29.6). In such cases, FDG PET-CT may be used as a complementary tool, as these aggressive tumours tend to have high glycolytic rates. Visual scales have been developed to help define the intensity of uptake of SSTR tracers, usually by comparing the tumour uptake to normal tissues such as spleen or liver. Such scales have been used mainly to select patients who may benefit from peptide receptor radionuclide therapy (PRRT).

Many benign or malignant pathologies are known to cause increased expression of SSTRs and may potentially be detected incidentally with an SSTR ligand on PET-CT. Common examples include vertebral haemangiomas (Fig. 29.7), vas-

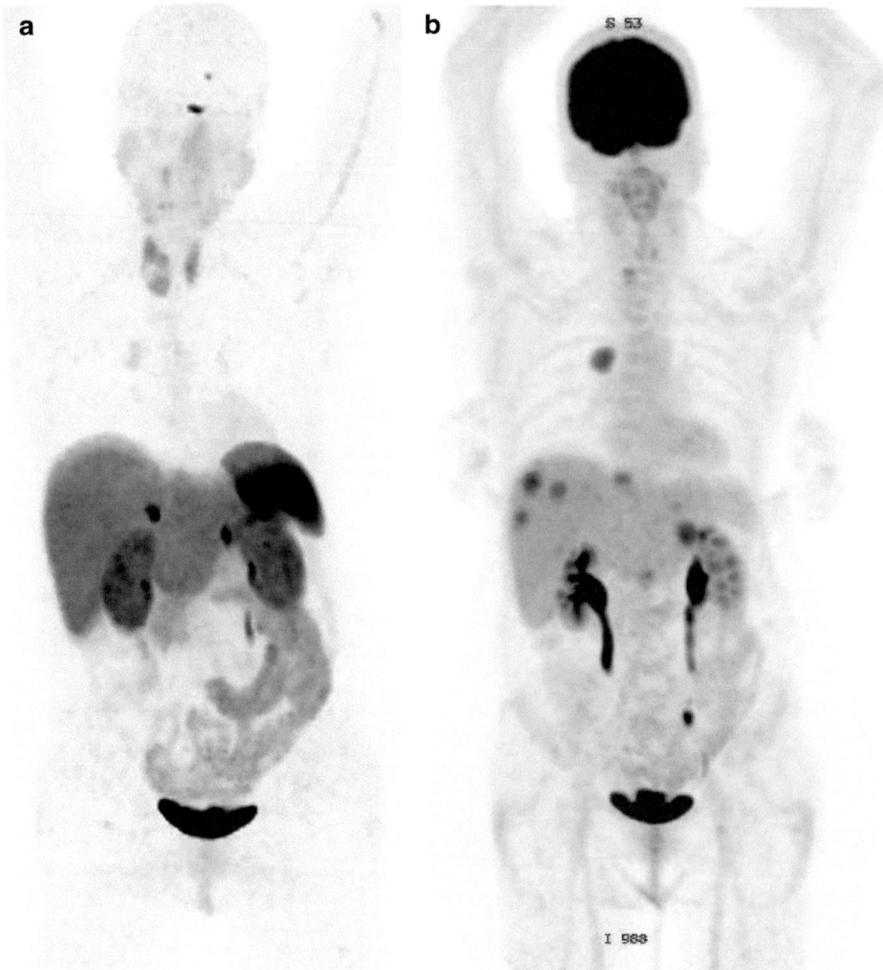

Fig. 29.6 Patient with high-grade neuroendocrine tumour with metastatic lung and liver lesions that are not visible on Ga-68-DOTATATE (**a**) but show high-grade uptake on F-18-FDG (**b**). Note a small incidental meningioma in the DOTATATE scan

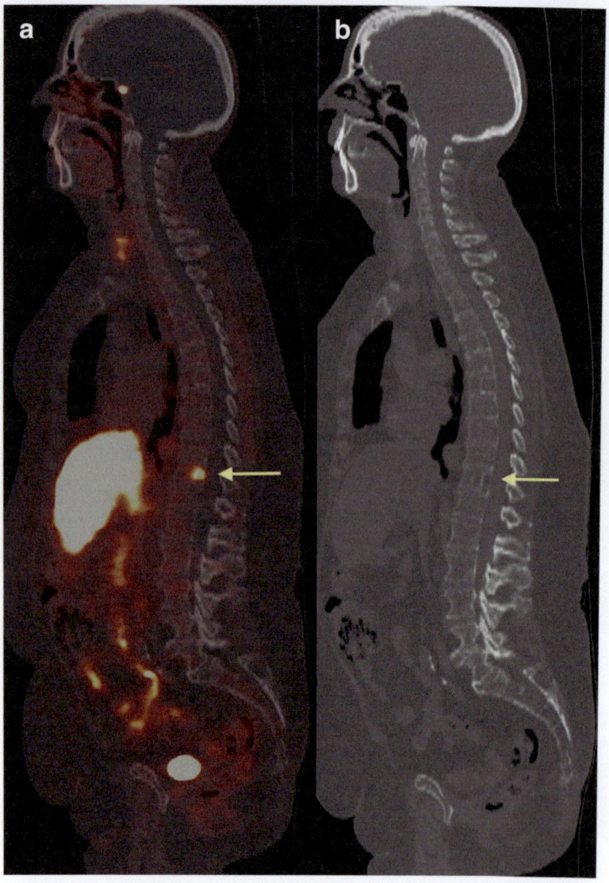

Fig. 29.7 Focal uptake of Ga-68-DOTATATE in T11 vertebral body (**a**) correlating with a CT lesion with thickened trabeculae (**b**) typical for a haemangioma

cular tumours, fibroadenomas in breast, Paget's disease and renal malignancies. Correlation with clinical history and biopsy confirmation of equivocal lesions when feasible is therefore essential.

Further Reading

1. Hofman MS, Lawrentschuk N, Francis RJ, et al. Prostate-specific membrane antigen PET-CT in patients with high-risk prostate cancer before curative-intent surgery or radiotherapy (proPSMA): a prospective, randomised, multicentre study. Lancet. 2020;395(10231):1208–16.
2. Huang S, Ong S, McKenzie D, et al. Comparison of ^{18}F-based PSMA radiotracers with [^{68}Ga] Ga-PSMA-11 in PET/CT imaging of prostate cancer – a systematic review and meta-analysis. Prostate Cancer Prostatic Dis. 2024;27:654–64.
3. Metser U, Ezzat S, Singh S, et al. 68 Ga-DOTATATE PET/CT in the initial diagnosis of patients with clinical, imaging, and/or biochemical suspicion of a neuroendocrine tumor. Clin Nucl Med. 2023;48:933–6.

30 Rubidium-82 (Half-Life 75 s; Decays 95.5% by Positron Emission and 4.5% by Electron Capture to Kr-82)

Rb-82 is a positron-emitting short-lived potassium analogue that is generator-produced from strontium-82 and used for myocardial perfusion scintigraphy (MPS) (Fig. 30.1). With such a short half-life, it can be administered on more than one occasion in the same imaging session, enabling routine same-session rest and post-stress MPS. The short half-life also enables high doses to be given, facilitating image resolution. The half-life of Sr-82 is 25 days, giving the generator a useful life span of about 1 month.

Rb-82 MPS illustrates the importance of the Crone-Renkin equation (Eq. 5.2) that defines the PS product of myocardial capillaries. Using a modelling approach, MPS with Rb-82 PET/CT measures regional Rb-82 clearance, which is converted to perfusion using an equation (Eq. 5.3) that gives perfusion as a function of clearance (Chap. 5).

Rb-82 is also a near-ideal tracer for measuring perfusion in a range of tissues using the Fick principle and theory summarised in Eq. 3.11 and Fig. 3.6. Exploiting the short physical half-life of the radionuclide enables measurement of the effects of interventions on blood flow. For example, it has been shown using a first-pass approach that regadenoson and adenosine have contrasting effects on renal and splenic blood flow, the for-

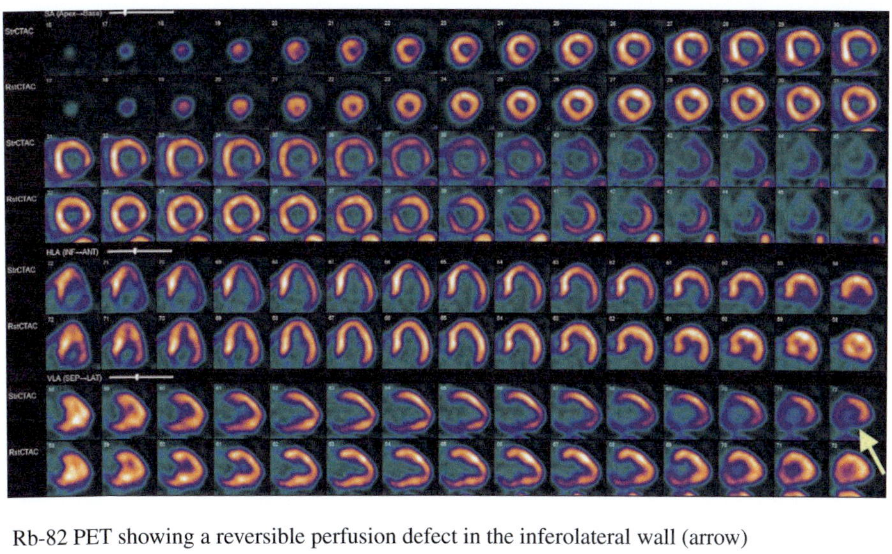

Fig. 30.1 Rb-82 PET showing a reversible perfusion defect in the inferolateral wall (arrow)

A. M. Peters, M. Vadrucci, *Introduction to Nuclear Medicine for Trainees in Imaging and Imaging Sciences*, https://doi.org/10.1007/978-3-032-18364-4_30

mer increasing both and the latter decreasing both, thereby highlighting the differential effects of A2A and A1 adenosine receptor stimulation.

Further Reading

1. Lortie M, Beanlands RSB, Yoshinaga K, Klein R, Dasilva JN, DeKemp RA. Quantification of myocardial blood flow with ^{82}Rb dynamic PET imaging. Eur J Nucl Med Mol Imaging. 2007;34:1765–74.
2. Sciagrà R, Lubberink M, Hyafil F, et al; Cardiovascular Committee of the European Association of Nuclear Medicine (EANM). EANM procedural guidelines for PET/CT quantitative myocardial perfusion imaging. Eur J Nucl Med Mol Imaging 2021; 48:1040-1069.

MIX
Papier aus verantwortungsvollen Quellen
Paper from responsible sources
FSC® C105338

If you have any concerns about our products,
you can contact us on
ProductSafety@springernature.com

In case Publisher is established outside the EU,
the EU authorized representative is:
Springer Nature Customer Service Center GmbH
Europaplatz 3, 69115 Heidelberg, Germany

Printed by Libri Plureos GmbH
in Hamburg, Germany